The Nutrition Crisis: a reader

The Nutrition Crisis:
a reader

THEODORE P. LABUZA
University of Minnesota

WEST PUBLISHING CO. | St. Paul • New York • Boston
Los Angeles • San Francisco

Library of Congress Cataloging in Publication Data

Main entry under title:

The Nutrition crisis.

  Bibliography: p.
  Includes index.
  1. Nutrition—Addresses, essays, lectures. 2. Diet—Addresses, essays, lectures. 3. Cardiovascular system—Diseases—Nutritional aspects—Addresses, essays, lectures. 4. Food—Addresses, essays, lectures. I. Labuza, T. P. [DNLM: 1. Nutrition. QU145 N973]

RA784.N845   641.1   75-20459
ISBN 0–8299–0063–2

Several years ago
Students had a crisis
They yelled, demonstrated, fought
Mine this year could have done the same
I work too hard, am hard to find
I dedicate this book
To their patience
Thank you
  Liz
    Pat
      Karen
        Felix
          Sue
        Hank
      Ray
    Sam
  Kathy

Preface

Recently, while reading a book on the energy crisis, I found the Chinese meaning of the word *crisis*. The ideograms used to compose the word are a combination of the symbols for *danger* and *opportunity*. This gave me the idea for the thread that runs through this reader on nutrition.

In teaching a beginning course on nutrition to liberal arts students, I have been confronted continuously in my lectures with the crisis of widely divided viewpoints on the same supposed fact. A problem existed in compiling a list of articles for the students to read which gave the opposing viewpoints on each of the topics in question. The articles were in quite diverse journals, which would make it difficult for students to find. Thus, I felt that it would be helpful to compile a reader of not-too-technical articles which would cover some of the controversial areas in the field of nutrition. A student of mine made it possible since her husband was a publisher.

The book covers a wide range of topics. It begins with an explanation of the Recommended Dietary Allowances (RDA), and a discussion of the nutritional status of the U. S. population with respect to this RDA follows. The malnutrition observed in this country has, in fact, led to a 1974 Senate hearing on nutrition. It has become clear that a danger exists for members of our population who are malnourished, but many opportunities exist to eliminate this crisis.

Other danger areas covered include the misuse of vitamins, the unwarranted prejudice against sugar cereals which possibly is depriving some children of breakfast, the misconception that organic foods are better than processed foods, the relation of diet to heart disease, and the interest in fad diets. In each case, an attempt has been made to select articles that present the opposing viewpoints and draw conclusions which would lead to the opportunity of improved health. This controversy is no better related than in the chapter on heart disease and cholesterol.

The final articles peer to the future by examining our world status today. Will there be enough food, do we have enough energy to process it, and are the chemicals we add to it safe? These are just a few of the questions that must be answered. I have tried in each chapter to summarize the articles with my own opinions. The reader will see my obvious biases; something I cannot dispute but which I feel is valid based on my sixteen years of training in the areas of nutrition, bio-chemistry, and food processing.

This book is intended to be a supplement for those who have learned some basic nutrition and want to look at the problem areas in more depth as the experts see them.

Acknowledgements

Having written a book previously in which I acknowledged the whole
world because it was my first book, I found myself really looking
at who was responsible for this second. I have dedicated it to those
students of mine who put up with my continuous involvement in too many
things. I acknowledge their patience. I must thank Bette Zeigler,
who introduced me to her husband Ken. He is the publisher and gave
me the idea to put the book together. He also had the patience to
wait beyond his deadlines.

Jane Schleicher, a journalism student at the University of Minnesota,
was of invaluable assistance in selecting articles, editing, and handling
the tremendous amount of paperwork involved in compiling a collection
of readings. She was also partly responsible for initiating the book.
To her I owe very special thanks.

Contents

G.   The food-people-energy crisis—Continued

The Nutrition Crisis: a reader

†

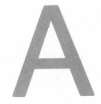

**Nutritional standards
for humans**

the scientific crisis

A Nutritional standards for humans

THE FIRST ARTICLE, by Dr. Hamish Munro, introduces the subject of nutritional standards. Munro discusses the impact of scientific research on the establishment of conditions for a healthy population. Although the field of nutritional research is relatively new, it already has lead to the eradication of many common diseases and the establishment of nutrient intake standards. Much more needs to be learned through nutritional research; Munro points out some of the questions that need to be answered.

One would think that experts could agree on man's nutritional requirements, but that has not been the case. However, as Dr. Alfred Harper points out in the next article, much of the misunderstanding among the experts results from semantic differences over what the word "requirement" means. Harper examines in detail the NRC/NAS 1973 revised Recommended Dietary Allowances (RDA) of nutrients, and responds to those critics who disagree with the prescribed levels. He explains how the levels were set and why the changes were made from the levels previously set. He shows the danger in setting levels too high or too low, and the difficulty in deciding which information is reliable and applicable before making a specific recommendation. The RDA, he points out, are for normal people, not those who are ill or have special needs, and he maintains that the distribution of needs of most healthy humans is well met by the RDA. Harper believes that the best way to ensure that nutritional needs are met is by variety of food choice. The RDA is one method of assessing the adequacy of the diet chosen, but not an ideal one. Harper also considers the subject of our last chapter: the effect of an energy crisis on formulating an adequate diet based on the RDA.

In the next article, Dr. Roger Williams takes issue with the RDA and the concept of the normal man. He argues convincingly that we all are not average men and thus have different requirements. However, after reading the previous papers, one could be convinced that only a few people have extremely high nutrient needs. Williams's experimental

evidence is, unfortunately, based on few subjects; with his evidence,
Williams contends that we all live at suboptimal nutritional conditions.
He assumes that requirements for individual nutrients are independent
variables. Actually, many nutrients are dependent on each other, a fact
that Williams, in another portion of the article, espouses to point out
the error of experiments which try to disprove the value of vitamins
in curing certain diseases. This confusion within one article written
by a scientist familiar with the field dramatically illustrates the very
real crisis confronting the average consumer who tries to interpret the
daily messages heard in the media. Dissemination of the wrong
material can lead to dangerous diet choices. It is my hope that in the
near future some sound information concerning nutrition and the
RDA can be made available to the public so they will have the opportunity
to improve their nutrition and health with this education.

The next article, by Dr. D. Hegsted and Dr. L. Ausman, analyzes some
fallacies in nutritional research and data interpretation. The authors
attack the "sole food" type experiment which tries to show that a
single food is not nutritious.

The last two articles in this chapter discuss specific components of the
diet. The first, by James Scala, reintroduces the "apple a day" concept
and points out that we have forgotten about fiber as a necessary dietary
component, especially in disease prevention. The second article questions
the "everybody needs milk" statement by showing that milk sugar
cannot be tolerated by all people.

1

IMPACT OF NUTRITIONAL RESEARCH ON HUMAN HEALTH AND SURVIVAL

Hamish N. Munro *

Let us begin by putting nutrition in its proper perspective, namely, as the central fact in the evolutionary history of animals. Animals emerged as distinct forms of life probably about 1 billion years ago, first as single cells and then as organisms made up of groups of cells, finally developing into the many species we now know, such as worms, insects, fish, birds, mammals, and the like. If we examine what these species have to obtain from their environment in order to survive, it is surprising to find that all types of animal from the simplest forms to the most sophisticated show basically the same needs for dietary constituents. For example, the proteins of their bodies contain 20 different species of amino acids as their structural components, but all species of animals, from single-celled types to man, can manufacture only half of these important compounds and are dependent on the environment for the remaining eight or ten amino acids, which thus become essential dietary components. This is quite different from the situation in bacteria, plants, and molds. Many bacteria and all plants are able to synthesize all the amino acids from simple precursors. It can be concluded that the branch point at which the plant and animal kingdoms

Reprinted from *Federation Proceedings*, Vol. 30, No. 4, July–August 1971. Printed in U. S. A.

Symposium on "Contributions of Basic Biomedical Research to Human Welfare" presented at the National Biological Congress, cosponsored by FASEB and AIBS, Detroit, Mich., November 8, 1970.

* Department of Nutrition and Food Science, Massachusetts Institute of Technology, Cambridge, Massachusetts.

evolved separately from more primitive cells was also the point at which the animal cells lost the capacity to make these eight or ten essential amino acids. Part of the DNA carrying the information for making these compounds became deleted from the genetic information of the cells and all subsequent forms of animal cells perpetuate the defect. Consequently, the most characteristic feature of animals is their dependence on outside sources of carbon compounds, including the essential amino acids. In other words, the basic feature that distinguishes animals from plants is that the animal needs to have a supply of food and this demand has largely determined subsequent evolutionary developments in animals.

Presumably the earliest single-celled animals survived by feeding on the dead bodies of their next door neighbors; any cell that was able to move had a considerable advantage in enlarging the area of its food supply. In this way early animal forms that developed the contractile structures we call muscles would have a tremendous advantage over their competitors and thus would win in the evolutionary competition. To control these muscles and coordinate their action, animals that developed the capacity to transmit messages through a primitive nervous system had a further advantage. Neither muscles nor nervous systems have evolved in plants, which in general are satisfied with the mineral elements they can get from the adjacent soil. Consequently, man has emerged as a thinking animal because he possesses a nervous system that has evolved as part of his ancestor's equipment for regulating movement in the search for food. Furthermore, the ideas that man conceives can only be communicated through muscular movements, originally favored because of their evolutionary advantage in the hunt for food.

The process of evolution of animals still continues and represents the matching of the genetic endowment of the organism to its environment. In this respect, man has done well. Emerging some 2 million years ago, probably in Africa, he has spread to the more remote areas of the globe in quite recent times. Thus, the Mediterranean was probably colonized 500,000 years ago, but Northern Europe received its first human visitors only a few thousand years ago, North America 20,000, and the date of human arrival in Iceland is precisely known; it is A.D. 874. In spite of this short period of human expansion, much of it within the past 300 generations (10,000 years), many adaptations have taken place. For example, Loomis has provided an interesting theory to account for the emergence of the light-skinned races. He suggests that vitamin D, which is made by sunlight falling on the skin, was not made in sufficient quantity by dark-skinned races who migrated to the less sunny northern climates. Because they made insufficient vitamin D, they developed rickets and childbirth became impossible because of deformities of the bones of the pelvis. Only variants of primitive man with somewhat lighter skin had a chance of survival, because their lighter skins allowed sufficient sunlight to penetrate.

In this way, evolutionary pressure resulted in the emergence of the light-skinned races.

What then is the lesson from all this? It is that, as man has spread around the earth, he has undergone adaptation to his environment. The ultimate function and justification of all science is, I believe, to promote human evolution as man adapts to his surroundings. The physical sciences, chemistry, and physics, offer control of the environment, while the biological sciences not only offer potential regulation of the living things in man's surroundings, but also permit changes in the evolutionary potential of man himself. The challenge to science is thus to participate in the completion of man's adaptation to his environment, and the environment to man. Since nutrition has been a fundamental factor in animal evolution, it must therefore continue to play a significant role in the future evolution of man.

SCIENCE OF NUTRITION AS A MEDICAL SUCCESS STORY

How far has nutritional research contributed to improving man's lot up till now? A survey of some of the major successes during the past half-century is very impressive. Rickets, a disease of young children resulting in softening and deformities of the bones, is seldom seen nowadays in this country, thanks to our knowledge of vitamin D. Pellagra was once the cause of a large amount of illness among corn-eating groups in the southern United States and was the cause of half of the cases in the insane asylums of the South; it is seldom seen nowadays, because of the knowledge that one of the vitamin B complexes can prevent and cure it. Pernicious anemia was once a fatal disease, now curable with vitamin B_{12}. In 1915, an experiment involving iodine treatment in the prevention of goiter reduced the frequency in one Ohio town from 29% to less than 1% of the school-children. It may be that the use of fluorine in appropriate amounts will have a similar action on the frequency of dental caries. All these are diseases with a long history, some stretching back into the medical writings of antiquity. Nutritional research has conquered them during this century. Indeed, from here on we can expect few further basic discoveries of this kind involving new and unsuspected food components needed by man. Does this mean that no further research needs to be done on nutritional diseases? Of course not!

First of all, there is much profit for human medicine in continued study of how each of the essential components of the human diet affects bodily function. Take the case of vitamin D. This substance is found in certain foods and is also formed by sunlight falling on the skin. Recent studies show that vitamin D (chemically referred to as cholecalciferol) has first to be transformed in the liver to a derivative named 25-hydroxycholecalciferol.[1]   This substance then causes the cells lining the intestine to make a protein that carries calcium into the body, thus promoting calcium absorption; it also probably stimulates the bone to lay down more calcuim.   Now it so happens that, although most children with rickets respond readily to treatment with vitamin D, there is an infrequent form of rickets that is resistant to vitamin D except in very high, somewhat toxic doses.   It has been found that transformation of vitamin D to 25-HCC is much less efficient in these patients than in normal people.   It is also not surprising that, in cases of cirrhosis of the liver, vitamin D is not efficiently transformed to 25-HCC and there is consequently loss of calcium salt from the bones.   It is thus a logical step to treat cases of resistant rickets and cases of liver damage with 25-HCC instead of vitamin D itself. The uses of this recently discovered derivative of vitamin D are only now being exploited, but it is obvious that exploratory basic research of this kind can have many forms of payoff.   In selecting vitamin D for such an illustration, I have taken only one of many areas that could be so used. The lesson to be learned is that, the more we know about the function of food constituents in the body, the more rational therapy of human diseases emerges.

A second and very important reason why research in nutrition must continue to be done is to provide better ways of detecting malnutrition. The importance of this is strikingly illustrated by the recent large-scale surveys carried out in several parts of the United States by Dr. Arnold Shaefer for the National Nutrition Survey in accordance with the provisions of the Health Amendment Act of 1967, in which Congress directed the Secretary of Health, Education and Welfare to "conduct a survey to determine the location, cause, and prevalence of hunger and malnutrition in the U.S.A."   These surveys made use of a variety of ways of determining whether individuals in the U. S. population were receiving adequate amounts of different food constituents, including medical evidence of deficiency and biochemical tests of blood and urine.   Ten states were surveyed in such a way as to highlight groups that might be likely to show malnutrition.   Although the data dealt primarily with low-income groups, the results of these surveys shocked the American public by revealing serious and humiliating degrees of malnutrition in an affluent nation. For example, one-fourth of the subjects examined had anemia due to iron deficiency, and many also showed evidence of lack of other essential components of the diet.   Such a discovery means that ways have to be found for adding extra iron and other components to the deficient diets of these Americans.   To do so, one must first have a reasonable knowledge of the amount of each dietary component needed for health.

This brings me to the third objective of nutritional research, namely, to provide reliable estimates of the requirements of man for various

---

[1] Abbreviations used are: 25-HCC, 25-hydroxycholecalciferol; PKU, phenylketonuria.

food components. This has not proved to be easy. Take for example the question of how much protein is required by an adult, an important question in view of the low intake of protein in many parts of the world. For more than a century, scientists have been trying to decide what is an adequate intake. In 1865, the professor of chemistry at the University of Edinburgh considered the minimum amount compatible with survival to be 57 g/day, since this was the quantity of protein in the subsistence diet given to patients in the University hospital. Thirty years later a German investigator examined the diet taken by the working man and found in it an average of 118 g/day. Since the German laborer of that time worked well, it was concluded that what was good for him must be good for everyone. Shortly thereafter, an American nutritionist conceived the idea that people were being poisoned by too high a protein intake and borrowed a platoon of soldiers from the U. S. Army, and fed them on a diet low in protein for many months. Not only did they survive but it is claimed that their physical fitness surpassed that of their colleagues who ate large amounts of meat. Public nutrition policy cannot, however, be based on such individualistic viewpoints. Consequently, the responsibility for determining requirements of individual components of the diet such as protein has passed out of the hands of individual scientists into the anonymity of national and international committees of scientists. Even so, we still display great areas of ignorance. For example, in the case of the requirement for protein in the diet, we still do not know whether physical work imposes a need for more protein, an important question in underdeveloped countries where poor nutrition is combined with much physical labor. Progress in developing more precise ideas on requirements for protein and other nutrients is limited by the cost of such experiments on man, and does not in general command much support from government agencies. Even meetings of the Food and Nutrition Board, the American committee that periodically reviews new knowledge of human requirements, are much restricted in frequency because of lack of funds.

NEW AREAS FOR FUTURE NUTRITIONAL RESEARCH

While all these established areas of nutritional research—mechanism of action of nutrients, diagnostic tests of deficiency, and standards for requirements of dietary components—will continue to provide valuable applications as more knowledge is gained from further research, nutritional studies are continuously breaking new ground. One area in which I anticipate much more excitement in future nutritional research is that of the early development of the animal. It is becoming increasingly evident that the environment into which an animal is born conditions its subsequent development. This has been demonstrated with rats receiving different amounts of mother's milk until weaned. If you change the sizes of litters of rats at birth so that some mothers have only 2 or 3 infant rats and others have 12 to 18 rats, you will find at the time of weaning that, of course, those animals from the large litter have not grown as well because the milk supply has been divided among a much greater number of mouths. However, if the different litters of rats are now weaned onto the same adequate diet, those that were in the small litters continue to grow faster than the members of the large litters. Early nutrition has thus had a permanent effect. This general picture has been examined recently in more detail. It has been found that different organs of the body are programmed at birth to achieve a given number of cells and then stop; if a period of undernutrition is applied while the organ is still adding to its population of cells, the final size of the organ will be smaller than normal. If, on the other hand, the maximum cell population of the organ has already been achieved, a period of undernutrition may cause shrinkage of that organ, but it will subsequently return to its full size when the period of underfeeding ceases. This means that, after birth, nutrition can alter the programming in the nucleus of a cell, so that its predetermined pattern of cell division and final shutoff is altered. An important example of this principle is the growth of the brain, which attains its adult number of brain cells quite early in life—in the case of man, this occurs at about 2 years, in the case of the rat at 2–3 weeks. Lack of adquate food during pregnancy or lack of sufficient milk during lactation, each result in a permanent restriction in the brain cell population in the rat. A combination of malnutrition during pregnancy and lactation has the most severe effect on brain cell number. Restriction of food intake after weaning fails to affect brain cell population in rats, since the number of brain cells has by now become static. These changes in brain cell number have been correlated with mental behavior. In the case of animals, evidence of mental retardation has been demonstrated, but in the case of children, it is much more difficult to separate the effects of malnutrition on subsequent intelligence from the effects of social environment, which is usually bad where malnutrition is present. The suspicion nevertheless remains that malnutrition at an early stage of life has a permanent stunting effect on mental development of man.

Although the emphasis in such studies is on undernutrition, the development of the body can also be conditioned by early overnutrition. Just as the undernourished animal remains permanently stunted, so the animal overnourished during early development tends to put on excess fat. This has been shown to be due to the appearance at an early age of an excessive number of fat cells in its adipose tissue. The same is true of human subjects. The number of fat cells in the bodies of people who become obese in childhood remains permanently greater than the fat cell population in the bodies of normal adults. Consequently, people who first become obese in childhood develop additional fat cells which remain with them throughout life, even if food restriction is practiced. In that case, the extra fat cells lose some of their load of fat, but continue to signal for extra food, and the victim has a persistent desire to eat.

Obviously, we must pay much more attention to nutritional patterns laid down in early childhood. We must find ways of assessing the individual as a metabolic machine, and then prescribing a personalized program for the optimum conditions of development for that individual. This question of individuality in requirements for food components is emerging in many ways. An increasing number of congenital diseases are being recognized in which dietary constituents—notably amino acids—are not utilized properly by the body, and abnormal products are accumulating in the body and causing damage, especially to the brain of the young child. A good example is PKU (phenylketonuria), in which there is lack of normal removal of the amino acid phenylalanine. Phenylalanine and its derivatives therefore accumulate in the body of the child and cause brain damage. Consequently, the intake of the amino acid phenylalanine has to be kept down by feeding special diets; however, this has to be carefully arranged so that growth is not stunted by providing less than adequate amounts of this essential amino acid for the normal growth of the tissues. Such congenital errors of utilization of food constituents are comparatively rare. On the other hand, lesser degrees of variability in food utilization are probably common. Take for example the question of atherosclerosis. Everyone knows that diet is strongly suspected of playing a part in the high incidence of degenerative diseases of the arteries and heart. It has been concluded by many investigators in this important field that diet regulates the levels of cholesterol and other fats in the blood, and that people with high blood levels of cholesterol and fat run a high risk of coronary thrombosis. This has led to an extensive study of dietary factors that may be responsible for elevating blood cholesterol levels. For about 20 years, it has been known that populations who have a high fat intake suffer from a high frequency of heart attacks, and evidence has been gathered to show that the saturated fats are particularly injurious in this respect. More recently, there has been a campaign to demonstrate that coronary disease is related to the increasing intake of cane sugar by the population. Whatever the merits of these opinions, there is no doubt that individuals vary in the response of their blood fat levels when the diet is varied. Those with excessively high levels of blood fats fall into five classes, two of which predominate. One of these two groups shows an increase in blood fat level when a diet rich in fat is fed to them, whereas the other shows an increase in blood fat when given a diet rich in carbohydrate. This emphasizes the individuality of response which makes any statement about the role of diet in human health somewhat hazardous.

Finally, we come to the role of nutrition in ensuring the food supply of the future, not only in areas that are presently suffering from malnutrition, but also for expanding populations in advanced countries like the United States. To some extent, this is the province of the agricultural scientist who produces new "miracle" strains of wheat and rice with high yields. However, as the most recent Nobel Peace Prize recipient Dr.

Borlaug has emphasized, this will do little more than keep pace with the expanding population. Consequently, while attempting to restrict population growth, we should also look to the supply of food from unusual and novel sources, thereby liberating man from one major environmental hazard. Herein lies a real challenge to the skills and experience of a department studying nutrition and food science. It demands ingenuity in looking for likely new materials to act as sources of foodstuffs, and sophisticated methods of testing the products for usefulness and for potential dangers. This area of new research has received considerable stimulus from the Space Program. In long-distance space travel, it is not possible to transport enough foods for the journey, and this has taxed the ingenuity of scientists from various areas of biology on how best to utilize the waste products of the astronauts in order to synthesize edible products. Solutions to this problem include the chemical synthesis of carbohydrates from carbon dioxide and water, and the growth of various types of bacteria, yeasts, molds, and primitive plants on excretory products. This has provided a considerable incentive to the more general cultivation of these unusual food sources, such as photosynthetic algae, which use sunlight much more efficiently than higher plants and can be maintained under conditions where you get crops continuously, and not seasonally. This plant synthesizes protein and vitamins as well as serving as a source of energy in the diet, and it has been computed that 1 m^2 of algal crop can renew itself at a rate sufficient to maintain one man. At Massachusetts Institute of Technology, scientists are looking into other sources, particularly yeasts and bacteria as sources of protein for man. This demands all the resources of a large department, utilizing methods of pilot-plant growth of the organism, processing, examining for hazardous components, and testing on human subjects with the help of facilities for human studies. Another group has been working on new compounds that can be used as sources of energy for the body. The eventual success of such programs will depend on the harnessing of these processes of artificial food production to industrial resources. For a number of years now, the oil companies have been interested in the possibility of using their by-products, such as gas oil and paraffins, on which to grow yeasts and bacteria. There is evidence that, in the near future, a safe and useful protein ingredient of animal feedstuffs will be achieved. This has already represented only about 10 years of research. There is reason to believe that a product suitable and acceptable for human consumption will soon follow. The important point to recognize is that, by using oil wastes, the product shows a prospect of becoming economically desirable. If this can be achieved in other areas of industry, then the incentive for producing new and novel sources of food will quicken. Once more, the environment in which man is evolving is being subject to control.

I am glad to think that the scientist is nowadays a respected, if sometimes feared, member of the community. The public knows that much can be expected of him. I have tried to show that science is a form of organized evolution directed toward the perfection of physical man in his environment. Within this objective, nutritional control of man and his environment at all stages of his development plays an important part. The study of man's nutritional well-being involves a complex operation in which we have to combine knowledge of his requirements, the biochemical factors in food utilization, clinical evidence of malnutrition in populations, food sources for missing dietary components, and surveys of dietary intakes.

2

RECOMMENDED DIETARY ALLOWANCES

are they what we think they are?

Alfred E. Harper, Ph.D.*

The Recommended Dietary Allowances (RDA) are not to be confused with the "U. S. RDA'S" devised by the Food and Drug Administration (FDA) as standards for regulating the labeling of foods for nutrient content. The FDA standards are derived from the Recommended Dietary Allowances, but of necessity are based on only a few broad age groups.

What constituted major problems for the Committee on Dietary Allowances in revising the allowances? *Energy*—how low is it rational to set the allowance? *Protein*—what are the relative merits of high vs. low allowances? *Ascorbic acid*—what is the logical allowance in the heat of the current controversy about this nutrient? *Calcium*—what are appropriate criteria on which to base an allowance? *Vitamin E*—is it rational for the allowance to exceed estimated intakes of healthy individuals? *Trace minerals*—is it possible to develop allowances for more of these? The Committee made decisions on these controversial problems for the eighth revision. However, in describing the decisions, I must say that I like the British usage of a plural verb with a collective noun, for the Committee agreed—not as a unit—with varying degrees of enthusiasm from individual members on different decisions. Knowledge of human nutritional needs is not adequate for decisions about allowances for several nutrients to be unanimous.

Reprinted from *Journal of The American Dietetic Association*, Vol. 64, No. 2, February 1974. © The American Dietetic Association. Printed in U. S. A.

* Professor, Nutritional Sciences and Biochemistry, University of Wisconsin, Madison; and Chairman, Committee on Dietary Allowances, Food and Nutrition Board, National Research Council–National Academy of Sciences, Washington, D. C.

As other papers in this series deal with problems relating to specific nutrients, I shall confine my comments to some of the more general aspects of dietary allowances.

The new revision of the Recommended Dietary Allowances (1) includes two new sections: an introduction in which the basis for estimating an allowance is explained, together with some discussion of factors affecting the allowances, and a section detailing some of the cautions to be observed in using the allowances for different purposes. The Food and Nutrition Board, because of their concern with misconceptions about, and misuse of, Recommended Dietary Allowances, constituted a "Committee on Uses of RDA" under the chairmanship of Helen Walsh. This Committee assembled information which the present Committee on Dietary Allowances used freely in preparing these new sections. Hopefully, these will reduce the probability of misunderstanding about what the Recommended Dietary Allowances represent and their appropriate uses.

Misconceptions about the allowances begin either through misinterpreting the term "Recommended Dietary Allowances" or misunderstanding the objectives of formulating allowances. To some, this is "merely semantics," but I contend that knowledge of semantics is a key-stone of a scientific education. There can be no meaningful discussion if some participants assume that any word they use means just exactly what they want it to mean.

HISTORIC BACKGROUND: DEFINITION OF ALLOWANCES

The origin and objectives of the Recommended Dietary Allowances have been described in this Journal (2) by Lydia J. Roberts, who chaired the first Committee. These objectives have been reiterated in abbreviated form by succeeding committees (3). She stated that the National Nutrition Program, forerunner of the Food and Nutrition Board, the body responsible for development of the first Recommended Dietary Allowances during World War II, "was initiated . . . to insure that the nutrition of the people would be safeguarded" and went on to say that the Recommended Dietary Allowances, which were developed as part of the effort to accomplish this, were meant to be "goals at which to aim in providing for the nutritional needs of groups of people."

From the beginning, the Recommended Dietary Allowances, except that for energy, have been recommendations for levels of intake of nutrients sufficiently in excess of average nutritional requirements to meet the needs of nearly all of the population—a public health or statistical concept. They are intakes that, on the basis of the available scientific evidence and in the judgment of the Committee developing them, are compatible with maintenance of the health of most people. As Dr. Roberts emphasized, they are not amounts required by all individuals; they are not absolute nutritional standards; they are not recommendations for an ideal diet, as many assume. They are "goals at which to aim in providing for the nutritional needs of groups of people." Yet, the term "Recommended Dietary Allowances" connotes to many people recommendations for the ideal, best possible, diet. Such terms as "acceptable nutrient intake" or "acceptable levels of nutrient intake" are probably more descriptive of the original concept and less open to misinterpretation.

This brings us to the phrase "goals at which to aim," a second source of misunderstanding and a phrase that should be examined critically. The ultimate goal of the National Nutritional Program was to insure that the food supply would contain enough of each of several critical nutrients to insure that there would be no threat to the health of the population from inadequate supplies of these nutrients. The Recommended Dietary Allowances were not intended to be goals for the amounts of nutrients that should be present in some vaguely defined ideal diet. They were to be goals in the sense that they were estimates of amounts of nutrients great enough to meet *the physiologic needs of most people*, quite independently of the amounts that could be provided readily from the available food. This is clear from reading about the objectives of the original Committee.

The Recommended Dietary Allowances are recommendations for intakes of specific chemical compounds. The published bulletin does not deal with foods and preparation. Rather, it is a guide to human nutritional needs for those who prepare and for those who use diet manuals. The introduction emphasizes that diets are more than combinations of nutrients. They are composed of foods that should satisfy social and psychologic needs, as well as nutritional needs. Formulation of a diet must, therefore, begin with selection of a combination of foods that will be palatable and appetizing. If a diet is palatable, and if sufficient in quantity, any healthy individual will ordinarily eat enough to satisfy his energy needs. If foods are not eaten, we do not have a diet—just an assemblage of natural products. Also, it is an axiom of dietetics, repeated several times in the new bulletin, that the best way to insure that nutrient needs are met is to formulate diets from as wide a variety of foods as is possible. With these objectives accomplished, the diet can then be assessed from food composition tables and the Recommended Dietary Allowances to determine whether it contains less than the recommended amount of any particular nutrient (for which recommendations are made).

ENERGY ALLOWANCES

Allowances for energy are estimated on an entirely different basis from those for specific nutrients. Energy allowances are estimates of the requirements of average persons in each age group and approximate the average need of the population group; they are not intended to be recommended intakes for individuals. Thus, about half the individuals in a population group may be expected to consume less than the average. Nevertheless, as energy consumption is determined primarily by energy expenditure, few are likely to consume less than they need as long as there is no barrier, such as poverty or crop failure, to obtaining a palatable diet.

The low energy expenditure of the United States population has begun to be of concern to the Committee on Dietary Allowances. We have been confident that consumption of a diet composed of a wide variety of foods will meet all specific nutrient needs when consumed in an amount sufficient to meet energy needs. However, the current pattern of low energy expenditure, coupled with a rather high intake of such foods as sugars and oils that provide energy but only small quantities of essential nutrients, is a situation with potential for creating nutritional problems. There is no assurance that persons with low energy intakes have low requirements for essential nutrients, and it is unlikely that anything short of a critical fuel shortage will increase the energy expenditure of most people in this country. Therefore, the problem of devising low-energy diets that will provide the recommended quantities of specific nutrients is likely to remain with us for the foreseeable future.

ALLOWANCES BASED ON NORMAL NEEDS

Anyone who has reviewed information on human nutritional requirements is aware that it is impossible to formulate recommended dietary allowances for various age groups for many nutrients solely on the basis of the available scientific information, and that an element of judgment is needed to make any estimate. Nevertheless, it would seem that judgments should not be so divergent as to preclude the possibility of devising allowances or acceptable nutrient intakes that would be valid for any healthy population anywhere, i. e., values that would require adjustments only for differences in environmental conditions, body size, and physiologic state of the population group. This has been the aim of FAO/WHO, but differences between FAO/WHO recommendations and various national standards indicate that, to date, success in achieving this aim is limited. Some of the reasons for this become evident from reviewing the procedure used to estimate allowances.

It should first be emphasized, however, that the Recommended Dietary Allowances are estimates of amounts of nutrients that, if *consumed* daily by each individual in a specified population group, should insure that the needs of nearly all individuals in the group who are well will be met. The Recommended Dietary Allowances are not formulated to cover the needs of those who are ill—they are not therapeutic needs—nor do they take into account losses of nutrients that occur during the processing and preparation of food.

Labuza—Nutrition Crisis CTB—3

VALUE JUDGMENTS

The logical starting point for estimating allowances for nutrients other than those that are consumed solely for their energy content is to assemble information about estimated requirements. However, requirements differ with age and body size; among individuals of the same size owing to differences in genetic make-up; with the physiologic state of the individual—growth rate, pregnancy, lactation; and with sex. They may also be influenced by a person's activity and by environmental conditions. Information about all of these factors cannot be included in tables of allowances, although the values are presented for selected age, weight, and sex groups, as physiologic state and body size are the most important factors that influence nutritional needs.

Table 1: Selection of heights and weights for age groups *

Age	Body weight at 50th percentile		Height at 50th percentile	
	male	female	male	female
	kg.		*cm.*	
11 yr.	36.7	37.7	146.9	148.1
12 yr.	40.2	42.3	152.3	154.3
13 yr.	45.5	47.0	158.9	158.4
14 yr.	51.7	50.3	165.3	160.4
average	44	44	156	155

* Based on information from Vaughan *et al.* (4).

The age-weight-sex groups have been changed in the new edition. After the first year, the age groups are for three- or four-year intervals. Up to age ten, no distinction is made between the sexes; beyond age ten, allowances are listed separately for males and females. The heights and weights for the groups were calculated by averaging the values for the fiftieth percentile of each year in the group. This is shown for the eleven-to-fourteen-year-old groups (Table 1). The age groups are inclusive, so the eleven-to-fourteen-year groups represent the age range from eleven years to fifteen less one day. A table included as an appendix to the Bulletin gives information about the ranges of heights and weights that may be encountered in each age group.

Once the age groups have been selected, the initial problem in estimating an allowance is to establish values for average requirements. If sufficient data are available from human experiments, an average requirement can be calculated. If not, information from studies on other species or about minimum nutrient intakes of individuals in good health may have to be used.

Even when knowledge of human requirements is available, agreement about the criterion for judging when the requirement has been met may still be a problem. The requirement for a nutrient is the minimum intake that will maintain normal function and health. For infants and children, the requirement may be equated with the amount that will maintain a satisfactory rate of growth; for an adult, with the amount that will maintain body weight and prevent depletion of the nutrient from the body as judged by balance studies or the maintenance of acceptable blood and tissue concentrations. For some nutrients, the requirement may be assessed as the amount that will just prevent the development of specific deficiency signs, an amount that may differ by several fold from that required to maintain maximum body stores. A substantial element of judgment is involved in deciding where, between these extremes, the requirement has been met. The problem is illustrated for ascorbic acid in Figure 1(4).

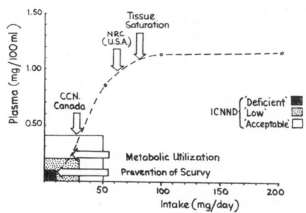

Figure 1: Relationships among intake of ascorbic acid, blood plasma concentration, tissue saturation, 1968 allowances, and standards of the Interdepartmental Committee on Nutrition for National Defense (after Arroyave [5], based on data in [6, 7]).

FROM REQUIREMENT TO ALLOWANCE

To derive an allowance from a requirement, variability among the requirements of individuals must be considered. The ideal way to do this is to determine the variability of the individual values used in estimating the average requirement. Assuming that individual requirements fit a statistically normal distribution pattern, 95 per cent of the population should have requirements that fall within plus or minus twice the standard deviation of the average requirement as shown in Figure 2(8, 9). Thus, if an allowance is set at two standard deviations above the average, that amount should be sufficient to meet the needs of 97.5 per cent of the individuals in a population. For many biologic measurements, this is from 30 per cent to 40 per cent above the average.

The probability that human requirements are skewed, as some would have us believe, to cover a range tenfold or more above the average seems highly unlikely. Were this common in biologic systems, biologic measurements would not show the consistency they do. Genetic defects, unique diseases, and severe trauma can greatly increase nutritional needs. Some drugs may also increase needs for specific nutrients. Claims that a variety of diseases respond to treatment with amounts of nutrients 100 to 1,000 times the accepted requirements, because nutritional needs are so high that they cannot be met by many United States diets, are based on subjective observations that are rarely reliable. It should also be recognized that nutrients, like other chemicals, may, when administered in large doses, have pharmacologic effects. So, in my view, even those claims that appear to have some basis in fact have about as much to do with nutritional needs as treatment of excess gastric acid with sodium bicarbonate has to do with sodium requirements.

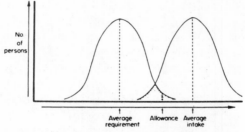

Figure 2: Schematic representation of relationship between requirement, allowance, and intake. Intake is represented as following a statistically normal distribution; in actuality, intake is usually skewed toward the right, with the average exceeding the median. Thus, more than half of the individuals surveyed have intakes below the average [10] (adapted from Lorstad [9] and Beaton [8]).

In setting allowances, it is also necessary to consider any factor that influences efficiency of utilization of the nutrient. For some nutrients, a part of the requirement may be met by a precursor which is converted to the essential nutrient within the body. In setting the allowance for vitamin A, for example, which is met in part by carotenes, consideration is given to the efficiency of conversion of carotenes to vitamin A. For some nutrients, absorption is incomplete and the allowance must reflect the proportion of the ingested nutrient that fails to gain entrance to the body. This is of major importance in setting allowances for several minerals, especially iron.

DIFFERENCES OF OPINION

With such problems, it is perhaps not surprising that there are differences of opinion about the validity of values for requirements and allowances. It is not overly difficult to obtain agreement on the selection of the scientific literature pertinent to requirements and, where there are enough values for individual requirements, an estimate of variability can be made mathematically. However, because of the paucity of information about requirements for some nutrients and because of differences of opinion concerning the criteria of nutritional adequacy for others, "in the judgment of the Committee" is the key to understanding why there may be differences of opinion on a value for the requirement and in extrapolating from the requirement to an allowance.

Few would fault the procedure of review by a committee, with further review of committee recommendations by consultants, before reaching conclusions. However, a psychologic element enters here. The evidence must be culled (I prefer this word to the modern one, "collated"—a vague term used so widely by administrators and committees); some of the information must be discarded out of hand because of its inadequacy; some must be given greater weight, some less; this requires judgment. And collective judgment—be it committee judgment, corporation judgment, or public judgment—can result in an action that would not be taken by any individual alone. A committee with a majority of optimists may be confident that a low allowance is fully adequate while one with a majority of pessimists will feel that a high allowance is inadequate. A single dominant consultant or member of the organization charged with making the decision may influence the judgment of a majority of others. Committee judgments are far from infallible; differences among the United Kingdom, Canadian, FAO/WHO, and U. S. recommendations testify to this. It is well to keep in mind that the best efforts of a conscientious committee—which I assure you this one was—do not create data to fill the many existing voids and do not eliminate human fallibility.

Despite obstacles, Committees on Dietary Allowances derive values that are useful guides for practical nutrition. But what do they mean and what are their limitations?

LIMITATIONS OF ALLOWANCES

If all members of the population group have intakes equal to or in excess of the allowances, the likelihood of any individual having an inadequate intake is small. Even if an individual has a low intake on one day, this is not of particular concern if it is compensated by a high intake on another. The Committee concluded that if intakes fluctuated, but average intakes over five to eight days met the allowances, there was little cause. for concern.

However, if the average intake of a population exceeds the average allowance, it is not valid to assume that all members of the population have adequate intakes. Intakes, like requirements, vary among individuals. They are not usually distributed normally, as is assumed in Figure 2, but are usually skewed toward the upper end of the range. Information from the Ten-State Nutrition Survey (10) indicates that the average intake of a nutrient commonly exceeds the median, so that considerably more than half the population may have intakes below the average. Beaton (8) and Lorstad (9) have calculated, assuming a normal distribution, that inadequate intakes must be anticipated in a population, even if the average is greatly in excess of the allowance.

On the other hand, if intakes of some nutrients are habitually less than the allowances, it does not necessarily mean that an individual consuming such amounts has an inadequate diet. The Recommended Dietary Allowances, except that for energy, are estimated to exceed the requirements of most individuals in a population. Nevertheless, with no way of predicting whose needs are high and whose are low, it does mean that the farther habitual intake falls below the allowance, and the longer the period of low intake, the greater is the risk of deficiency.

CRITICISMS REFUTED

Two opposing criticisms of the Recommended Dietary Allowances, both of which I find disturbing, are voiced frequently. The first relates to statements that the allowances are not meaningful because they are excessive. I would re-emphasize that many such statements result from a misunderstanding of the objectives of the allowances. They are not requirements; *they are recommendations directed toward insuring the nutritional health of groups.* They must, therefore, be high enough to meet the needs of those with the highest requirements and, hence, must exceed the needs of most people.

On the other hand, some allowances may be higher than they need to be. Committees given the responsibility for developing the Recommended Dietary Allowances, when in doubt, tend to select the higher of alternative values because there is no evidence that small surpluses of nutrients are harmful, whereas small deficits, over time, lead eventually to depletion and deficiency. If allowances are unrealistically high, observations that many diets fail to meet the high allowances raise unnecessary concern about the adequacy of the food supply. Some eminent nutritionists have concluded that if there is no evidence that the health of the population is at risk when the allowance for a nutrient is not met, one should probably examine critically the allowance rather than the diet. This is a sound reason for regular revision of the Recommended Dietary Allowances.

The other criticism that disturbs me even more represents the other side of the coin; it is the assumption that the Recommended Dietary Allowances are inadequate and do not represent the amounts of nutrients that should be provided by an ideal diet. We do not know the ideal nutrient intakes for longevity, resistance to chronic diseases, and maximum physical and mental performance in old age. While it may be true that requirements for these differ from those for a satisfactory rate of growth and for prevention of depletion of a nutrient from the body, there is no evidence to support such views. For energy, there is evidence that more is not better—and there is reason to question whether this does not hold also for protein for older age groups. Vitamins A and D in excess are toxic.

Proposing unrealistically high intakes of nutrients, on the assumption that if meeting needs is good, exceeding them is better, is like doing a cost-benefit analysis without being able to quantify the benefit—it is a meaningless exercise. Decisions concerning nutritional recommendations based on opinion rather than on scientific evidence and judgment are grist for the food faddists' mill. We should be aware that, although we do not have methods for proving absolutely what is true, we are able to detect what is false—and the more we discard what is false, the greater is the probability that what remains approaches truth. This has been the objective of successive Committees on Dietary Allowances.

Another, not uncommon, assumption that disturbs me is that bulletins in which the Recommended Dietary Allowances are presented are sociopolitical documents. As I have emphasized, they are scientific documents, developed to the best of the ability of those concerned with their preparation; nevertheless they are also documents that have social and political uses. This makes it critical that they be as scientifically sound as possible. If allowances were to be adjusted or modified for social or political reasons, the recommendations would soon lose their value—both as guides for dealing with nutritional problems and as a source of information for those dealing with social and political problems. With the current danger of the food supply becoming limited, and with the likelihood of even greater limitations in the future, it is especially important that allowances be based on realistic estimates of physiologic needs and that we do not allow ourselves the luxury of proposing high allowances just because the amounts of nutrients currently available in the food supply are in excess of nutritional needs.

COMMENTS ON SPECIFIC NUTRIENTS

While most of the major problems of the present Committee have been discussed in other articles in this series, a few additional points should be mentioned.

The calcium allowance posed probably the greatest difficulty for the Committee in preparing the eighth revision. The United Kingdom, Canada, and FAO/WHO all recommend 400 to 500 mg. calcium per day for the adult man, whereas in the United States, the allowance is 800 mg. Discussions of calcium allowances, like those for ascorbic acid, tend to generate more heat than light. The Committee found that consultation on requirements and allowances for this nutrient reflected the firm conviction that the allowance should be high, despite evidence that healthy people in many parts of the world have low intakes and that many people in this country have intakes well below the allowance without there being evidence of calcium deficiency in the population. In fact, one must search the literature with a microscope to find that dietary deficiency of calcium has been reported.

In its review of calcium allowances, the Committee emphasized observations at Wisconsin and at Berkeley on the influence of protein intake on calcium balance. These studies indicated that as protein intake rose, urinary calcium loss increased. With protein intakes in the range of the protein allowance, calcium equilibrium was maintained in adults with calcium intakes of 500 mg. per day. However—and here the Committee was not consistent with its own guidelines—the recommendation for calcium was left at 800 mg. per day in view of the relatively high average protein intake in this country. A statement is included in the text indicating that adults with intakes of protein below the customary United States intake will maintain calcium equilibrium on intakes well below the allowance.

The Committee was also concerned that the term "niacin equivalents" carried the implication that 60 mg. tryptophan were used for each milligram of niacin formed. Although on the average, 1 mg. niacin is derived from each 60 mg. tryptophan in the diet, values in the literature for efficiency of conversion of tryptophan to niacin are quite variable. How efficiency of conversion varies with tryptophan intake is not clear, but as tryptophan used for protein synthesis is not available for conversion to niacin, and as this use is greatest during growth, the niacin allowance has been expressed as niacin with a footnote indicating that each 60 mg. tryptophan in the diet may contribute approximately 1 mg. niacin.

With folic acid, the major problem was: "How well are the conjugated forms of this vitamin utilized?" There is evidence that folate conjugates may be better utilized than has heretofore been considered, but the Committee was not satisfied that there was enough evidence to alter the allowance at this time. Therefore, the folacin allowance remains at 400 mcg. for adults, with the stipulation that less than 25 per cent of this will be required if free folic acid is provided.

For vitamin B_{12}, the allowance was reduced by 40 per cent, from 5 mcg. to 3 mcg. per day for adults on the basis of new information supporting the lower value and re-interpretation of some of the previous information about requirements. This value is also more in line with FAO/WHO recommendations.

REFERENCES

1. Food & Nutr. Bd.: Recommended Dietary Allowances. 8th revision. Washington, D. C.: Natl. Acad. Sci.-Natl. Research Council, in press.

2. Roberts, L. J.: Beginnings of the Recommended Dietary Allowances. J. Am. Dietet. A. 34: 903, 1958.

3. Miller, D. F., and Voris, L.: Chronologic changes in the Recommended Dietary Allowances. J. Am. Dietet. A. 54: 109, 1969.

4. Nelson, W. E., Vaughan, V. C., and McKay, R. J.: Textbook of Pediatrics, 9th ed. Philadelphia: W. B. Saunders Co., 1969.

5. Arroyave, G.: Standards for the diagnosis of vitamin deficiency in man. *In*: Metabolic Adaptation and Nutrition. Sci. Pub. No. 22. Washington, D. C.: Pan Am. Health Organ./WHO, 1971.

6. Lowry, O. H., Bessey, O. A., Brock, M. J., and Lopez, J. A.: The interrelationship of dietary, serum white blood cell, and total ascorbic acid. J. Biol. Chem. 166: 111, 1946.

7. Ralli, E. P., Friedman, G. J., and Sherry, S.: Vitamin C requirement of man. Prolonged study of daily excretion and plasma concentration of vitamin C. Proc. Soc. Exp. Biol. Med. 40: 604, 1939.

8. Beaton, G. H.: The use of nutritional requirements and allowances. *In*: Proc. Western Hemisphere Nutr. Congress, 1971. Mt. Kisco, N. Y.: Futura Publishing Co., 1972.

9. Lorstad, M. H.: Recommended intake and its relation to nutrient deficiency. FAO Nutr. Newsletter 9: 18, 1971.

10. Ten-State Nutrition Survey, 1968–70. I. Historical Development and II. Demographic Data; III. Clinical, Anthropometry, Dental; IV. Biochemical; V. Dietary; and Highlights. DHEW Pub. Nos. (HMS) 72–8130, –8131, –8132, –8133, –8134, 1972.

Food and Nutrition Board, National Academy of Sciences—National Research Council Recommended Daily Dietary Allowances, Revised 1973

(Designed for the maintenance of good nutrition of practically all healthy people in the U.S.A.)

	(years) From up to	Weight (kg)	Weight (lbs)	Height (cm)	Height (in)	Energy (kcal)[2]	Protein (g)	Vitamin A activity (RE)[3]	Vitamin A activity (IU)	Vitamin D (IU)[2]	Vitamin E activity (IU)[5]	Ascorbic Acid (mg)	Folacin[6] (ug)	Niacin[7] (mg)	Riboflavin (mg)	Thiamin (mg)	Vitamin B$_6$ (mg)	Vitamin B$_{12}$ (ug)	Calcium (mg)	Phosphorus (mg)	Iodine (ug)	Iron (mg)	Magnesium (mg)	Zinc (mg)
Infants	0.0–0.5	6	14	60	24	kg×117	kg×2.2	420[4]	14,400	400	4	35	50	5	0.4	0.3	0.3	0.3	360	240	35	10	60	3
	0.5–1.0	9	20	71	28	kg×108	kg×2.0	400	2,000	400	5	35	50	8	0.6	0.5	0.4	0.3	540	400	45	15	70	5
Children	1–3	13	28	86	34	1300	23	400	2,000	400	7	40	100	9	0.8	0.7	0.6	1.0	800	800	60	15	150	10
	4–6	20	44	110	44	1800	30	500	2,500	400	9	40	200	12	1.1	0.9	0.9	1.5	800	800	80	10	200	10
	7–10	30	66	135	54	2400	36	700	3,300	400	10	40	300	16	1.2	1.2	1.2	2.0	800	800	110	10	250	10
Males	11–14	44	97	158	63	2800	44	1,000	5,000	400	12	45	400	18	1.5	1.4	1.6	3.0	1200	1200	130	18	350	15
	15–18	61	134	172	69	3000	54	1,000	5,000	400	15	45	400	20	1.8	1.5	2.0	3.0	1200	1200	150	18	400	15
	19–22	67	147	172	69	3000	54	1,000	5,000	400	15	45	400	20	1.8	1.5	2.0	3.0	800	800	140	10	350	15
	23–50	70	154	172	69	2700	56	1,000	5,000		15	45	400	18	1.6	1.4	2.0	3.0	800	800	130	10	350	15
	51+	70	154	172	69	2400	56	1,000	5,000		15	45	400	16	1.5	1.2	2.0	3.0	800	800	110	10	350	15
Females	11–14	44	97	155	62	2400	44	800	4,000	400	10	45	400	16	1.3	1.2	1.6	3.0	1200	1200	115	18	300	15
	15–18	54	119	162	65	2100	48	800	4,000	400	11	45	400	14	1.4	1.1	2.0	3.0	1200	1200	115	18	300	15
	19–22	58	128	162	65	2100	46	800	4,000	400	12	45	400	14	1.4	1.1	2.0	3.0	800	800	100	18	300	15
	23–50	58	128	162	65	2000	46	800	4,000		12	45	400	13	1.2	1.0	2.0	3.0	800	800	100	18	300	15
	51+	58	128	162	65	1800	46	800	4,000		12	45	400	12	1.1	1.0	2.0	3.0	800	800	80	10	300	15
Pregnant						+300	+30	1,000	5,000	400	15	60	800	+2	+0.3	+0.3	2.5	4.0	1200	1200	125	18+[8]	450	20
Lactating						+500	+20	1,200	6,000	400	15	80	600	+4	+0.5	+0.3	2.5	4.0	1200	1200	150	16	450	25

1 The allowances are intended to provide for individual variations among most normal persons as they live in the United States under usual environmental stresses. Diets should be based on a variety of common foods in order to provide other nutrients for which human requirements have been less well defined.

2 Kilojoules (KJ) = 4.2 xkcal.

3 Retinol equivalents.

4 Assumed to be all as retinol in milk during the first six months of life. All subsequent intakes are assumed to be one-half as retinol and one-half as β-carotene when calculated from international units. As retinol equivalents three-fourths are as retinol and one-fourth as β-carotene.

5 Total vitamin E activity, estimated to be 80 percent as σ-tocopherol and 20 percent other tocopherols.

6 The folacin allowances refer to dietary sources as determined by *Lactobacillus casei* assay. Pure forms of folacin may be effective in doses less than one-fourth of the RDA.

7 Although allowances are expressed as niacin, it is recognized that on the average 1 mg of niacin is derived from each 60 mg of dietary tryptophan.

8 This increased requirement cannot be met by ordinary diets; therefore, the use of supplemental iron is recommended.

3

A RENAISSANCE OF NUTRITIONAL SCIENCE IS IMMINENT

**Roger J. Williams, James D. Heffley,
Man-Li Yew, and Charles W. Bode ***

INTRODUCTION

There is a wide spectrum of uninformed inexpert opinion regarding the practical importance of quality nutrition in our daily lives. At one extreme are the food enthusiasts, including faddists; at the other is the majority of practicing physicians who through the fault of their medical school training tend to ignore all but the most elementary aspects of nutrition, and to avoid becoming involved in a field so characterized by intricacies, uncertainties, and ignorance.

Those who have medical training are in a unique position; they alone have the background necessary to grasp fully the deep-seated significance of nutrition in relation to health and disease. Uufortunately, however, medical science has not developed and nurtured nutritional science [1], and the public has all too often discovered that those who should know the most about nutrition know very little.

There have been, of course, far-sighted physicians who have been interested in nutrition and have contributed a substantial part of what is presently known. They have often chided their colleagues—generally, but not always, with soft voices—largely to no avail. These physicians who are really interested in nutrition often lack prestige and tend to operate outside the mainstream of medicine. In addition, an increasing number

Reprinted from *Perspectives in Biology and Medicine*, Vol. 17, No. 1, Autumn 1973. © 1973 by The University of Chicago. All rights reserved. Printed in U. S. A.

* Department of Chemistry. Clayton Foundation Biochemical Institute, University of Texas, Austin, Texas 78712.

of those who are medically trained carry out investigations which impinge strangely on nutrition, yet because of their training they are not nutritionally oriented.

As a result of decades of neglect of nutritional science by medical science, what we would regard as sophisticated well-rounded nutritional science does not exist. Senator Schweiker, a layman, has recognized this severe deficiency and has introduced a bill authorizing the appropriation of $5 million annually to provide nutritional education in medical schools.

Expert sophisticated nutritional science necessarily involves a basic understanding of biochemistry, physiology, and pathology and an ability to deal in depth with the functioning and interrelationships of all the nutrients—minerals, trace minerals, amino acids, vitamins, etc. Not only this, but it must also encompass the biological nature of the human beings who are to be nourished, including the inheritance factors which affect their nutrition. As with other branches of science, its development must depend on interdisciplinary interest and intercommunicating specialized experts. Many tools, including those of mathematics, are now available with which to study human beings and their biological uniqueness. What is needed is the incentive, interest, and support of such investigations.

Sophisticated nutritional science, when developed, will recognize four basic facts which have not entered the mainstream of medical thinking. These four facts will be presented briefly, not with the claim that they are completely new or previously unheard of, but rather that they are crucial to the development of nutritional science and are commonly neglected.

I. Food is a part of our environment

Once stated, the above proposition becomes so obvious as not to require defense. We get oxygen from the air we breathe, water from the fluid we drink, and an assortment of about 40 or more essential nutrients from the food we consume. These all become a part of our internal environment, the *milieu intérieur* that Claude Bernard talked about in the last century.

The mere recognition of this fact raises serious questions. What happens to cells and tissues if this nutritional environment is not well adjusted? May not the quality of the nutritional environment have a profound effect on health [2]? Can we afford to monitor carefully and scientifically other aspects of our environment like air and water, at the same time giving inexpert stepmotherly attention to the most complex part? From a practical standpoint, in what ways is this complex nutritional environment most subject to damaging deterioration?

II. Suboptimal nutrition prevails in nature

Because nutritional science has been neglected, another crucial consideration has not been grasped. It is the fact that it is very common indeed for organisms in nature to live continuously under suboptimal nutritional conditions. This may happen during embryonic stages of development, but is most certainly the rule during postembryonic stages of life.

Among higher organisms, those receiving the best nutrition are the very young, the sprout nurtured by the seed, the embryos of mammals and fowls, and the suckling young. Nature has ordained it so that good nutrition is often furnished; otherwise the young would not survive. When, however, organisms pass from these early stages to become corn growing in a field, partially grown fowls or mammals, children of school age or younger, there is no automatic way in which they get what they need, and suboptimal nutrition prevails.

That suboptimal nutrition is common throughout the biological kingdom can be made clear by a few examples. A half-ounce cake of compressed yeast, if given good nutrition continuously, will yield in 1 week over a billion tons of yeast. This kind of nutrition is not supplied to yeast cells in nature. Corn growing in a field may produce all the way from less than 1 bushel up to 150 or more bushels per acre, depending on the quality of the environment furnished. Practically speaking, this environment is always suboptimal. Young weanling rats fed grain diets which were thought "normal" 50 years ago develop slowly, gaining weight at the rate of 1–2 grams per day. Now, when we know more about rat nutrition, they may be expected to develop rapidly and gain, if well fed, 5–7 grams per day. Some organisms commonly get in nature better nutrition than others, but in general adult organisms do not get nutrition of such high quality that it could not be improved.

No doubt the same principles apply to human beings. Large segments of the world population subsist on nutrition which is very far from optimal. The cells and tissues of our bodies (like those of other species, including all plants and animals) commonly compete for food essentials, and it certainly cannot be assumed that even in more advanced countries these cells and tissues automatically get precisely the right assortment of individual nutrients. This is a particularly dangerous assumption when applied to a highly industrialized culture in which processed and preserved foods are consumed and scientific nutrition is neglected.

We often get passable nutrition for the cells and tissues of our bodies because we are surrounded by plants and animals which furnish us food. These plants and animals have in their metabolic machinery the very same building blocks—minerals, amino acids, and vitamins—that we have in our cellular machinery. The removal of some of these building blocks during processing and preservation can only cause damage, and this damage cannot be repaired by partial replacement.

The acceptance of the idea that suboptimal nutrition is universal is enough by itself to change one's entire outlook. Nutrition now becomes something that is always subject to improvement. "Normal nutrition" becomes a relatively meaningless expression; if it means anything, it is some level of suboptimal nutrition. If nutrition were optimal, it certainly would not be "normal."

III. Individuality is a crucial factor in nutrition

A third vital consideration neglected by a backward nutritional science, in spite of its tremendous practical importance, is individuality in nutrition. Lucretius wrote about 2,000 years ago: "What is one man's meat is another's poison," but medical science in its general neglect of realistic nutrition has not sought to explore the roots and determine the full significance of this ancient saying.

The bearing of individuality on the practical application of nutrition can be indicated by this illustration. The following five statements are probably true. (1) The majority of adults require 750 mg or less of calcium per day. (2) The majority of adults require 10 mg or less of iron per day. (3) The majority of adults require 800 mg or less of lysine per day. (4) The majority of adults require 1 mg or less of thiamine per day. (5) The majority of adults require 1.5 mg or less of riboflavin per day.

If we attempt to collect and tabulate these five bits of information, we may arrive at the following table. This, however, is completely spurious.

Daily needs of the "majority of adults" (spurious)

Calcium	750 mg or less
Iron	10 mg or less
Lysine	800 mg or less
Thiamine	1 mg or less
Riboflavin	1.5 mg or less

To explain how this collective tabulation is invalid and that the collective data do not necessarily apply to not more than about 3 percent of the supposed population, we may start with an imagined population of 1,000 adults. If the first statement regarding calcium needs is strictly and literally true, 499 out of the 1,000 adults may have calcium needs higher than 750 mg and, hence, strictly speaking must be excluded from the tabulation. If the second statement is likewise strictly true, 250 more may have iron needs above 10 mg and, hence, cannot with strictness be included. If the third, fourth, and fifth statements are likewise true, 125, 62, and 31 additional individuals may be successively eliminated from the collective estimates, leaving a residue of only 33 out of 1,000 to whom all five estimates must apply.

If our illustration had included a large number of nutrient items, the percentage for whom the collective estimates certainly apply would decrease to the vanishing point, regardless of the exact method of calculation. If 30 nutrients were involved, for example, calculating on the same

basis as above shows that all but about five members of the entire estimated world population would be excluded from the collective estimates.
If the five original estimates were correct for "80 percent of adults" instead of the "majority of adults," the collected estimates would apply
not to "80 percent of adults" but to about 33 percent. If in this case there
were 30 nutrient items involved, the collected estimates would apply to
only one adult in 806 instead of "80 percent of adults."

Those who neglect this principle may concern themselves unwittingly
with the nutrition of a minuscule part of the whole population—those
whose needs are about average in each of dozens of respects.

This discussion would be merely academic if individual needs were
clustered around narrow limits, but this is very far from the case. When
the Food and Nutrition Board considered several years ago the desirability
of publishing the ranges of human needs, they were confronted by the
fact that these ranges were not known. The studies essential to such determinations had not, in many cases, been made.

The situation is about the same at the present time. We have found
definitive, though not necessarily ample, evidence with respect to range of
needs of 10 nutritional items as presented in table 1.

For 10 other items—magnesium, iron, copper, iodide, vitamin A, vitamin D, vitamin E, ascorbic acid, pyridoxine, cobalamine—there is some
indirect evidence about differences in requirements but little about ranges.
In the cases of vitamin A [14, pp. 143–146; 15; 16], vitamin D [17, 18, 19],
ascorbic acid [20, 21, 22], and pyridoxine [23, 24, 25], the evidence is
that the ranges are probably very wide if the entire population is included.
For 16 other nutrients, about which there can be no serious question, we
find no information whatever regarding ranges of human needs. The
presumption, on the basis of the definitive information available, is that
the needs for all nutrients vary on the average over a fourfold range.

These data cannot be neglected in any intelligent realistic approach to
human nutrition. To do so can result only from living in a dream world

Table 1: Ranges of daily human needs for certain nutrients

Nutrient	Range	No. subjects	Reference
Tryptophan	82–250 mg (3–fold)	50	3,4
Valine	375–800 mg (2.1–fold)	48	3,5
Phenylalanine	420–1,100 mg (2.6–fold)	38	3,6
Leucine	170–1,100 mg (6.4–fold)	31	3,7
Lysine	400–2,800 mg (7–fold)	55	3,8,9
Isoleucine	250–700 mg (2.8–fold)	24	3,10
Methionine	800–3,000 mg (3.7–fold)	29	3,9
Threonine	103–500 mg (4.8–fold)	50	3,11
Calcium	222–1,018 mg (4.6–fold)	19	12
Thiamine	0.4–1.59 mg (3.9–fold)	15	13

where the "hypothetical average man" is of most vital concern and real individuals are banished.

An inspired writer in the *Heinz Handbook of Nutrition* wrote 13 years ago as follows:

> Individual organisms differ in their genetic makeup and differ also in morphologic and physiologic aspects, including their endocrine activity, metabolic efficiency, and nutritional requirements. . . . It is often taken for granted that the human population is made up of individuals who exhibit average physiologic requirements and that a minor proportion of this population is composed of those whose requirements may be considered to deviate excessively. Actually there is little justification in nutritional thinking for the concept that a representative prototype of *Homo sapiens* is one who has average requirements with respect to all essential nutrients and thus exhibits no unusually high or low needs. In the light of contemporary genetic and physiologic knowledge and the statistical interpretations thereof, the typical individual is more likely to be one who has average needs with respect to many essential nutrients *but who also exhibits some nutritional requirements for a few essential nutrients which are far from average.* [26] [Italics supplied]

This statement, however, has barely rippled the waters of the dyed-in-the-wool nutritionists. The time has come, we believe, when far more serious attempts will be made not only to know more about the ranges of human needs, but also to determine for individuals what needs they may have which are "far from average." In the case of some nutrients, this can be done now, but to make substantial progress in this area will require a major effort. Medical science must come to the rescue, applying to the job a substantial proportion of the resources it has been furnished. Automated equipment and computerized techniques will be widely used in this effort.

Acceptance of the facts of individuality greatly magnifies the possibilities of improving the suboptimal nutrition which is so widespread. People who are regarded as in relative good health may be living with suboptimal nutrition in a generalized sense; more pointedly, however, they are very likely to be functioning at a low level of efficiency because their nutrition is suboptimal in specific ways which can be not only determined but also corrected.

These considerations lay the groundwork for a grand eye-opening with respect to the importance of expertly monitored nutrition for people in general as well as the tremendous role it can play in medical practice. Instead of assuming, as physicians are prone to do, that patients automatically are well nourished, it will become accepted as common knowledge that generally speaking they are not, even if they do escape beriberi, pellagra, scurvy, and kwashiorkor. It will be realized that with human beings as with experimental animals [27], there is an enormous variability on the part of individuals to subsist on diets of mediocre or poor quality.

The genetotrophic concept, now 23 years old, is of vital concern in this discussion [28]. The basic idea may be simply expressed as follows: Diseases which have hereditary roots (this may be a widely inclusive category) may exist because the individuals concerned have unusual nutritional needs that are not easily met. If this is so, then meeting these needs should abolish the diseases in question.

It is well recognized in biological science that specific organisms require suitable environments if they are to thrive. The genetotrophic concept is an application of this principle. Certain individuals, it proposes, must have special nutritional environments if they are to thrive.

In spite of the fact that genetotrophic diseases may well include most noninfectious diseases, the validity or nonvalidity of this postulate has received practically no attention. The word genetotrophic is in medical dictionaries, but that is about as far as the matter has progressed. This could not possibly have happened if medical science were alert to the principles of nutrition. The soundness of the genetotrophic idea has never been questioned; it simply has not been tested for its applicability to any common disease.

It has been found inadvertently to be valid in some cases. In phenylketonuria, for example, fully adequate diets low in phenylalanine are not found naturally, but when these are compounded and furnished children suffering from phenylketonuria, the difficulty is controlled.

Certain rats with a hereditary need for high levels of manganese develop on ordinary diets severe inner ear difficulties. When these animals are artificially furnished high manganese diets, the inner ear difficulties do not appear [29–31]. There are probably a number of other isolated examples that could be cited, but what medical science needs to ascertain, by using expertise that is not generally cultivated, is whether individuals who are peculiarly susceptible to heart disease, obesity, arthritis, dental disease, mental disease, alcoholism, muscular dystrophy, multiple sclerosis, and even cancer, can be benefited by nutritional adjustments. How can we possibly know if medical science, taking the vital facts of individuality into account, does not try seriously to find the answer?

IV. In nutrition, teamwork is essential

The fourth basic fact in nutrition which has been sadly neglected by medical science is that of the essential "teamwork" among nutrients. Because this principle has been neglected, a wholly unscientific concept has been widely accepted with respect to what a nutrient may be expected to do.

The basic error, tacitly accepted, may be expressed as follows. Nutrients—amino acids, minerals, and particularly vitamins—are potential "medicines," and should be tested accordingly, using statistical methods and suitable placebo controls to determine their efficacy in combating diseases. If they prove to be "specifics" for particular diseases, well and good; if not, they must be regarded as medically worthless. In defense of this way of thinking is the historical fact that individual nutrients have in some cases acted like medicines—thiamine for beriberi, ascorbic acid for scurvy, niacinamide for pellagra. However, the parallel between these vitamins and "medicines" is more apparent than real, as careful consideration will show.

Following this erroneous reasoning, it is concluded that since specific individual nutrients are ineffective when tested in this way against specific common ailments, these nutrients are worthless for combating disease. It is easy to conclude also that there should be no substantial concern regarding the intake of these nutrients on the part of patients.

The joker in the argument is that while no nutrient by itself is an effective remedy for any common disease, the nutrients acting as a team are probably effective in the prevention of a host of diseases. Against infective diseases, the teamwork may serve to increase resistance. The reasonableness of this broad claim becomes apparent if we accept the postulate that when the environment of our body cells and tissues is adequate and perfectly adjusted, the cells and tissues will perform all their functions well, and a disease-free condition will be promoted.

It must be emphasized that adequate nutrition must involve the complete chain of nutrients. If a diet is missing one link in the nutritional chain, it may be as worthless for supporting life as if it were missing 10 links. One nutrient—mineral, amino acid, or vitamin—added as a supplement to a food can bring no favorable effect unless the food contains some of all the other nutrients or unless they are available from the reserves of the person being nourished.

It is now well recognized, for example, that while thiamine does act as a remedy for beriberi, it does so because in the diet of polished rice the weakest link in the chain is its thiamine content; thiamine alone will do no good if the other members of the nutrition chain are absent. It is a well-authenticated fact that to bring back health to a victim of beriberi, pellagra, or scurvy, complete nutrition—the complete chain or team—is essential. Manifestly, the nutritional chain is as strong as its weakest link. Every nutrient in the list acts like a gear in a complicated machine. There are no nutrients (or gears) which are dispensable.

To seek to educate the public as the Wheat Flour Institute has done [32, p. 14] by teaching that vitamin A, thiamine, niacin, riboflavin, vitamin C, vitamin D, protein, calcium, and iron are the "key nutrients" is to miseducate. Is there any evidence to suggest that phosphate, magnesium, zinc, vitamin B_6, vitamin B_{12}, and pantothenic acid are not key nutrients? Actually, the list of key nutrients is a long one. Every essential nutrient is a separate key which operates only when the other keys are also available.

The development of nutritional science will reveal, we believe, a clear-cut distinction between medicines and nutrients. The physiological effects of medicines can be ascribed to their ability to enter into metabolic machinery and interfere with enzyme systems. This can happen to the detriment of parasites, and presumably in a beneficial way when the host tissues are concerned. Nutrients, on the other hand, act constructively as building blocks for enzyme systems. If a medicine were to act constructively, it would cease to be medicine. It would be a nutrient.

Those who would lightly dismiss the teamwork principle as exemplifying the "shotgun approach" fail to appreciate that biologically every kind of organism in existence derives from its environment all of its nutritional essentials as a team. An organism typically derives whatever nutrients it needs simultaneously, not *ad seriatim*. If the teamwork principle exemplifies the "shotgun approach," it can hardly be condemned on this basis. This approach has a very long and honorable history. It has been used consistently and universally ever since life on earth began.

It is no coincidence that those nutrients so often stressed in elementary "nutritional education" of the past include conspicuously those which have historically acted like "medicines." These are undeniably important, but to think of them as "*the* key nutrients" is to deny the teamwork principle.

Nutrients as physiological agents must be judged on the basis of how they participate in teamwork. A substance suspected of being an indispensable nutrient cannot be excluded on the basis of its ineffectiveness when tested as a "medicine." Nutrients can be extremely valuable, particularly in preventive medicine, but not unless they are used with intelligent appreciation of how they work as members of a team.

Those who recognize fully the validity of the teamwork principle cannot be complacent about the possible existence of nutritional "unknowns." If there are still unrecognized cogs, they must be identified before the operation of the whole machinery can be adequately controlled and studied. Unless there are important alternative ways in which organisms bring about metabolism, the furnishing of each of the nutrients we know about depends upon all the other nutrients being available. Laboratories that are pharmaceutically oriented tend to be interested in any new "medicine," but the search for unknowns in human nutrition is relatively quiescent. That these may exist is suggested by our inability to grow cells at will in chemically defined media in tissue culture. If medical science were fully alert, it would be very much concerned with the problem.

A reflection of the lack of appreciation of the teamwork principle is the reliance placed upon food composition tables. These tables as ordinarily presented in government publications and elsewhere give no hint of the existence of a large indispensable team of coordinated nutrients. They give only fragmentary information which is easily misleading. Judgments as to the nutritional value of a food based on such tables are subject to serious error, especially when processed foods are involved and when nutrient items listed include prominently those which have commonly been added as fortification—thiamin, riboflavin, niacin, and iron.

"Nutrition surveys" [33] reflect the same neglect of the teamwork principle. The nutritional adequacy of the food consumed in different localities cannot be judged adequately on the basis of its content of thiamin, riboflavin, niacin, and iron, particularly when these are the nutritional elements used to "enrich" bread and cereals.

In our laboratories we have recently studied an alternative criterion for judging food values [34]. This is by measuring what we call the "trophic" or beyond-calorie value. Experimentally we ascertain how much new tissue the food in question can produce, beyond that produced in control animals where carbohydrate is supplied in place of the tested food. This method, which inevitably involves biological testing, measures the effective presence of the entire team necessary for tissue building and repair, including the unknowns if they exist.

BROAD SIGNIFICANCE OF THESE FOUR CRUCIAL FACTS

The four facts we have outlined—food is a part of our environment; suboptimal nutrition is ubiquitous; individuality is crucial in nutrition; and teamwork is essential in nutrition—cannot be seriously disputed, and they are far from trivial. When they are accepted, as they must be, there will be a revolution not only in nutritional science, but also in all of medicine, particularly when it is concerned with prevention.

When these four facts are duly considered and nutritional science developed, many currently accepted ideas will be weighed in the balance and found wanting, as either meaningless or misleading and essentially false. Such statements as the following are often made or tacitly accepted. "People in America get good nutrition." "Food contains an abundance of all the minerals, vitamins, etc. that are needed." "Food composition tables adequately reveal food values." "Nutrition surveys will tell us wherever there is malnutrition." "The recommended daily allowances of the Food and Nutrition Board are a safe guide to all nutrient needs." "If you want nutritional advice, ask your physician."

In the light of the four facts we have emphasized, these statements are puerile and are accepted only in ignorance. The fact, which must be faced, is that nutrition is an involved and intricate matter, and at present no one knows just what optimal nutrition is or how precisely to find out. Abundant incentives exist for attempting to reach this goal [35]. Such an objective must await the further development of nutritional science.

The general acceptance of the four facts we have outlined will result in far more intelligent regulations on the part of the Food and Drug Administration. This body is naturally influenced greatly by current medical opinion, and it will change its attitudes as medical thinking changes. At present the Food and Drug Administration credits physicians with an expertise they should possess but do not. Their regulations too often reflect the backwardness of nutritional science.

The four facts we have discussed are simple ones. They can be and need to be understood even by adolescents. The menace of faddism and charlatanism can only be overcome by education, but it has to be education at a much higher level than has been customary. When the public is reasonably well informed, and medical science has adopted nutritional science as its own, faddism will tend to disappear, and people can get dependable nutritional advice from their physicians.

The prevention of disease, an objective which is inherent in better nutrition and the development of nutritional science, is as old as Hippocrates, who advocated nutrition first, then drugs, then surgery.

Prevention of disease—by every means at our disposal—is the wave of the future in medicine. The expertness medical science has developed in preventing infectious disease will spread to the prevention of non-infective disease. The economies resulting from prevention in terms of health and wealth will be enormous [36]. Prevention of a disease in an individual, when the means are known, may cost only a few cents or a few dollars, while if the disease is allowed to strike, the cost in money alone may easily run into the thousands of dollars. A gram of prevention is worth a kilogram of cure. The development of nutritional science is the principal highway that will lead to the prevention of non-infective disease.

Scientifically, nutritional science is a mere shadow of what it will be when medical science throws its weight behind its development by promoting a health-oriented instead of a disease-oriented discipline.

One relatively open area for scientific investigation is that of intercellular symbiosis [37]. There are probably many substances, of which glutamine, other "nonessential" amino acids, inositol, lipoic acid, and coenzyme Q are examples, which are considered nonessential for the "normal human being" who produces them endogenously. In the light of our discussion of individuality and the genetotrophic concept, however, these nutrients may be crucially needed by certain individuals whose endogenous processes may be somewhat impaired. It appears, for example, that victims of heart disease often are unable to produce enough coenzyme Q to keep their heart muscle unimpaired [38].

All the nutrients we have mentioned above, as well as others, are potential additions to the armamentarium of future physicians who wish to prevent and treat disease by sophisticated nutritional means.

A well-developed nutritional science which recognizes the hard facts of individuality will also delve into many other problems such as the matter of imbalances, the role of intestinal microorganisms in the nutrition of individuals, the question of the incidence and importance of defective enzymatic systems in the digestive tract [2, pp. 189–190], the large problem of malabsorption as it relates to the nutrition of individuals, and the broad question of the overall effects of slow or rapid development during youth on future health and well-being during adulthood.

Another area of great concern to those who would embrace sophisticated nutritional science is that of the basic functioning of some of the well-established nutrients like vitamin A acid, vitamin E, and vitamin C. Because enzymology is a relatively active field, the functioning of many of the B vitamins is relatively well understood, but the physiological function of the vitamins which were originally designated by the first, third, and fifth letters of the alphabet, still presents serious enigmas.

Another area of great scientific interest is the relationship of nutrition to hormone production. It is well known, for example, that thyroid hormone production may be limited by the availability of dietary iodine. Is insulin production, for example, ever limited by dietary lack of sulfur-containing amino acids, or are there other hormones the building of which may be impaired because of nutritional lacks? Development of sophisticated nutritional science will inevitably help solve the major problem of the biochemical functioning of hormones and the general problems of endocrinology.

Of great practical interest is the question of how expert nutritional adjustments can come into play in protecting against pollution. The well-recognized fact that ascorbic acid protects animals against lead poisoning and the recent finding that vitamin E protects animals against atmospheric pollutants [39, 40] call attention to this important potentiality. The broad problem of pollution includes iatrogenic pollution of the internal micro-environments and that produced by self-medication and self-indulgence in tobacco, marijuana, caffeine, and alcohol. All of the foreign elements which enter into the *milieu intérieur* are capable of affecting the nutritional status of the individual concerned.

Still another area of great practical interest and one that cannot be explored without regard for the facts of individuality and the other facts we have discussed is that of the self-selection of food.

Some nutritionists have stated dogmatically that there is no instinct which guides one in his choice of food. This extreme position in our opinion is just as untenable as the opposite one, namely, "instinct always guides us to select the right food." Somewhere between these two extremes lies the truth, and it needs to be ascertained. It is known that in healthy animals total food consumption (also water consumption) is often well controlled by internal forces. It is also known that impairment of the adrenals greatly affects salt consumption and the ability to taste salt [41, 42]. Some recent studies show that rats have a mechanism in which the brain is involved for selecting essential amino acids [43, 44]. Their food consumption is also affected by the amino acid levels in the blood [45]. It is known that in humans excessive sugar or fat or salt consumption may lead to nausea and rejection.

Experiments have shown that healthy young children given a wide selection of wholesome foods will provide themselves with reasonably good nutrition. Such experiments beg the question of how well the selection will work if some of the foods are not so wholesome! It is a common observation that if children are given a choice of beverage—milk, sweetened chocolate milk, or a cola drink—a large percentage will choose most unwisely. It seems probable this unwise selection is based, in part at least, upon previous poor nutrition of that portion of the brain which plays a role in food selection. Body wisdom is probably not fostered by the consumption of deficient foods. The whole problem of whether and to what extent human beings have internal mechanisms which help them select food wisely needs exploration, along with the question of whether nutritional adjustments can improve faulty choice mechanisms.

The problem of prenatal nutrition requires, in our opinion, special attention, taking into account all of the four facts we have stressed. Nutrition during the reproductive period is more exacting than at other times. It has been found consistently that diets which will successfully maintain adult animals may not be adequate for reproduction. This has been demonstrated in rats, mice, dogs, cats, foxes, monkeys, chickens, turkeys and fish. For this reason one might suspect that in a world where suboptimal nutrition generally prevails, pregnant women are often inadequately nourished. Nature tries to provide growing fetuses with good environments, but it is powerless to do so if the necessary raw materials are absent from the food consumed. Prenatal nutrition merits extensive and careful study because for reasons we cannot detail here it is probable that infertility, miscarriages, "spontaneous" abortions, premature births, birth deformations, minor birth defects, and mental retardation often have their roots in the suboptimal environment pregnant women furnish the embryos when they eat carelessly or follow inexpert advice [2, chap. 4]. Even if the hereditary cards are stacked somewhat against one, this does not mean in the light of the genetotrophic concept that expert nutritional help could not obviate the potential difficulty.

SUMMARY AND PROSPECTS

Up until recent years interest in nutrition had been waning, but there is now evidence of resurgent interest. In 1967, for example, there was a projected national nutrition survey which resulted finally in a 10-state survey (1968–1970). This indicated a substantial interest on the part of what we may call "the establishment."

There is also a rapidly growing grass roots interest in better nutrition on the part of millions of people as is evidenced by the multiplication of health food stores, the sale of food supplements, and the publication of numerous books and magazine articles dealing with health and nutrition. Misinformation is common, of course, but how could it be otherwise when the majority of physicians are themselves so untutored. Faddism has its roots in interest, accompanied by inadequate basic knowledge. It cannot be corrected by lack of interest accompanied by inadequate knowledge. It will be corrected when more physicians are both interested and reasonably competent in the area of nutrition.

Thousands of physicians and medical students are becoming interested in nutrition and in the possibilities which have been missed up to the present. This groping on the part of physicians and medical students, of course, leads to error, but in the end the groping will pay off. Four new medical societies have been formed in the past year or two, all of them leaning strongly toward nutrition and its use in the prevention and treatment of noninfective disease. They are the International Academy of Preventive Medicine, the Academy of Orthomolecular Psychiatry, the Society of Biologic Psychiatry, and the International Academy of Metabology.

Many encouraging signs indicate that at long last a renaissance of nutritional science is imminent.

REFERENCES

1. R. J. Williams, Persp. Biol. Med., 14:608, 1971.

2. R. J. Williams, Nutrition against disease. New York: Pitman, 1971.

3. W. C. Rose, Nutr. Abstr. Rev., 27:631, 1957.

4. R. M. Leverton, N. Johnson, J. Pazur, and J. Ellison, J. Nutr., 58:219, 1956.

5. R. M. Leverton, M. R. Gram, E. Brodovsky, M. Chaloupka, A. Mitchell, and N. Johnson, J. Nutr., 58:83, 1956.

6. R. M. Leverton, N. Johnson, J. Ellison, D. Geschwender, and F. Schmidt, J. Nutr., 58:341, 1956.

7. R. M. Leverton, J. Ellison, N. Johnson, J. Pazur, F. Schmidt, and D. Geschwender, J. Nutr., 53:355, 1956.

8. E. M. Jones, C. A. Baumann, and M. S. Reynolds, J. Nutr., 60:549, 1956.

9. S. G. Tottle, S. H. Bassett, W. H. Griffith, D. B. Mulcare, and M. E. Swendseid, Amer. J. Clin. Nutr., 16:229, 1965.

10. M. E. Swendseid, I. Williams, and M. S. Dunn, J. Nutr., 58:495, 1956.

11. R. M. Leverton, M. R. Gram, M. Chaloupka, E. Brodovsky, and A. Mitchell, J. Nutr., 58:59, 1956.

12. F. R. Steggerda and H. M. Mitchell, J. Nutr., 31:407, 1946.

13. L. B. Pett, J. Public Health, 36:69, 1945.

14. R. J. Williams, Biochemical individuality. New York: Wiley, 1956.

15. R. J. Williams and R. B. Pelton, Proc. Nat. Acad. Sci., 55:125, 1966.

16. M. Z. Rodriguez and M. I. Irwin, J. Nutr., 102:909, 1972.

17. T. D. Spies and H. R. Butt, *In:* G. D. Garfield (ed.). Diseases of metabolism, p. 473. Philadelphia: Saunders, 1953.

18. F. Albright et al. Amer. J. Dis. Child., 54:529, 1937.

19. C. I. Reed, et al. Vitamin D. Chicago: Univ. Chicago Press, 1939.

20. A. B. Kline, J. Nutr., 28:413, 1944.

21. R. J. Williams and G. Deason, Proc. Nat. Acad. Sci., 57:1638, 1967.

22. Man-Li Yew, Proc. Nat. Acad. Sci., 70:969, 1973.

23. C. J. Malory and A. H. Parmelee, J. Amer. Med. Ass., 154:405, 1954.

24. A. D. Hunt et al. Pediatrics, 13:140, 1969.

25. L. E. Rosenberg, New Eng. J. Med., 281:145, 1969.

26. B. T. Burton (ed.). The Heinz handbook of nutrition. New York: McGraw-Hill, 1959.

27. R. J. Williams and R. B. Pelton, Proc. Nat. Acad. Sci., 55:126, 1966.

28. R. J. Williams, E. Beerstecher, Jr., and L. J. Berry, Lancet, 1:287, 1950.

29. R. M. Hill et al. J. Nutr., 41:359, 1950.

30. C. W. Asling et al. Anat. Rec., 136:157, 1960.

31. L. S. Hurley and G. J. Everson, Proc. Soc. Exp. Biol. Med., 102:360, 1959.

32. Eat to live. Chicago: Wheat Flour Institute, 1970.

33. Interdepartmental Committee on Nutrition for National Defense. Manual for nutritional surveys. 2d ed. Bethesda, Md.: Nat. Inst. Health, 1963.

34. R. J. Williams, J. D. Heffley, M.-L. Yew, and C. W. Bode, Proc. Nat. Acad. Sci., 70:710, 1973.

35. R. J. Williams. Paper presented to Nat. Acad. Sci., October 1971.

36. C. E. Weir. An evaluation of research in the United States on human nutrition. Benefits from nutrition research. Washington, D. C.: U. S. Dept. Agr., 1971.

37. R. J. Williams, Tex. Rep. Biol. Med., 19:245, 1961.

38. K. Folkers et al. Inter. J. Vitamin Res., 40:380, 1970.

39. B. D. Goldstein, R. D. Buckley, R. Cardenas, and O. J. Balchum. Science, 169:605, 1970.

40. J. N. Roehm, J. G. Hadley, and D. B. Menzel, Arch. Intern. Med., 128:88, 1971.

41. C. P. Richter, Amer. J. Psychiat., 97:878, 1941.

42. G. C. Supplee, R. C. Bender, and O. J. Kahlenberg, Endocrinology, 30:355, 1942.

43. Q. R. Rogers and A. E. Harper, J. Comp. Physiol. Psychol., 72:66, 1970.

44. P. M. B. Leung and Q. R. Rogers, Life Sci., 8:1, 1969.

45. Y. Peng and A. E. Harper, J. Nutr., 100:429, 1970.

4

SOLE FOODS AND SOME NOT SO SCIENTIFIC EXPERIMENTS

D. M. Hegsted, Ph.D., and Lynne M. Ausman, Sc.D.*

The abundant and relatively inexpensive food supply which we enjoy in the United States is due to the success of modern agriculture. The production, harvesting, processing, and distribution of this food requires a system that is quite different from that which was possible when people relied largely upon food produced in their own locality. An increasingly large proportion of the food we eat must be processed in order to preserve it and make it available to the consumer. Most American consumers demand and are willing to pay for as much freedom as possible from the work of preparing food in their own kitchens. The wide acceptance of prepackaged, convenience foods is adequate evidence that few housewives are willing to pluck the feathers off chickens, bake their own bread, or spend as much time in the kitchen as their mothers did.

It is clear that if a large proportion of our food supply is preprocessed and prepackaged, the housewife has little control over the nutritional content of the diet her family eats. It is also clear that the availability of many of these foods in the market depends upon the use of various materials such as food additives in their manufacture. Since food processing is a rather recent development, it is not surprising that we have not had time in which to learn the actual long-term consequences of living on a diet

Reprinted with permission of *Nutrition Today.* Copyright November/December 1973 by Nutrition Today Inc.

* Dr. Hegsted is Professor of Nutrition, School of Public Health, Harvard University. Dr. Ausman is Research Associate in Nutrition, also at the School of Public Health, Harvard University.

of such foods. Vigilance is, of course, required. However, there is no reason to assume *a priori* that living off processed food is detrimental to health. Indeed, if we know what should and what should not be in foods and how much of each is permissible, a food supply of this nature provides the opportunity to "tailor make" and actually improve the nutritional quality of our diets.

Concern over the complex problems involved in providing an adequate and safe food supply for all Americans is legitimate, but it has led to many ill-conceived and illogical recommendations, many of which could be dismissed if they had not misled so many people. Apparently experiments labeled "scientific" are the most impressive to the lay reader who is unable to distinguish between the good ones and bad ones. We wish to present here the results of a "scientific experiment" similar to some of those that have been presented to the public in recent years and have been widely discussed. It is hoped that the reader will be able to discern the illogical conclusions that have been drawn from such experiments.

A popular type of research consists in feeding one food to test animals until they die, then crying, "Ah ha! So and so will kill you." The conclusions may be right, but in too many cases the experiment is wrong. The results, taken out of context or improperly interpreted, could be entirely misleading. We tested a number of single foods commonly consumed by the American public, none of which proved capable of supporting normal growth and development in young rats!

Young growing rats are the most popular species for nutritional experiments. This deserves some comment. The nutritional needs of rats are better known than those of any other species. As a model for man, nevertheless, it should be noted that the species has serious deficiencies. It is instructive to note that a well-nourished child of 2 to 3 years of age who consumes about 300 gm of food per day, weighs about 14 kg (31 pounds) and gains from 4 to 6 gm per day. Five gm of body tissue contain about 1 gm of protein, and the child's diet must provide enough protein to maintain his body structure and deposit an additional gm of new protein each day. A young rat weighing 50 to 100 gm (0.1 to 0.2 pounds) and consuming only 10 to 15 gm of food per day, also gains about 5 gm a day. Thus, this little animal must make the same amount of new tissue protein every day as the child, but its food intake is much smaller. The level and quantity of protein in the diet is enormously more important for the young rat than for the young child. Many foods that are seriously inadequate in protein for the young rat are less so, or perhaps adequate, for the young child. In this regard, we should note that there is little dispute over the fact that, although only 6 to 7 percent of its calories are protein, breast milk is an adequate and appropriate food for babies. This level of protein is not adequate for young rats. Because of its rapid growth, the young rat also has greater needs for several other nutrients than do infants and children.

On the other hand, a young rat will grow very well on a diet that contains no vitamin C, folic acid, or some other nutrients, which are essential for man. The fact that a young rat fed on a particular diet shows good growth is no assurance that the diet will also be adequate for the human species. It is clear that the results of an experiment must be interpreted in the light of what is known about the nutritional requirements of the species used and of the nutritional requirements of man.

Finally, it should be noted that growth experiments in rats provide no information about the long-term effects of various diets. Williams, Hefley and Bode (*Proc. Natl. Acad. Sci.* Vol. 68, p. 2361, 1971), after feeding various foods to young rats, concluded that "eggs proved to be a remarkably complete food." These authors ignore the abundant evidence that, for man, coronary heart disease is a major health problem that is associated with elevated plasma cholesterol levels and that plasma cholesterol levels are partially determined by the dietary level of cholesterol. Furthermore, the rat is little affected by dietary cholesterol and is very resistant to atherosclerosis. Almost everyone agrees that it is wise for Americans to limit their consumption of saturated fat and cholesterol. Thus, conclusions based upon the rat can be misleading.

SOLE FOODS

One 13-week experiment involved 54 young male rats which were obtained from a commercial source. They had previously received a good diet and weighed, on the average, 75 gm. They were divided into groups of 6 animals each of approximately the same average weight. Each group then received water and one of the following commonly-acknowledged nutritious foods as its sole diet:

Group 1—a commercial dog food which long experience has shown to allow good growth in young rats and dogs. We consider this the normal or "control" group.

Group 2—whole pasteurized milk.

Group 3—hamburger steak, medium-well-done.

Group 4—commercial skim milk powder.

Group 5—commercial enriched white bread.

Group 6—one of the highly enriched breakfast cereals.

Group 7—frozen french fried potatoes, cooked according to the instructions.

Group 8—frozen orange juice concentrate.

Group 9—fresh spinach.

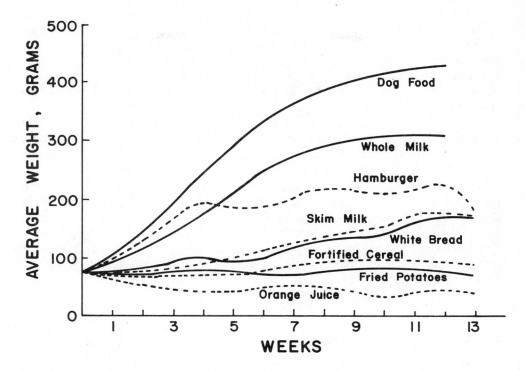

All of the animals were weighed twice weekly and their condition noted. Animals that became terminally ill were anesthetized with ether and killed.

The reader might test his nutritional knowledge by guessing what happened to the animals in the various groups.

As expected, those receiving the commercial dog food grew very well and remained normal in all respects. This was not true of any of the other groups.

The most striking result was that none of the animals fed fresh spinach survived more than 3 days. The cause of these casualties was probably the rather high oxalic acid content of spinach, since this precipitates calcium as an insoluble salt. The kidneys were not examined microscopically, but it is known that diets containing excessive oxalate cause crystals of calcium oxalate to form in the kidneys, blocking their usual function.

The growth of the other groups of animals varied. Those on the milk diet showed a rather satisfactory rate of gain during the first several weeks but ceased to gain after approximately 9 weeks, while those consuming only orange juice showed a loss of weight during the entire experiment. Of the group on the orange juice and that on the hamburger diet, only one animal survived the 13 weeks of the experiment. Two of the 6 animals fed skim milk powder died during this time.

In addition to the observations on weight, it should be noted that the rats fed only whole milk became pale and anemic; those fed hamburger became severely paralyzed; those fed nothing but skim milk soon became blind with cataracts. All the animals maintained on white bread, enriched breakfast cereal, french fried potatoes, or orange juice showed loss of hair to varying degrees and had an unkempt appearance.

Milk is known to be a relatively complete food, except that it is a very poor source of iron. In fact, feeding a whole-milk diet is one of the classic ways of producing iron deficiency for experimental purposes. Therefore, it was not unexpected that the animals living on milk became iron-deficient and developed anemia.

Skim milk powder is similar to whole milk, except that the fat has been removed. This process, it should not be forgotten, also removes the fat-soluble vitamins. Thus, skim milk is much lower in calories than whole milk and lacks the vitamins A and D in whole milk. However, the development of cataracts in the rats fed skim milk resulted from the high content of lactose in this diet. Lactose is the sole source of carbohydrate in milk. It breaks down into two simpler sugars, glucose and galactose, in the body. Since skim milk contains no fat, considerably more of it than of whole milk must be consumed to obtain the proper calorie supply. This high consumption overloads the capacity of the body to metabolize galactose, which accumulates in the body tissues and causes cataracts. This phenomenon has been known for many years. However, there was a report in the June 12, 1970 issue of *Science* that the feeding of yogurt to rats also caused cataracts and blindness. Characteristically, this was duly reported in *The New York Times* and elsewhere with the implication that there is something wrong with yogurt and it might be a dangerous food.

Although the animals forced to live on hamburger alone grew well initially, every one of them eventually developed paralysis. This also was expected. Meat is very low in calcium so, as these animals grew, they had to fall back of the calcium already present in their bones. The depletion resulted in longer, but very thin and fragile, bones that eventually collapsed and caused the paralysis. It is of some interest to note that meat is very high in the essential nutrient, phosphorus, but that this is a disadvantage rather than an advantage, because the high intake of phosphorus inhibits the utilization of the small amount of calcium that meat does contain.

The growth performance of the remaining groups, those receiving white bread, breakfast cereal, french fried potatoes, and orange juice, was most likely influenced by the quantity and quality of protein each food contained, although their content of other nutrients varied greatly. For example, the animals on white bread grew better than those on breakfast cereal, even though the breakfast cereal had relatively high levels of many of the vitamins added to it. Those fed orange juice alone could not possibly grow, because their diet contained practically no protein. Orange juice is a good source of vitamin C but since rats, unlike man, monkeys, and some other species, can synthesize vitamin C in their bodies, this nutrient is of no use to them. Of all the foods fed, only spinach and orange juice contain significant quantities of vitamin C. It is pertinent to point out, that had this experiment been done with a species requiring vitamin C in the diet, the outcome of these experiments would have been quite different.

It should also be noted that although hamburger, white bread, french fried potatoes, and skim milk are all poor sources of vitamin A, our experiments did not provide any clear-cut evidence of vitamin A deficiency. An animal that is not growing well requires lesser quantities of most nutrients, and this is especially true of such fat-soluble vitamins as vitamin A. The young animals we used, having received an adequate diet prior to the time the experiment was begun, had some vitamin A stored in their livers. But, when it did begin and they grew less well, their requirement for most nutrients was reduced and the vitamin A in their livers sufficed to prevent the development of vitamin A deficiency. Studies of this kind do not necessarily identify which of the various nutrients may be most deficient under other conditions. The outcome depends upon which nutrient the animal needs during the time of the study.

Animals remaining alive in various groups at different times (six animals in each group originally)

Weeks on diet	Spinach	Source of Food				
		Orange juice	Skim milk	Hamburger	Breakfast cereal	All other foods [1]
1	0	5	6	6	6	6
2		5	6	6	5	6
3		5	6	6	5	6
4		4	6	6	5	6
5		4	6	6	5	6
6		4	6	5	5	6
7		4	5	5	5	6
8		4	5	3	5	6
9		3	4	2	5	6
10		2	4	2	5	6
11		1	4	2	5	6
12		1	4	1	5	6
13		1	4	1	5	6

[1] Animals which received either dog food, whole milk, white bread or french fried potatoes.

WHICH FOOD IS BEST

One is tempted to ask "Which is the best food for man?" Clearly, this is a nonsense question since none of the splendid foods we eat every day is wholly adequate nor is it meant to be. Therein lies the fallacy of "scientific experiments" such as ours. With the exception of the commercial dog food, all of the foods fed the rats were deficient, to one degree or another, and in one or more of the nutrients required. Drawing a conclusion about the nutrient value of any one of them is like asking whether one would prefer to be deficient in vitamin A, protein, iron, or some other nutrient. Since a severe deficiency of any essential nutrient eventually causes death or serious disability, there is little purpose in making such a decision.

Milk is the only one of the foods used in the experiment that approaches nutritional adequacy when fed alone. It is designed as a sole source of food for very young animals, even though it is an inadequate source of iron. Nature overcame this inadequacy by assuring that young animals, human and non-human, born to adequately fed mothers have enough iron stored within their bodies to last until they are ready to consume other foods to supply the iron they need. Since milk does contain a rather generous supply of protein and most of the vitamins and minerals, its inclusion in the diet provides a safeguard against nutritional deficiencies. It is not an essential food, however, since necessary nutrients can be provided by many types of mixed diets.

What does one conclude about the nutritional value of spinach? Clearly, a diet consisting solely of spinach is toxic. The spinach-fed animals died sooner than they would have if they had had no food at all. Some years ago it was suggested that the Food, Drug and Cosmetic Law be amended to extend the provisions of the Delaney Clause to include "any toxic materials." In essence, the Delaney Clause says that no food containing any material known to produce cancer shall be sold. The extension of this clause would thus prohibit the sale of any food which contains toxic materials. The difficulties in this are exemplified by the feeding of spinach, which is "toxic," alone. The definition of "toxicity" depends upon the conditions of the test.

Probably few people would be willing to have spinach banned from the market. Every diet contains toxic materials (and carcinogens) and, on top of that, everything in the environment is toxic. Excessive amounts of essential nutrients are toxic, and excessive consumption of vitamins A and D has been known to cause serious disease. Excessive consumption of sugar or water, excessive oxygen in the atmosphere, excessive exposure to sunlight, excessive consumption of brown rice (the Macrobiotic Diet) are all lethal. Yet rigid prohibitions on any of these are not logical or possible.

NO ABSOLUTES

This is not to say, of course, that there are no dangers in the modern foods. In our increasingly complex society we have to use a variety of chemicals and other materials if we are to produce enough acceptable food and distribute it to the population of this country and to the world, and this clearly requires vigilance. However, there are no absolutes.

Caution combined with judgment based upon experience is the only procedure that can be followed.

Finally, we should like to mention the recent controversy over cereals and bread which has had considerable exposure in the public press. The breakfast cereal that was fed in our experiments was one of the "most nutritious" cereals, according to the rating chart prepared by Mr. Choate and presented to the Subcommittee on the Consumer, Committee of Commerce, United States Senate, July 23, 1970. Therefore, it might surprise some people to learn that rats fed this material were less well nourished than those that subsisted on white bread alone. However, from what has been said, it should be clear that we feel such comparisons are meaningless.

FAVORITE WHIPPING BOY

White flour has been a favorite whipping boy of the food activists for a long time. Consider what's been said about it: John Lear writing in the *Saturday Review* emphasized that the milling of flour removed a wide variety of minerals and vitamins and quotes such values as "40 percent of the chromium, 86 percent of the manganese, 60 percent of the calcium, 78 percent of the sodium, 77 percent of the thiamin, most of the vitamin A", and so forth. Then Roger J. Williams of the University of Texas has pointed out that young rats do not grow well on bread alone, but if one adds a variety of nutrients including protein or amino acids, vitamins and minerals, they do grow well. But from this does one cry out, "Ergo! Bread is a bad food!?"

The results of this kind of an experience should surprise no one. All foods when consumed alone are inadequate and could be improved by the addition of the specific nutrients required.

What then do we do? Require that all meat be fortified with calcium and vitamin A; orange juice (which probably cannot be fortified with enough nutrients to make it nutritionally complete and still be edible) be prohibited; skimmed milk be kept off the market: This is obvious nonsense.

Roger Williams in his book, *Nutrition Against Disease*, Putnam Publishing Co., Boston, 1970, also uses another kind of illogic which should be recognized. He points out that when he feeds rats a diet containing inadequate amounts of a vitamin, they do very poorly. When he doubles the amount of the vitamin in the diet, they do much better. Thus, Dr. Williams implies that if the vitamin content were quadrupled or more, they would be still better. One could as reasonably argue that since a child receiving 50,000 units of vitamin A per day will become ill but does not when he receives 5,000, he should be still healthier if he received only 500 units or, better still, 50 units. The trouble with this logic is that a child receiving only 500 units of vitamin A per day, would probably become deficient in vitamin A, and if he were receiving only 50 units a day he would certainly die.

A simpler example might be to recall that most of us need about 2,000 calories per day in order to remain healthy. Do we then conclude that if we had 3,000 or 4,000 calories per day we would be better still? Even the least sophisticated recognize that this is not true.

The addition of nutrients to foods is a well-established public health measure. Those that should be added, however, depend upon the particular food and the circumstances under which it will be consumed. The sole food of very young infants is likely to be the formula the pediatrician prescribes, and, quite obviously, it should be complete with regard to all nutrients. Such completeness may be accomplished by adding specific nutrients to the product from which it is constructed, usually a milk product. In contrast, the objective in most other fortification programs is simply to select a vehicle which will be effective in providing those nutrients which are low in a relatively large number of diets. In order to do this job, the food fortified must be one that is consumed by most people, and the fortification process must be technically feasible and relatively inexpensive. It was because bread meets those specifications that its fortification with certain B vitamins and iron was proposed many years ago. The fortification of bread or of salt with iodine, of water with fluoride, of milk with vitamin D, and of margarine with vitamin A clearly is not an attempt to make these complete foods. They have been chosen because they are effective carriers of nutrients.

Various cereal products are often reasonably satisfactory as carriers of nutrients, not only because they are widely consumed but because they are relatively inexpensive. They provide a mechanism for the delivery of nutrients to those with limited income, the population group most likely to be living on inadequate diets.

FORTIFICATION QUESTIONS

The question is often asked whether nutrients other than those now included in fortification programs should be added to bread and cereals and perhaps other foods. This question deserves continuing review. As we have indicated, the answer should be determined not by the effect observed when bread is the sole food consumed but rather by the nutritional needs of the population. If it is determined that a certain nutrient is generally low in a significant proportion of diets and if the addition of that nutrient to some food is technically feasible and economic, then it may be wise to add it. However, these are dangers in relying too heavily upon the addition of specific nutrients to foods as a primary means of protecting the nutritional quality of the food supply. The trend toward increased reliance on food fortification encouraged by the recent laws on nutrition labeling, may not be advantageous. We do stress that our knowledge of the nutritional needs of man is limited. Studies with rats and other species, if properly interpreted, are informative on that point but rarely definitive.

The consumption of a wide variety of foods, selected with some knowledge of their nutritional characteristics, is the best way to assure that a diet is safe, adequate in nutrients and low in undesirable materials. Heavy reliance upon any particular single food source should be avoided. Vigilance on the part of government, industry, and the consumer is necessary but we should not be misled by over-simplified or "scientific" experiments, with emphasis on the quotation marks.

5

FIBER

the forgotten nutrient

James Scala *

"AN APPLE A DAY . . . ." I've often wondered how the old saying "an apple a day keeps the doctor away" originated. The fact is, apples have very little vitamin or mineral content and practically no protein or fat. How, then, did they gain the widespread reputation for being so good for us?

Perhaps some old-timer, asked to explain the secret of his longevity and good health, recalled that many years earlier he had started eating apples and noticed when he did that he had regular bowel habits. When he had regularity, he felt good. Hence, "an apple a day" became his formula for good health. As far as he went, he was right. The apple provides "roughage" or, to be more specific, the "fiber" contained in fruits, vegetables, and cereals. Fiber does indeed promote regular elimination. But modern science has suggested a far more vital role for fiber: its potential in helping to deal with some of the most insidious enemies of man—atherosclerosis, diverticular diseases, and cancer of the large intestine.

FIBER IN THE DIET

Plant materials which are indigestible by the secretions of the human digestive system are loosely defined as dietary fiber. It consists mostly

Reprinted from *Food Technology*, January 1974, pp. 34–36.

* Director of Nutrition, Thomas J. Lipton, Inc., 300 Sylvan Ave., Englewood Cliffs, N. J. 07632.

of nondigestible carbohydrates, such as pectin, celluloses and hemicelluloses, and usually contains some noncarbohydrate substances such as lignin. These materials should not be considered crude fiber—a time-honored term in food composition tables. Crude fiber is what remains after treatment with hot sulfuric acid, alkali, alcohol, and other non-physiologic materials. For this reason, crude fiber and dietary fiber are not strictly interchangeable expressions; in fact they differ markedly—only one-fifth to one-half of the total dietary fiber is actually crude fiber.

It is difficult to accurately evaluate "fiber" consumption in our diet due to lack of interest in its recognition as a nutrient. The confusion is increased by the use of crude fiber as an index.

This century has seen a marked decline in the consumption of whole wheat flour and cereals from 160 lb per capita in 1900 to less than 100 lb in 1970. Fresh fruit and vegetables have declined precipitously in use, going from 250 lb per capita in 1940 to under 180 lb in 1970. But the consumption of processed fruit and vegetables has increased in the same period from 65 lb to almost 110 lb per capita. This is a minimum net decrease of 25 lb per capita.

One can evaluate consumption tables *ad nauseam*, but one conclusion is inescapable—fiber from fruits and vegetables (fresh and processed) has declined by about 20%, and fiber from cereals and grains has decreased by as much as 50% in this century. Due to the discrepancy between crude fiber and dietary fiber any more precision would be impossible.

Another means of obtaining trends in the fiber consumption is to assess groups of people with dietary similarities. Rural Africans have a diet similar to Western man in the mid-19th century in contrast to the urban African whose diet is similar to Western man in 1970. The difference in the diets of these two groups of people is 4 to 1 in crude fiber; and one can estimate that it is as much as 6 to 1 in dietary "fiber." From these and other evaluations (e. g., vegetarians vs non-vegetarians) we can conclude that our dietary fiber has declined by about 5 to 1 in the past century.

WHAT DOES FIBER DO?

Fiber ingestion promotes regularity, softer stools, more frequent elimination, (Holmgren et al., 1972) but in the case of certain vegetables (e. g., legumes) it increases flatulence (Steggerda et al., 1966). It also increases the excretion of bile acids, sterols, and fat (Stanley, 1970).

Many of the bulk effects on regularity are the result of the high water binding capacity of fiber which increases stool weight by about 15 g for each g of fiber added to the diet.

FIBER AND ATHEROSCLEROSIS

Atherosclerosis, the cause of most cardiovascular diseases, is Western man's greatest scourge. Fifty percent of all deaths past the age of 45 can be directly attributed to it. It is characterized by material deposited on and within the arterial walls called "plaque," which consists of fat, protein, and cholesterol (its major component).

Cholesterol is not only ingested with foods, but is produced in large quantities by our own body tissues—especially the liver. Cholesterol is converted to the bile acids which are secreted into the small intestine where they help with the digestion and absorption of fat and dietary cholesterol.

Studies with human volunteers (Mathur et al., 1968 and de Groot et al., 1963), confirmed by animal research (Vijayagopal et al., 1973), indicate that in a low-fiber/high-blood-cholesterol population, an increase in dietary fiber will reduce blood cholesterol significantly, especially over a long period of study. When volunteers are put on a high-fiber, hypercholesteremic diet they almost never exhibit cholesterol levels as high as the low-fiber, hypercholesteremic diet controls.

The mechanism by which fiber exerts this influence involves the bile acids. People on a high-fiber diet excrete more bile acids, more sterols and fat. This implies that fiber sequesters the bile acids and sterols, thereby preventing bile acid re-absorption, cholesterol and fat absorption.

Since bile acid excretion is the main elimination pathway of internally produced cholesterol, the increase in excretion reduces the cholesterol pool. This reduction is followed by a lowering of blood cholesterol.

Heart disease is relatively rare in people who eat a vegetarian diet, either in Western countries or in countries where meat is scarce (Groen et al., 1962; Shaper, 1970; Trowell, 1972). Vegetarians often have a low fat consumption, but in the case of many vegetarians fat consumption is similar to a control urban population due to consumption of a great deal of dairy products. These factors emphasize the fiber correlation.

FIBER AND DIVERTICULAR DISEASE

Diverticulitis will result in major surgery for 500,000 Americans in 1973—9 women for every 7 men. Probably 4 to 6 times that number will be treated at home and won't undergo surgery. Since the surgery often includes a temporary colostomy, it's not trivial. To add insult to injury, the incidence of the disease is increasing, the rate has been estimated as high as 16%. Therefore, it's surprising that most people have never heard of the disease.

Diverticular disease is characterized by small "blow-out type" protrusion lesions on the large intestine—usually in the upper regions (ascending and transverse colon) which become inflamed and often burst, producing infection. Statistical correlations indicate that people who have diverticular disease are likely to have appendicitis, polyps of the bowel, hemorrhoids and vericose veins. These associations indicate the hereditary role, but fiber apparently also plays a role.

In some societies these diseases simply don't exist. Indeed, the rural African never has diverticular disease, but his city relative does—with frequency similar to Western man (Painter et al., 1971; Painter, 1969; Kim, 1964; Kyle et al., 1967). Other comparisons can be made with Oriental groups in which similar differences exist.

Clinical studies show that dietary fiber, more specifically cereal fiber, is very effective in relieving the symptoms of diverticulitis (Painter et al., 1972). Indeed, the looser, softer stools of a high fiber diet often relieve the pain associated with diverticular problems and, in many cases, obviates the need for surgery. "Straining," which is characteristic of diverticular patients, causes undue pressure in the venous system of the large intestine and legs. This increases the development of hemorrhoids and varicose veins—both of which can to some extent be relieved by an increase of dietary fiber, and the concomitant decrease in the need for "straining."

To summarize at this point, fiber has two distinct effects; a biochemical effect on the absorption and reabsorption of cholesterol and bile acids respectively, and a physiological effect on the gastrointestinal function which promotes a reduction of intracolonic pressure and therefore is beneficial in diverticular disease. Neither can be evaluated quantitatively.

FIBER AND INTESTINAL CANCER

Intestinal cancer is the second ranked killer among cancers in adults (lung cancer is first), accounting for 47,000 deaths a year in the United States in 1972. The American male is six times more likely to contract intestinal cancer than his counterpart in lesser developed societies. Surgery for the disease is drastic and usually results in a permanent colostomy. Probably 5 to 10 patients survive surgery each year for each death.

Epidemiologists continue to search for the relationships which probably exist between dietary factors and cancer of the alimentary canal (Saxon et al., 1972; Morton, 1973; Nutrition Reviews, 1973). Although clearly established correlations have not been observed, it is reasonable to postulate a role for fiber. Since fiber consumption has decreased by a considerable proportion in the past 25 years, the frequency and volume of fecal elimination has undoubtedly decreased in proportion (Burkitt et al.,

1972). Therefore, it follows that if cancer of the intestine is caused by a foreign material which has access through the diet it has more time to do its harm than previously. In short, if virus A or chemical B causes cancer of the intestine it spends a longer time in the intestine on a low fiber diet than a high fiber diet.

In addition to the simple consideration of residence time, fiber also increases the amount of water, sterols, bile acids, and fat which pass through the large intestine (Burkitt, 1971; Hill et al., 1971). These materials have a combined solvent-like effect which could remove a wide variety of chemical factors.

THE PROMISE OF PROCESSED FOOD

All the information on dietary fiber still doesn't permit the assignment of a nutritional requirement as we do with vitamins. Certainly "an apple a day" won't suffice and we can't expect a reversion to a diet similar to that of the 1870s.

But it is certain that a substantial increase of our dietary fiber would be very beneficial. Hence, an increase of crude fiber consumption from about 6 g per day to 12, or a little more—yielding a total dietary fiber intake of about 20 to 36 g per day would be beneficial. Clinically this is no problem—the patient can be told to eat about two tablspoons of bran with each meal. But that won't work in the everyday world, so fiber offers a new challenge.

Perhaps the Food and Nutrition Board will someday recommend the equivalent of an RDA for fiber. Does that mean they will, in effect, be instructing us to eat so much fresh fruit, vegetables and cereals each day? Definitely not, especially when the cost of natural foods will continue to rise disproportionately to that of processed foods. Rather, it is processed food which holds the greatest promise. Supplementation of food with fiber represents a minimal challenge in a breakfast food, but is certainly a formidable task in meal replacements or entrees which utilize highly processed components.

Because fiber would have to be added to a food formulation in much higher amounts than are vitamins and minerals, its addition would have a more significant effect on the organoleptic characteristics of the food product than does the addition of vitamins and minerals. Fiber could be used as a carrier for other products; as a binder to impart shape; or as the vehicle for texture.

If the food technologist is going to meet the challenge expected of processed food it appears certain that he will have to think of enrichment in more extensive terms than vitamins, minerals, and proteins.

REFERENCES

1. Burkitt, D. P. 1971.　Epidemiology of cancer of the colon and rectum.　Cancer (Philad.).　28:3.

2. Burkitt, D. P., Walker, A. R. P. and Painter, N. S. 1972.　Effect of dietary fibre on the stools and transit times, and its role in the causation of disease. Lancet.　2:1408.

3. de Groot, A. P., Luyken, R. and Pikaar, N. A. 1963.　Cholesterol-lowering effect of rolled oats.　Lancet.　2:303.

4. Graham, S., Schotz, W. and Martino, P. 1972.　Alimentary factors in the epidemiology of gastric cancer.　Cancer.　30:927.

5. Green, J. J., Tijong, K. B., Koster, M., Willebrands, A. F., Verdonek, G. and Pierloot, M.　1962.　The influence of nutrition and ways of life on blood cholesterol and the prevalence of hypertension and coronary heart disease among Trappist and Benedictine monks.　Amer. J. Clin. Nutr.　10:456.

6. Hill, M. J., Crowther, J. S., Drasar, B. S., Hawksworth, G., Arles, V. and Williams, R. E. O.　1971.　Bacteria and actiology of cancer of large bowel. Lancet. 1:95.

7. Holmgren, G. O. R. and Mynors, J. S.　1972.　The effect of diet on bowel transit times.　S. Afr. Med. J.　46:918.

8. Kim, E. H.　1964.　Hiatus hernia and diverticulum of the colon.　Their low incidence in Korea.　New. Eng. J. Med. 271:764.

9. Kyle, J., Adesola, A. O., Tinckler, L. F. and de Beaux, J.　1967.　Incidence of diverticulitis.　Scand. J. Gastrognt.　2:75.

10. Mathur, K. S., Khan, M. A. and Sharma, R. D.　1968.　Hypocholesterolaemic effect of Bengal gram; a long term study in man.　Brit. med. J. 1:30.

11. Morton, J. F.　1973.　Plant products and occupational materials ingested by esophageal cancer victims in South Carolina.　13(1):2005.

12. Nutrition Reviews.　1973.　Diet and cancer of the colon.　4:110.

13. Painter, N. S. and Burkitt, D. P.　1971.　Diverticular disease of the colon; a deficiency disease of western civilization.　Brit. med. J.　2:450.

14. Painter, N. S.　1969.　Diverticular disease of the colon: a disease of this century.　Lancet.　2:586.

15. Painter, N. S., Almeida, A. Z. and Colebourne, K. W.　1972.　Unprocessed bran in treatment of diverticular disease of the colon.　Brit. med. J.　2:137.

16. Shaper, A. G.　1970.　In atherosclerosis: Proceedings of the second international symposium.　Edited by Jones, R. L.　314.

17. Stanley, M. M.　1970.　Quantification of intestinal functions during fasting: estimations of bile salt turnover, fecal calcium and nitrogen excretions. Metabolism.　19:865.

18. Steggerda, F. R. and Dimmick, J. F.　1966.　Effects of bean diets on concentration of carbonic dioxide in flatus.　Amer. J. Clin. Nutr. 19:120.

19. Trowell, H. C.   1972.   Ischemic heart disease and dietary fiber.   Amer. J. Clin. Nutr. 25:926.

20. Vijayagopal, P., Saraswathi, D. and Kurup, P. A.   1973.   Fibre content of different dietary starches and their effect on lipid levels in high fat-high cholesterol diet fed rats.   Atherosclerosis.   17:156.

6

LACTOSE
one of nature's paradoxes

G. G. Birch *

Lactose is the major carbohydrate of mammalian milk but its concentration in milks from different species varies considerably. Dietary lactose is responsible for a number of ill-effects in many species including man, both in normal and abnormal conditions of the organism. Although etiologically perplexing, certain distinct nutritional advantages have been attributed to lactose, and technologically we already know how to harness its properties to advantage.

Lactose, or milk sugar, is practically speaking the only carbohydrate in cow's milk and constitutes 4 to 5% of the total weight of the milk. The amount of lactose in milk varies from species to species and reaches levels between 6 and 7% in human milk. This is not in itself nutritionally advantageous, however, because the ability to digest lactose properly varies, not only among different mammalian species, but also among different human races.

LACTOSE IN FOODS

Lactose is not a very sweet sugar, always tastes very gritty, and won't dissolve very well. In some of our foods these properties are

Reprinted from *Journal of Milk and Food Technology*, January 1972, Vol. 35, No. 1 (pp. 32–34).

* National College of Food Technology, University of Reading, Weybridge, **Surrey**, **England.**

harnessed to useful advantage. The texture of sweetened condensed milk depends on exactly the right amount of lactose being present. Too much can cause a sandy feeling in the mouth and too little will result in a slimy product. Lactose interacts with milk protein when heated to form brown colored substances. This is useful in toffee manufacture but can be a nuisance in dried milk manufacture, when heat has to be applied in the process. Generally, all those technological difficulties make purification and use of lactose uneconomical and each year, therefore, thousands of tons of waste liquor from dairies are dumped into the sea. Whey contains a lot of lactose, but it is not normally wasted. After concentrating in evaporators, creameries sell it for use in confectionery or pharmaceutical products, or in cruder preparations for animals feeds.

PHYSIOLOGICAL CHARACTERISTICS OF LACTOSE

If we want to know why lactose differs from other sugars we must examine it, first at the molecular level and then in terms of its biochemical functions. Molecules of lactose are formed out of galactose joined by a β-D-(1,4) linkage to glucose and before we can absorb milk sugar it must be hydrolyzed in the brush border region of the small intestine, to glucose and galactose, by lactase. The subsequent fates of the glucose and galactose depend on a number of utilizable metabolic pathways and galactose does exist as a permanent feature of many tissues. Brain cells for example contain galactose joined to other groupings, and indeed the brain would not be able to function properly without its galactose. However, it is by no means certain that we need to eat lactose or galactose for this purpose, and probably our bodies convert all the galactose which we absorb into glucose. Galactose is then resynthesized out of glucose whenever it is needed for nervous tissue.

LACTOSE IN MILK

The milk of mammals contains all the essential vitamins, minerals, fats, and proteins which are needed for healthy living. What is not clear, however, is why the milk of so many species should contain over 4% of carbohydrate. More particulaly, why should it be lactose?

If we look more carefully at the composition of milk in the different mammalian species we find that there is considerable variation in lactose content not only between species, but also between individuals. Furthermore, although only a limited amount of research has so far gone into it there is also a considerable variation in the amount of the enzyme lactase in the intestine of individuals *(7)*. There may possibly be a relationship between the lactose content of the milk and the lactase content of the intestine. In the California Sea Lion, for example, whose milk contains no lactose, there is no intestinal lactase.

PROBLEMS WHEN MILK IS CONSUMED

During the past decade it has become clear that the majority of the world's adult population cannot very easily drink milk and this may be caused by the absence of the enzyme lactase in their intestines, so that they cannot digest lactose. As a result adults who drink milk develop cramping pains, sometimes within minutes of drinking the milk, followed frequently by flatulence and diarrhea *(2)*. In several surveys 70–90% of adult Africans, Thais, Chinese, and other Oriental races were found to suffer from the complaints, which are typical of many rare food sugars *(1)*. In such individuals the unhydrolyzable lactose (or other sugar) draws water osmotically from the walls of the intestine, and is attacked by gut microflora producing acids. Fortunately for most of us in the U.K. and U.S.A. only 5–10% of the population or less suffer in the same way. Why should this racial difference exist? The answer is still obscure and scientists are divided in their opinion over whether the difference is genetic or environmental. In other words either we inherit the ability to digest lactose normally, or we may develop the inability to do so by failing to drink enough milk after weaning, so that the level of the enzyme lactase decreases in the intestine.

Babies and children may also suffer from the same type of symptoms after drinking milk and the collective syndrome is referred to specifically as *lactose intolerance*. In surveys among Bantu populations doctors have fed lactose to children and produced very violent intestinal disturbances, so that in some instances death has resulted following the tests *(5)*.

Another way of proving lactose intolerance is to feed lactose to the patient and subsequently to take blood tests every few minutes for the next hour. If the blood sugar level rises normally, as after the ingestion of sucrose, the patient is normal. If, however, the blood sugar level does not rise, this means that the patient is lactose intolerant. Consequently the lactose in the intestine is not digested, bacteria will attack it, and all the usual symptoms of cramping pains, flatulence, and diarrhea will result.

Lactose intolerance is encountered all over the world, but a rarer and much more deadly disease is glactosaemia. This disease is inherited but only affects about one baby out of 40,000 due to the lack of the enzyme glucose 1-phosphate: galactose 1-phosphate uridyl transferase. Galactose builds up in the liver (as its phosphate) because it cannot be converted to glucose, and the babies become very ill and frequently die *(11)*.

Almost all surviving galactosaemics are mentally retarded and the only way to treat the disease known to doctors is to recognize it quickly and remove all galactose and lactose from the babies' diet. Obviously, since babies drink only milk, we cannot do this without special dietary preparations being made available in the hospitals to meet such emergencies. Fortunately food manufacturers in the developed countries are already able to produce substitute milk powders sweetened with substances such as corn sugars or fructose. There are several products of this type now available *(6)* and the demand for similar commodities tailored for clinical purposes will probably increase in the future. A typical preparation for use in cases of galactosaemia, lactose intolerance, or gastroenteritis is shown in Table 1, but these substitute milks are not complete foods and should therefore only be used under medical supervision.

Table 1: Composition of substitute milk powders

Approximate analysis	Dry food (g per 100g)
Vegetable fat	22.3
Unhydrogenated coconut oil	15.0
Unhydrogenated maize oil	7.3
Protein (washed casein)	22.3
Carbohydrates (liquid glucose)	50.2
Mineral salts	3.0
Moisture	2.0
Calcium	0.720
Phosphorus	0.480
Lactose (approx.)	0.098
Meso-inositol	0.313
Choline chloride	0.067
Calories	503

As well as the inability of some humans to digest lactose properly there are several known cases of animal species which are also unable to tolerate milk sugar in quantity as a nutrient. If weanling rats, for example, are fed lactose at a level of 30% of their diet, in addition to diarrhea they rapidly (within a few days) develop cataract *(8)* or opacity of the lens of the eye. This must result from the galactose part of the lactose, because if rats are fed either galactose or human milk alone, they also develop cataract, but they do not if they are fed glucose alone. Galactose-cataract formation in rats is not reversible. A more alarming experiment along these same lines has recently been carried out at the Johns Hopkins Hospital, Baltimore *(9)*. Every single member of a colony of rats fed yogurt as an exclusive diet developed cataract. Evidently galactose, part of the lactose structure, constitutes 22 to 24% of the caloric value of yogurt. Chicks also develop a peculiar syndrome if they are fed galactose or lactose, which is characterized by shivering and shaking and general debilitation *(10)*.

FURTHER USES FOR LACTOSE

Since some human beings cannot tolerate lactose as a food we are left with the problem of harnessing some of the lactose which we produce for some other useful purpose. One which has already been discovered is to use it as a fermenting medium for penicillin production, as the sugar is fermented slowly and conveniently by penicillin moulds.

It must not be thought that because lactose has certain drawbacks for some human beings that the majority of us in the western world cannot enjoy it as a normal food component. It is clearly of great use as a health food in special diets when decreased sweetness is required and some have claimed that diabetics can tolerate lactose levels far in excess of what might be expected compared with sucrose or glucose. Some accepted diabetic ice-creams have relatively large levels of lactose. In normal health lactose may exert considerable nutritional benefit in the diet. In a recent experiment it was shown that when lactose was ingested by normal adult volunteers the fecal and urinary calcium and phosphorus fell, with a striking improvement in calcium and phosphorus balance. In lactose intolerant patients no such improvement in mineral balance occurred *(4)*.

In most food products lactose probably exists as milk or milk products rather than as the refined sugar. Lactose is a large component of dry coffee cream preparations, for example, and concentrated whey is used in many of our chewy confections. Whey lactose interacts with the milk protein, casein, and on heating, brown substances are formed with attractive flavors that are essential ingredients in toffee making *(3)*. Sogginess in pie crusts can be reduced by applying a lactose solution wash to the surface before baking. Potato chips and French-fried potatoes can be given a deeper, more uniform golden color if they are dipped into a lactose solution before cooking in deep fat. For more of us lactose taken as a normal balanced constituent of milk products in our diet is probably a beneficial nutrient, encouraging us not to hunt for immoderate levels of sweetness which may result in obesity and related dietary problems. Probably the racial differences in regard to lactose intake described in this paper reflect acquired dietary needs, resulting from generations of national food preferences. Provided that we take care to note any physiological disorders recurring after a particular food intake and seek medical advice where necessary, we may with some safety, accept the old adage 'a little of what you like is good for you.' As in many other aspects of our diet it appears that Nature has deliberately concealed her purpose in providing lactose as the milk sugar of so many different species. We must be careful how we use it, so that we may be sure its applications can be extended further.

REFERENCES

1. Birch, G. G. 1969. Rare food sugars. Food World. March 5–7.

2. Bolin, T. D., and A. E. Davis. 1970. Primary lactase deficiency: Genetic or acquired? Digestic Diseases 15:679–692.

3. Call, A. E. 1958. Utilization of lactose. J. Dairy Sci. 41:332–334.

4. Condon, J. R., J. R. Nassim, A. Hilbe, F. J. C. Millard and E. M. Stainthorpe. 1970. Calcium and phosphorous metabolism in relation to lactose tolerance. Lancet: 1027–1029.

5. Cook, G. C. 1968. Some observations on racial lactase deficiency. Proc. Roy. Soc. Med. 61:1102–1104.

6. Cow and Gate. 1970. Handbook for the use of the medical profession, p. 24.

7. Dahlqvist, A., J. B. Hammond, R. K. Crane, J. V. Dunphy, and A. Littman. 1968. Intestinal lactase deficiency and lactose intolerance in adults. Gastroenterol. 54:807–810.

8. Korc, I. 1961. Biochemical studies on cataracts in galactose-fed rats. Arch. Biochem. Biophys. 94:196–200.

9. Richter, C. P., and J. R. Duke. 1970. Cataracts produced in rats by yoghurt. Science 168:1372–1374.

10. Wells, H. J., and S. Segal. 1969. Galactose toxicity in the chick: tissue accumulation of galactose and galactitol. FEBS Letters 5:121–123.

11. Woolf, L. I. 1968. Recent studies on galactosaemia, phenylketonuria and homocystinuria. Proc. Nutri. Soc. 27:88–95.

B

**Nutritional status
of humans**

the crisis

B Nutritional status of humans

IN THE FIRST CHAPTER we introduced the concept of nutritional requirements in terms of the RDA. Various food guides have been developed to translate such dietary standards into food choices which would lead to a balanced diet. The first article, by Drs. Hertzler and Anderson, traces the history of such food guides in the United States and how they have evolved into the present "Basic Four," a food education concept. Many people, including consumer advocates and legislators, feel that the "Basic Four" is inadequate and have demanded that nutrition education be incorporated into food education. Recently, the Food and Drug Administration (FDA) has responded to these pressures by requiring the food industry to increase information about the nutrient content of their foods on the labels. The second article, by Dr. Ogden Johnson, former director of nutrition for the FDA, discusses the potential value of this labeling to consumers. In a report on how consumers presently use this information, L. Klinger discusses various consumer-use surveys. He concludes that the average consumer still does not use the data in any tangible educational manner. Thus, we still have a nutrition education crisis.

The results of the U. S. Dept. of Health, Education, and Welfare 1970 Nutrition Survey of low and high income groups is presented graphically in the next article. The 1970 survey found the same results for low income groups as a 1965 survey: deficiencies in iron, vitamin A, vitamin C, and Riboflavin. In addition it was discovered that members of high income groups, especially females also had nutritional deficiencies for intake of vitamins A and B_2 and a high, incidence of iron deficiency.

Based on this, many food consumer activists and nutritionists feel that American diets are getting worse regardless of income. The challenge for nutritional researchers then, lies in trying to find out whether this is due to unrealistically high standards, a change in the food environment, or to poor education. We already have seen discussion on standards; the next article, by Dr. Henderson, examines the changing food environment.

Henderson discusses the change in food consumption patterns based on food disappearance data that has occurred since the early 1900s. The average data show no significant reduction in vitamin and mineral intake; however, a shift to more fats in the diet and a lower total caloric consumption is indicated. This shift is interesting since it would seem to indicate fewer overweight problems. On the contrary, over 20 percent of the population now suffers from obesity, the major over-nutrition problem in the United States. The fact that food disappearance data show no reduction, on the average, in nutrient intake of vitamins and minerals points out the problem of inferring too much from averages. Many people today do not make the proper food choice; a smaller percentage cannot afford the proper choice. Poor education about nutritional needs is partially to blame, but the United States food environment also is a factor. Food choice for most people is based not only on availability, but also on acceptability. Some scientists stress the need for more public nutrition education, while others believe that all snacks and processed foods should be fortified to supply a balanced nutrient intake since these foods have grown to such a large proportion of the average diet. Henderson's article sets the stage for the debate on the problem.

Ruth Leverton writes in the following article that we have to be careful about how we apply the RDA a point that Dr. Harper also made earlier. In fact, the new 1974 RDA indicate less of a vitamin A problem and, if Canadian standards are used, no iron problem for females is indicated. In a recent survey I made of more than 1500 college students no severe nutritional deficiencies were found.

Drs. Thomas and Call continue the debate in an article on teenagers' between-meal eating. They discuss whether such snacking is dangerous and should be stopped, and whether snack foods should be fortified. Although they believe that overeating and unbalanced meals are problems within the teenage population they support better education rather than outright fortification.

The last article in this chapter presents a debate on supplementation of foods versus nutrition education. It should be clear to the reader that education is our most important weapon against malnutrition, but it must be started at a young age and continued throughout the school years. It also must be nutrition education, not just food education as the "Basic Four" provides. However supplementation of some foods is necessary to alleviate problems that have been created by our new food habits.

We now can see the crisis that could arise from a concerted attempt to improve human nutrition. For example, we have the opportunity and knowledge to supplement ketchup with vitamin A, but we have little control over ketchup consumption. Although the supplementation could alleviate the cases of low vitamin A intake, could it also create a danger for those who eat ketchup but already consume sufficient vitamin A from other sources?

7

FOOD GUIDES IN THE UNITED STATES

**Ann A. Hertzler, Ph.D., R.D., and
Helen L. Anderson, Ph.D., R.D.**

Dietary standards, defined as "quantitative recommendations for essential nutrients and calories," have been developed in the United States for the purpose of promoting optimal nutritional status in the population (1–4). One means that has been used to accomplish this goal has been the translation of standard recommendations into suggested servings of foods from groups arranged according to primary nutrient contributions. The re-

Reprinted from *Journal of The American Dietetic Association*, Vol. 64, No. 1, January 1974. © The American Dietetic Association. Printed in U. S. A.

Contribution from the University of Missouri Extension Division. Journal Series Number 6663.

* Department of Human Nutrition, Foods, and Food Systems Management, College of Home Economics, University of Missouri, Columbia. The authors are grateful to Franklin Bing, Mary Hill, Ruth Leverton, Ethel Austin Martin, the late Leonard Maynard, Louise Page, W. H. Sebrell, Hazel K. Stiebeling, Daniel Swope, E. Neige Todhunter, and Helen E. Walsh who contributed helpful information for this review. Also appreciated is the correspondence from Esther Batchelder, Robert S. Goodhart, Charles G. King, Helen S. Mitchell, and Leroy Voris.

The development of the five food groups of the early 1900's and the four food (basic 4) groups currently in use are documented in the literature. However, that of the food guides issued in the 1940's is not well documented. Therefore, historical information for this time period has been provided by short news items in periodicals, Food and Nutrition Board members in strategic positions during the development of the wartime nutrition programs, and confirmation by "written communication" of the early thinking of some of the people who pioneered in this area.

sulting food guides have been designed to assist the public in selecting foods that provide the recommended intake of essential nutrients.

The purpose of this paper is to review the evolution of our national food guides in order to broaden the understanding of the guides and their nutritional objectives. No attempt is made to incorporate the many and varied food plans developed for emergency feeding situations, state and community nutrition programs, agricultural purposes, or food industry programs.

GUIDES BASED ON THE ATWATER STANDARD

Atwater was the first to develop dietary standards for the United States population (5). By studying Americans of different socioeconomic levels, he was able to relate food composition and utilization to fulfillment of physiologic needs. His dietary standards emphasized protein for building muscle and fuel for providing energy and discussed food cost, preparation, and wastage. Tables of food composition, published (6) with the assistance of C. D. Woods, H. B. Gibson, and C. F. Langworthy at the Agricultural Experiment Station, were the basis for translating the standards into foods.

In the 1890's, when Atwater was publishing his work, Ellen Richards was applying this new knowledge of nutrition to menu planning. As part of her educational efforts, Mrs. Richards planned two or three lunches for the Massachusetts Exhibit of the Rumford Kitchens at the Chicago World's Fair in 1893. These meals approached one-fourth of the day's ration of protein, fat, carbohydrate, and calories; the amounts of each were listed on the menu (7).

The five food groups of 1916–1923. In 1916, under the direction of C. F. Langworthy, Atwater's successor as chief of nutrition investigation and the first Director of the Office of Home Economics in the Department of Agriculture (8), Caroline Hunt, a scientific assistant, authored the first national food guide; foods were classified in five groups and presented in simple, short discussions, using homemakers' terms (9). About the same time, Langworthy presented similar information to the scientific community. His lecture, delivered at the 1916 annual meeting of the American Association for the Advancement of Science, was published in *Scientific Monthly* (10) and in the *Journal of Home Economics* (11).

Langworthy's food groups were: (a) protein, (b) starch and similar carbohydrates, (c) fat, (d) mineral substances and organic acids, and (e) sugars. Hunt's groups were (a) milk, meat, fish, poultry, eggs, and meat substitutes, (b) bread and other cereal foods, (c) butter and wholesome fats, (d) vegetables and fruits, and (e) simple sweets. In 1918, Langworthy combined his and Hunt's designations when presenting the five food groups at the Tenth Annual Meeting of the American Home Economics Association (12).

Although it was being debated whether two recently recognized food constituents—fat-soluble A and water-soluble B "vitamines"—should be given special consideration in meal planning, Langworthy felt that regrouping foods to provide for these vitamins was not feasible because of insufficient knowledge of their relationship to body building and body fuel. However, he indicated that major food sources of these nutrients were distributed throughout the five food groups. Therefore, "to be satisfactory, meals must be truly varied if they are to supply the needed body fuel and the building and repair materials, including the 'unknown' essentials" (12).

In 1921, the five food groups were published as a family food guide (13). This publication was slightly modified in 1923 (14) for use by teachers, extension workers, club leaders, and social service workers in teaching "housekeepers" (15); the information subsequently appeared in college home economics texts (16).

The 1923 Farmers' Bulletin 1313 (14) continued the earlier method of labeling each of the five groups with the names of common foods. To simplify presentation and to emphasize the selection of wholesome food, the Bulletin pictured a week's supply of food for the average family from each of the five groups and described amounts of food by weight, volume, or count and 100-kcal portions in order to accommodate the knowledge of different "housekeepers" (13). Similar illustrations were prepared for cereal foods, vegetables and fruits, fats and fat foods, and sugar and other sweets (13).

The major nutritive contributions of each food group as noted in the Bulletin are summarized in Table 1. Since fuel is derived from protein, starch, sugar, and fat, these foods were grouped accordingly. In addition to this method of classification—and with mention of vitamin contributions—fruits, vegetables, and cereal grains were recognized for their ash, while animal foods and cereal grains provided nitrogen for growth and repair. Sugars and sweets for quick energy and fat for concentrated energy were the groups that primarily provided flavor and assured adequate caloric intake.

Underlying assumptions were: (a) ordinary food habits would provide a variety of foods in liberal quantities; (b) 3,000 to 3,500 kcal per man per day would almost inevitably supply necessary protein, ash, and other constituents; and (c) a reasonable amount of milk, green vegetables, and fruit should be consumed each day. The need for more information about (a) kinds and quantities of protein; (b) functions, sources, and availability of minerals; and (c) the nature of "vitamines" or other regulatory substances was recognized (11).

Energy needs of the average family were the basis for recommended amounts of food from each group. The family was defined as a mother

Table 1: Nutritive contributions of the five food groups *

Food group	Fuel (energy) †				"Vitamines"			Ash		Amounts for an average family for one week
	Protein	Starch	Sugar	Fat	A	B	C (ascorbic acid)	Iron	Lime	
Group I: Vegetables and fruits										70 lb. fresh produce
Green leafy: spinach, lettuce, kale; dandelion, turnip, radish, and salad greens										*or*
All vegetables and fruits		x	x		x	x			x	160 100-kcal portions (since "vitamines" are thought to
Lemons, oranges, tomatoes, cabbage, turnips, and potatoes		x	x			x				be destroyed by drying, cooking, and the addition of soda, some raw fruits and green leafy vegetables are recommended)
nips, and potatoes		x	x		x	x				
Group II: protein										14 qt. milk + 10½ lb. flesh
Milk, cheese	x				x				x	foods, cheese, eggs, and peanuts
Eggs	x				x			x		*or*
Flesh foods										160 100-kcal portions (half from milk)
Lean and medium-fat meats	x							x		
Fish, poultry, game, and seafood	x									
Peanuts and soybeans	x									
Group III: Cereal grains and their products										15 lb. dry cereal
Wheat, corn, rye, rice, barley, and oats (whole grain)	x	x				x	"mineral substances"	x		*or* 240 100-kcal portions (if white bread is used instead of whole grain cereal products, larger proportions of fruits and vegetables should be included)
Group IV: sugars and sugar foods										4½ lb. sugar
Sugars, molasses, honey, sirups, candy, sweet chocolate, rich preserves, jellies, jams, and marmalades			x							*or* 80 100-kcal portions
Group V: fats and fat foods										4 lb. pure fat
Butter				x	x					*or*
Cream	x			x	x					160 100-kcal portions (if a food contains two and a
Oil, lard, suet, and other cooking fats				x						half times as much fat as protein, it is classified in
Chocolate				x						the fat group)
Rich and oily nuts				x						
Bacon, salt pork, fat pork, sausage				x						

* Adapted from "A Week's Food for an Average Family " (13).

† Proportion of fuel to be provided by each group was: Group I, 20 per cent; Group II, 20 per cent; Group III, 30 per cent; Group IV, 10 per cent; and Group V, 20 per cent.

and father, with three children whose ages totaled twenty to twenty-four years, or as four average adults. Energy expenditures of adults were categorized as moderately active, or with one engaged in little or no muscular effort and the other doing hard muscular work, such as washing and cleaning. A chart indicated how to meet differing caloric requirements for additional family members (14).

The introduction of Farmers' Bulletin 1228 (13) stressed the guide's versatility in selecting foods for any family, at any season, and under any market condition. If families used the quantities of foods from the five food groups within a week, variation between meals or days would not matter, but the average family could save time and effort by selecting a food(s) from each group for each of the three daily meals. The proportions of foods from each group could be increased or decreased within certain limits. Although sweets could be completely eliminated, milk or green leafy vegetables should not be omitted and cereals, especially whole grain, could be increased.

THE DECADE OF THE 1930'S

During the twenties and thirties, some standards for vitamins and minerals were proposed. Sherman (17), McCollum (18, 19), and Roberts (20) were among those who adapted this information for the practical benefit of everyone. They shifted the focus in food selection from adequate calories to provision of the necessary vitamins, minerals, and protein.

As early as 1918, McCollum coined the phrase "protective foods," i. e., those often neglected foods which are rich sources of calcium, vitamin A, and ascorbic acid, and indicated that food patterns should consist of the equivalent of a quart of milk a day for everyone, a liberal serving of greens or potherbs daily, a salad with raw fruits and vegetables twice daily. He emphasized the importance of the protective foods, by saying: "Eat what you want after you have eaten what you should" (21).

Sherman stated that half of the required calories should come from protective foods (22). Harris, in his book on vitamins, stressed the relationship between good eating habits and improved physique, stature, and good health (23).

GUIDES BASED ON THE RECOMMENDED DIETARY ALLOWANCES

By 1939–40, nutrition had become an integral part of the nation's incipient defense program. In August 1940, representatives from the federal agencies concerned with nutrition were appointed to an overall Nutrition Policy and Planning Committee. M. L. Wilson, Director of Extension Work in USDA, served as Chairman, and Helen S. Mitchell, Research Professor of Nutrition, Massachusetts State College, as Secretary. With the United States' entry into World War II in December 1941, a Coordinator of Related Defense Activities (including nutrition) was established within the Federal Security Agency. The Nutrition Policy and Planning Committee, along with representatives from four national organizations concerned with nutrition, became the Nutrition Advisory Committee to the Coordinator. A Committee on Food and Nutrition within the National Research Council was established to advise on nutrition programs concerned with national defense.

To arouse nation-wide interest and cooperation in improving nutrition, President Franklin D. Roosevelt authorized the Nutrition Advisory Committee to convene a National Nutrition Conference. On the eve of this conference in May 1941, Dr. Russell M. Wilder, Chairman of the Committee on Food and Nutrition of the National Research Council, presented the first "Recommended Dietary Allowances" to the public via radio. These allowances for specific nutrients, designed to serve as goals in planning adequate nutrition for the civilian population in health, were published in the conference proceedings (24).

1941 food guides. The 1941 Recommended Dietary Allowances listed specific daily intakes of calories, protein, iron, calcium, vitamins A and D, thiamin, riboflavin, niacin, and ascorbic acid for healthy persons for seven-

Table 2: Comparison of three daily food guides issued in 1941

"Eat the Right Food to Help Keep You Fit" (26) *	"Recommended Dietary Allowances" (24) †	"A Guide to Good Eating" (31) ‡
Milk ¾ to 1 qt. for children; 1 qt. for an expectant or nursing mother; 1 pt. for other family members	**Milk** 1½ pt. to 1 qt. for children; 1 pt. for adults	**Milk** 2 or more glasses for adults; 3 to 4 or more glasses for children
Lean meat, poultry, and fish 1 or more servings (can use dried peas or beans several times a week)	**Lean meat, poultry, or fish** 1 3-oz. serving for adults; 1-oz. serving for one-year-old	**Meat, cheese, fish, or legumes** 1 or more servings
Eggs 1 (or at least 3 to 4 a week)	**Eggs** 3 to 4 a week	**Eggs** 3 to 5 a week (one daily preferred)
Leafy green or yellow vegetables 1 or more servings **Tomatoes, oranges, grapefruit, green cabbage, raw salad greens** 1 or more servings **Other fruits and vegetables** 2 or more servings	**Vegetables** 2 servings (one green or yellow) **Potato** 1 or more servings **Fruit** 2 servings (one citrus or tomato and one other, as apple, prunes, etc.)	**Vegetables** 2 or more servings besides potato (one raw; green and yellow often) **Fruit** 2 or more servings (one citrus or tomato)
Cereals and breads At least 2 servings of whole grain products or enriched bread	**Whole grain or "enriched" cereal and bread** At least half of intake	**Cereals and breads** Most should be whole grain or "enriched"
Fats Use butter or other vitamin-rich fat every day	**Butter or fortified oleo** 100 to 500 kcal	**Butter** 2 Tbsp. or more
Sweets In moderation	**Sugar and fat** To complete calories	
Water Regular habits; more with excessive perspiration		

* Bureau of Home Economics.

† Committee on Dietary Allowances, Food and Nutrition Board.

‡ National Dairy Council.

teen age and sex categories (24). Because the lay person could not translate these recommendations into foods, several committees designed food guides with seven to ten food groups. These were the first national guides to incorporate information on specific vitamins and minerals and to use the term "enriched" (Table 2).

At the time the first Recommended Dietary Allowances were officially accepted (May 1941), the food guide, "Eat the Right Food to Help Keep You Fit," was publishd by the Bureau of Home Economics, in cooperation with the Children's Bureau in the Department of Labor, the Office of Education, and the Public Health Service in the Federal Security Agency (24–28). The influence of the 1941 allowances is evident in this guide and is at least partially due to the fact that Lela Booher, Chief, Food and Nutrition, Bureau of Home Economics, from 1936 to 1941, was also a member of the first Food and Nutrition Board Committee on Dietary Allowances (29).

The nutritionally adequate dietary pattern given with the first Recommended Dietary Allowances (24) and the pattern prepared by the Bureau of Home Economics (26) were very similar (Table 2). The food groups in each plan and the suggested number of servings were basically the same, but with slightly different representation. In both guides, emphasis was on milk, animal protein foods, fruits and vegetables, and whole grain or enriched cereals and breads. Calories were considered in both plans with the use of fats and sweets to complete a day's energy needs. "Eat the Right Food to Help Keep You Fit" listed water as the tenth group. It also gave practical suggestions for selection and preparation of foods in each group.

About this time, an editorial on the National Nutrition Conference for Defense (30) listed the seven food groups proposed by Lydia J. Roberts, Chairman of the National Research Council's Committee on Dietary Allowances. This pattern was essentially the same as other patterns but potatoes and sweets were omitted.

Under the direction of Ethel Austin Martin, the National Dairy Council published "A Guide to Good Eating" (31) in 1941. This illustrated guide contained seven food groups (Table 2) and was developed, both in poster and handout form, as part of the Council's nutrition education program. Dr. Roberts served as consultant on the project and Dr. Wilder helped formulate the statement on selection of enriched cereal products (32).

1942—eight food groups. In 1942, Paul McNutt, Administrator of the Office of Defense Health and Welfare Services, announced a National Industrial Nutrition Program, designed to reach industry, homes, and communities and which introduced a new food guide. At this time, M. L. Wilson was the Assistant Administrator and W. H. Sebrell (U. S. Public Health Service) was Deputy Assistant Administrator of the Office of Defense Health and Welfare Services. Robert S. Goodhart, Mark Graubard, and Ernestine Perry also contributed to the development and coordination of this new program. State and local committees carried the program to the community (33). The war emergency and Wilson's leadership expedited the contributions of numerous committees in the development and presentation of the 1942 food guide (34).

The theme of the 1942 national industrial program became the title of the food guide: "U. S. Needs Us Strong—Eat Nutritional Food" (35). The overall objective of the program was to obtain "full health returns from the nation's food resources . . . for victory . . . and when the war is won" in order to promote optimal nutrition through wise food selection for war workers and the population at home. The scientific basis for the 1942 guide was undoubtedly the Recommended Dietary Allowances (24, 36, 37). The influence of nutritional status on the development of the guide is noted in the following:

> About one-fourth of the families in the United States have diets that could be rated good . . . more than a third, diets that might be considered fair . . . another third or more, diets that should be classed as poor . . . This national condition was highlighted when approximately a third of all men rejected by Selective Service were disqualified for reasons of physical disability and defects related to malnutrition (36).

The food groups in the 1942 guide were essentially the same as those in "Eat the Right Food to Help Keep You Fit." Sugar was omitted as a separate group, as was water, so that the protective foods were emphasized. Alternative choices were listed in view of the food shortages resulting from the war, and suggestions for meal planning (meal patterns, food examples, and cooking methods) were recommended to reduce food waste (35, 38). Special consideration was given throughout to workers who brought lunches from home (36).

The 1942 program solicited help from industry to promote the food guide. A "Plan of Cooperation" outlined procedures by which the eight-group plan could be incorporated into advertising. Advertisers of products not included in the food groups could use the information only if no other copy or illustrations were used and credit were given to the Office of Defense Health and Welfare Services (36).

In addition, the program was announced in the four June issues of the *Saturday Evening Post* (39–43). This information was considered basic to homemakers, teachers, dietitians, Red Cross nutrition aides, home demonstration agents, and community service workers (39).

1943—THE SEVEN FOOD GROUPS

The "Basic 7" food groups were developed through the efforts of many individuals and committees perhaps dating from 1940. Governmental agencies offering nutrition services contributed much to the development and approval of the guide, but the primary coordination was accomplished by a committee of members of the National Wartime Nutrition Program, (37, 44) (at that time, part of the Nutrition and Food Conservation Branch, Food Distribution Administration, USDA, of which Wilson and Sebrell, previous Directors of the National Nutrition Program, were Chief and Associate Chief, respectively [45, 46]).

The committee recommended that the food guide be based on the eight food groups of 1942, but that the wording be clarified and that the daily intake from each food group not be specified. Because of the war, the guide listed alternates for scarce, rationed, or unobtainable foods. Placing eggs with meat, fish, and poultry reduced the food groups from eight to seven. It was decided to arrange the seven groups in a circle to signify that no one group was more important than any other (37).

In the summer of 1943, Wilson and Sebrell announced that the "National Wartime Nutrition Guide" was available (47, 48). In August, a poster in color, "Eat the Basic 7 Every Day," was distributed to "post offices, banks, libraries, war plants, beauty parlors, housing projects, shipyards, retail stores, hotels, restaurants, drug stores, government agencies, and local nutrition committees" (49).

Although the seven food groups constituting the "National Wartime Nutrition Guide" were essentially a device for translating the first Recommended Dietary Allowances into foods (37), they are different from the seven groups in the 1941 and 1943 editions of the Recommended Dietary Allowances (50). The "National Wartime Nutrition Guide" included butter and fortified margarine as a separate group. The 1943 Recommended Dietary Allowances (50) did not contain additional sources of calories, such as the fats and sugars, but did list eggs as a separate group; it also stated that the need for iodine could be met by the regular use of iodized salt (50, 51).

Great effort was made to bring the food guide to public attention. A well known advertising firm served as liaison between the food industry and committees of the National Nutrition Program. As in the 1942 nutrition program, guidelines were established for using the "Basic 7" in advertisements and as handout brochures in groceries (37, 51, 52). In addition, a nutrition education program was planned for industrial workers, because many of them carried meals which furnished a substantial part of the day's food intake. It was recommended that lunches contain foods from the seven food groups so that one-third of the day's energy and essential nutrients would be provided. By December 1943, posters, folders, and table tents advertising the basic food groups were provided in industrial nutrition program materials (53).

The 1946 post-war version of the seven food groups was published as the "National Food Guide" by the Human Nutrition Research Branch of the Agricultural Research Service, USDA (54). The circular format, sometimes called the "Wheel of Good Eating," remained the key teaching device. The supporting information, although modified to include recommended servings, was basically the same as the wartime version with emphasis on conserving food by eating less of the scarce foods and more of the plentiful foods.

Probably the most readily available interpretation of the nutritional contributions of the seven food groups is found in Sherman's texts, especially *Chemistry of Food and Nutrition* (55). This philosophy was published when the 1946 version of the Basic 7 appeared while Sherman was Chairman of the Food and Nutrition Committee (29) of the National Research Council.

1954—THE FOUR FOOD GROUPS

In 1954, following a review of the discrepancies between nutrient intakes estimated from dietary surveys and recommended nutrient intakes, nutritionists began to consider the need for a new food guide (56). At the suggestion of the Interagency Committee on Nutrition Education and School Lunch, work began on a new guide (57). The development of the four food groups was initiated by USDA and preceded, roughly by a year, a 1955 publication which suggested dividing foods into two or four groups (58).

In 1956, the four food groups were presented in the USDA publication, "Essentials of an Adequate Diet," with Louise Page and Esther Phipard, nutritionists with the Institute of Home Economics, as the authors (59). The resulting food guide was issued in 1958 as USDA Leaflet No. 424, "Food for Fitness—A Daily Food Guide" (60). Before distribution, this leaflet was reviewed by the nation's leading nutritionists, as well as members of the Interagency Committee on Nutrition Education and School Lunch, the Food and Nutrition Advisory and the Home Economics Advisory Committees of the USDA, and by the Food and Nutrition Board of the National Research Council. Several food manufacturers and organizations that had prepared nutrition education materials based on the seven food groups, such as the National Dairy Council, Sunkist Growers, and the Cereal Institute, also reviewed the publication and offered comments (56, 59).

Several guidelines were used in developing the four food groups (59). Nutritional needs of individuals and families were based on the 1953 Recommended Dietary Allowances. The nutritional recommendations were translated into a food guide based on food groups weighted by U. S. food consumption studies in 1948 and quantities of food in the national food supply, 1953–54. Because of dietary inadequacies of calcium, vitamin A, and ascorbic acid in the American population, food sources of these nutrients were emphasized. The nutritive values of foods were derived from the 1950 edition of Agriculture Handbook No. 8 (61) and considered estimated losses of B vitamins during cooking. Since the trace elements used in enzyme systems were known to be essential but had not yet been quantitatively determinined, it was believed that a mixed diet of both plant and animal foods would provide these widely distributed nutrients (62, 63).

"Food for Fitness—A Daily Food Guide" was designed as a nutritionally reliable teaching device for individuals or families. Names of the food groups were those most likely to be used by homemakers in meal-planning and shopping: (a) milk, (b) meat, (c) vegetable-fruit, and (d) bread-cereal (59). This guide (60) differs from the Basic 7 (47, 54) in that the butter-fortified margarine group was eliminated and fruits and vegetables were placed in one group. However, the vegetable-fruit group comprised three sub-groups—vitamin A-rich, ascorbic acid-rich, and other fruits and vegetables—with explicit directions for selecting important sources of vitamin A and ascorbic acid. In addition, the minimum number of servings for each food group and serving sizes for all foods were defined.

"Essentials of an Adequate Diet" outlined (59) the development of the four food groups and indicated how the guide should be used. The milk, meat, and fruit-vegetable groups each provided one or two important nutrients and, in addition, supplied at least 25 per cent of the recommended intakes for two or more other nutrients. Although the guide specifies the minimum number of servings for everyone except infants, Table 3 presents the major nutrient contributions to adult diets of the recommended servings from each food group. Since vitamin A is concentrated in dark green leafy and deep yellow vegetables, the guide recommended one serving every other day. A daily serving of fruit or vegetable important for ascorbic acid intake was also recommended. The bread-cereal group, not a concentrated source of any one nutrient, contained low-cost foods with "steady amounts" of most of the calculated nutrients, provided whole grain, enriched, or restored products were selected (59). Although many of the synthetic and fabricated foods may be a concentrated source of one or more nutrients, they cannot replace foods in the four groups because they do not supply steady amounts of other nutrients (64, 65).

The minimum number of servings from each food group combined should provide a nutritionally sound diet that approaches the 1953 Recommended Dietary Allowances for protein, calcium, vitamin A, thiamin, riboflavin, niacin, and ascorbic acid (59). This is in contrast to earlier plans that outlined total food intake. The nutrient evaluation of the food guide which appears in "Essentials of an Adequate Diet" (59) is based on the

Recommended Dietary Allowances for an "average" adult. Through adjustments in serving sizes for young children, teen-agers, active adults, and pregnant and lactating women, the "Basic 4" (the popular name of the guide) can meet the differing nutritional needs of nearly all individuals.

Table 3: Nutrient contributions to diets of adults of recommended servings in "Food for Fitness"

Food group †	10 to 25 per cent of diet	25 to 50 per cent of diet	50 to 75 per cent of diet	75 per cent or more of diet
Milk	Calories Vitamin A Thiamin	Riboflavin Protein	Calcium	
Meat	Calories Vitamin A (if liver chosen)	Protein Thiamin Iron Riboflavin	Niacin	
Fruits and vegetables	Calories Calcium Iron Thiamin Riboflavin Niacin			Vitamin A Ascorbic acid
Bread	Calories Protein Iron Riboflavin Niacin	Thiamin		

Adapted from "Essentials of an Adequate Diet" (59).
† Based on minimum number and size of servings recommended for the adult.

Since the amounts of food advocated in "Food for Fitness—A Daily Food Guide" provide only half to two-thirds of the caloric recommendations for adults, additional calories can be obtained by choosing larger or more servings from among the four groups. Fats and sugars used in cooking or added at the table contribute substantially to the total caloric intake. Conversely, the use of skim instead of whole milk, trimming all visible fat from meats, and limiting additional fats and sugars permit the four food groups to be used as the basis for a reducing or limited-calorie diet.

Although modified slightly, the "Food for Fitness" guide has remained basically the same since original publication in 1957, the most recent revision appearing in 1971 (60). In 1966, the USDA's Agricultural Research Service urged that educators interpret the guide in terms of moderation in the total amount of fat and inclusion of food sources of linoleic acid in the diet (66). This recommendation has been used in at least one area nutrition program (67).

The 1968 Recommended Dietary Allowances have been used to assess the nutritional adequacy of the four food groups (56). Iron for women is particularly low when ordinary foods are selected from the "Food for Fitness" guide. The high allowance for iron is difficult to meet, even by using a variety of ordinary foods. Since information is limited on the content of certain nutrients in foods and on their requirements, Hill and Cleveland indicate that, "it seems premature to make major changes in the food guide based solely on trying to reach the current recommended levels for these nutrients" (56).

SUMMARY

The historical objective of national food guides for the United States has been to translate dietary standards into simple and reliable nutrition education devices for the lay person. Nutritional and dietary status, food patterns, food availability, nutritive value of foods, and food economics have been considerations in developing nutritionally reliable food guides from the first one of 1916 to the current guide. Simplicity has been attained by limiting the number of food groups in the plans and by using familiar names of foods.

REFERENCES

1. Leitch, I.: The evolution of dietary standards. Historical outline. Nutr. Abstr. Rev. 11:509, 1942.

2. Pett, L. B., Morrell, C. A., and Hanley, F. W.: The development of dietary standards. Can. J. Pub. Health, 36:232, 1945.

3. Connor, M. M.: A history of dietary standards. *In* Lydia J. Roberts Award Essays. Chicago: Amer. Dietet. Assoc. 1968.

4. Young, E. G.: Dietary standards. *In* Beaton, G. H., and McHenry, E. W., eds.: Nutrition, A Comprehensive Treatise in Three Volumes: II. Vitamins, Nutrient Requirements, and Food Selection. N. Y.: Academic Press, 1964, p. 299.

5. Atwater, W. O.: Food and Diet—Yearbook of the United States Department of Agriculture. Washington, D. C.: Govt. Prtg. Off., 1894, p. 357.

6. Atwater, W. O.: Methods and Results of Investigations on the Chemistry and Economy of Food. USDA Bull. No. 21, 1895.

7. Hunt, C. L.: The Life of Ellen H. Richards. 1842–1911. Washington, D. C.: Amer. Home Econ. Assoc., 1958.

8. Cofer, E., Grossman, E., and Clark, F.: Family Food Plans and Food Costs. USDA Home Economics Research Rept. No. 20, 1962.

9. Hunt, C. L.: Food for Young Children. USDA Farmers' Bull. 717, 1916.

10. Langworthy, C. F.: Food selection for rational and economic living. Sci. Monthly 2: 294, 1916.

11. Langworthy, C. F.: For the homemaker, food selection for rational and economical living. J. Home Econ. 8: 313, 1916.

12. Langworthy, C. F.: Teaching food values. J. Home Econ. 10: 295, 1918.

13. Hunt, C. L.: A Week's Food for an Average Family. USDA Farmers' Bull. 1228, 1921.

14. Hunt, C. L.: Good Proportions in the Diet. USDA Farmers' Bull. 1313, 1923.

15. Food charts. J. Home Econ. 14: 346, 1922.

16. Berry, P. G.: Chemistry Applied to Home and Community. 2nd rev. ed. Philadelphia: J.B. Lippincott Co., 1926.

17. Sherman, H. C.: Chemistry of Food and Nutrition. 8th ed. N. Y.: The Macmillan Co., 1952.

18. McCollum, E. V.: A History of Nutrition. Boston: Houghton-Mifflin Co., 1957.

19. McCollum, E. V.: Comment in Stefferud, A., ed.: Food—The Yearbook of Agriculture. Washington, D. C.: Govt. Prtg. Off., 1959, p. 458.

20. Roberts, L. J.: Nutrition Work with Children. Chicago: Univ. of Chicago Press, 1927.

21. McCollum, E. V.: The Newer Knowledge of Nutrition. N. Y.: The Macmillan Co., 1918, p. 82.

22. Sherman, H. C.: Chemistry of Food and Nutrition, 4th ed. N. Y.: The Macmillan Co., 1932.

23. Harris, L. J.: Vitamins in Theory and Practice, 2nd ed. N. Y.: The Macmillan Co., 1937.

24. Proceedings of the National Nutrition Conference for Defense, May 26, 27, and 28, 1941. Washington, D. C.: Govt. Prtg. Off., 1942.

25. Comm. on Food & Nutrition, Natl. Research Council: Recommended Daily Dietary Allowances. J. Home Econ. 33: 476, 1941.

26. Bureau of Home Econ., USDA: Eat the Right Food to Help Keep You Fit. (folder) Washington, D. C.: Govt. Prtg. Off., May, 1941.

27. What to eat. J. Home Econ. 33: 133, 1941.

28. Eat the right food to help keep fit. J. Home Econ. 33: 391, 1941.

29. Miller, D., and Voris, L.: Chronological changes in the Recommended Dietary Allowances. J. Am. Dietet. A. 54: 109, 1969.

30. National Nutrition Conference for Defense. J.A.M.A. 116: 2598, 1941.

31. A Guide to Good Eating. Chicago: Natl. Dairy Council, 1941.

32. Martin, E. A.: Personal communication, Nov., 1971.

33. National industrial nutrition program. J. Am. Dietet. A. 18: 596, 1942.

34. Bing, F. C.: Personal communication, Nov., 1971.

35. Off. of Defense Health and Welfare Serv.: U. S. Needs Us Strong—Eat Nutritional Food. (leaflet) Washington, D. C.: Govt. Prtg. Off. (0–457183), 1942.

36. Off. of Defense Health and Welfare Serv.: How Industry Can Cooperate with the National Nutrition Plan. Washington, D. C.: Information Serv., circa 1943.

37. Leverton, R. M.: Personal communication, Sept., 1971.

38. Maynard, L.: Personal communication, Sept., 1971.

39. National Nutrition Program of the Off. of Defense, Health and Welfare Serv.: U. S. needs us strong. Sat. Eve. Post 214: 91 (No. 49, June 6), 1942.

40. National Nutrition Program, Off. of Defense, Health and Welfare Serv.: Here's how to grow strong, America . . . Eat these foods every day. Sat. Eve. Post 214: 92 (No. 49, June 6), 1942.

41. National Nutrition Program, Off. of Defense, Health and Welfare Serv.: Food will build a new America. Sat. Eve. Post 214: 52 (No. 50, June 13), 1942.

42. National Nutrition Program, Off. of Defense, Health and Welfare Serv.: Only a healthy nation is a strong nation. Sat. Eve. Post 214: 98 (No. 51, June 20), 1942.

43. National Nutrition Program, Off. of Defense, Health and Welfare Serv.: America must eat right to work and fight right! Sat. Eve. Post 214: 62 (No. 52, June 27), 1942.

44. Sebrell, W. H.: Personal communication to Anthony, L. P. (J. Am. Dental Assoc.) Washington, D. C.: Natl. Archives & Records Serv., June, 1943.

45. Mitchell, H.: USA nutrition program: How it is organized. J. Home Econ. 35: 32, 1943.

46. Nutrition Division, Office of Defense, Health and Welfare Services, transferred to Food Distribution Admin., USDA. J. Am. Dietet. A. 19: 306, 1943.

47. War Food Admin., Nutrition and Food Conservation Branch: National Wartime Nutrition Guide. (folder) USDA NFC-4, 1943.

48. Nutrition program materials. J. Am. Dietet. A. 19: 600, 1943.

49. Postgraduate assembly on nutrition in wartime. J. Am. Dietet. A. 19: 728, 1943.

50. Food & Nutr. Bd.: Recommended Dietary Allowances. Natl. Research Council Reprint & Circ. Series No. 115, 1943.

51. Food Distribution Admin., USDA: Planning Meals for Industrial Workers. Washington, D. C.: Govt. Prtg. Off., 1943.

52. Benton and Bowles, Inc.: Working papers. Washington, D. C.: Natl. Archives & Records Serv., Feb., 1943.

53. Nutrition program materials. J. Am. Dietet. A. 19: 855, 1943.

54. Human Nutrition Research Br., Agric. Res. Serv.: National Food Guide. USDA Leaflet No. 288, 1946.

55. Sherman, H. C.: Chemistry of Food and Nutrition, 7th ed. N. Y.: The Macmillan Co., 1946, p. 534.

56. Hill, M., and Cleveland, L.: Food guides—their development and use. USDA, Nutr. Program News, July–Oct., 1970.

57. Leverton, R. M.: Personal communication, Jan., 1973.

58. Hayes, O., Trulson, M. F., and Stare, F. J.: Suggested revisions of the Basic 7. J. Am. Dietet. A. 31: 1103, 1955.

59. Page, L., and Phipard, E.: Essentials of an Adequate Diet—Facts for Nutrition Programs.   USDA Home Economics Research Rept. No. 3, 1957.

60. Food for Fitness—A Daily Food Guide.   USDA Leaflet No. 424, 1958; slightly revised, 1967; slightly revised, 1971.

61. Watt, B. K., and Merrill, A. L.: Composition of Foods—Raw, Processed, Prepared.   Rev. USDA Agric. Handbook No. 8, 1963.

62. Maynard, L.: An adequate diet.   J.A.M.A. 170: 457, 1959.

63. Phipard, E., and Page, L.: Meeting nutritional needs through food.   Borden's Rev. of Nutr. Res. 23: 30, 1962.

64. Leverton, R. M.: How to communicate food needs—and to whom.   Speech presented before 63rd Annual Meeting, Amer. Home Econ. Assoc., June, 29, 1972.

65. Leverton, R. M.: Tools for teaching food needs.   J. Home Econ. 65: 37, 1973.

66. "Food for Fitness" is guide to balanced diet.   J. Home Econ. 58: 352, 1966.

67. Conner, M. M.: A guiding star for modern nutrition.   J. Home Econ. 59: 734, 1967.

8

THE FOOD AND DRUG ADMINISTRATION AND LABELING

Ogden C. Johnson, Ph.D.*

Why should we label products? Some people may think this a silly question, since we all expect labels on products so that we can identify them before we buy them. We want information about what we are buying. Included in the labeling is the price and quantity—both items are essential if we are to make purchases appropriate to our needs and purses.

The Food and Drug Administration (FDA) has undertaken, during the past three years, a comprehensive review of food labeling and the regulations that control it. The result of this review has been a series of regulations on labeling. The first was published in the *Federal Register* in January 1973, and publication continued with surprising regularity—at least in the minds of some—during the next eight months (1–3). What does this new labeling mean? What benefit will it be? Is its usefulness sufficient to justify the anguish that some are reported to have over the various aspects of the regulations?

The new regulations are considered from four vantage points: the manufacturer's, the regulatory agency's, the educator's, i. e., those attempting to guide aspects of consumer purchasing, and the consumer's.

All four groups are, of course, so interrelated that what is said about one applies, at least in part, to the others. The success of the new nutri-

Reprinted from *Journal of The American Dietetic Association*, Vol. 64, No. 5, May 1974. © The American Dietetic Association. Printed in U. S. A.

* Hershey Food Corporation, Hershey, Pennsylvania. Formerly: Director, Office of Nutrition and Consumer Sciences, Food and Drug Administration, DHEW, Washington, D. C.

tion labeling, the use of a common or usual name rather than calling products that resemble traditional products "imitation," and more specific flavor labeling, depends in considerable measure on the willingness of all four parties to cooperate, to work together to understand what the new labeling means, and to apply it appropriately.

THE MANUFACTURERS OR PROCESSORS

The first group comprises those who manufacture and sell food products. The manufacturer has a responsibility to conform to the new regulations, which in some cases are mandatory and in others, voluntary. The three aspects of the new regulations all have a direct relationship to nutritional quality—a factor that is relatively new to FDA regulations.

Nutritional quality guidelines. In establishing "Nutritional Quality Guidelines," the FDA has presented a mechanism by which basic nutritional quality can be ascribed to a class of foods. In many cases, nutritional quality should be attained by good manufacturing practices, including the selection of ingredients and the handling of the product in a correct manner. It may require establishing nutritional quality standards for ingredients. In most instances, these guidelines will permit—in fact, require if the manufacturer wishes to conform—the addition of certain nutrients. It is an attempt to provide more uniform nutritional quality among foods in a class of food products known to be interchanged in the diet.

The Nutritional Quality Guidelines also provide a means by which manufacturers can establish nutritional identity for new products. With the continuing appearance on the market of new foods and foods which will, in many cases, displace traditional foods in the diet, the need to establish basic nutritional quality increases. We hope that manufacturers will take the initiative to include nutrition as part of their activities in product development. Some people assume that all actions by the FDA are internally initiated; we have, however, made it clear that companies, individuals, or organizations that feel a need for a Nutritional Quality Guideline can petition the Commissioner to establish such a guideline for a class of foods.

Imitation foods. Closely related to Nutritional Quality Guidelines is the regulation permitting a manufacturer that develops a food resembling a traditional food to establish a common or usual name for that food. To create an identity for the new product, it must be nutritionally equivalent to the food it replaces. For many years, manufacturers and consumers have been confused by the word "imitation" when applied to a food. "Imitation" could apply when an ingredient not permitted by the Standard of

Identity was used and also when the quantity of a permitted ingredient was either less or more than the Standard indicates.

The simple description, "imitation," provided no clear-cut picture of the product. In instances in which the nutritional quality of the food being imitated is important in the diet of the population, consumers need to know if the imitation product is nutritionally inferior or equal. The new regulation covering products that resemble traditional foods spells out how manufacturers may achieve nutritional equivalency and develop a common or usual name.

Since information on nutritional content and ingredients will appear on the label, consumers will be able to judge for themselves whether a new product is one they wish to eat.

Nutrition labeling. Nutrition labeling, the third regulation, provides for telling consumers about the nutrient content of the food. Many persons have raised questions about the usefulness of nutrition labeling—not only from the consumer's standpoint but also in relation to the dietitian seeking to assist patients in modifying their diets. Nutrition labeling should be given a fair chance, since, for the first time, it offers a mechanism by which manufacturers can honestly state the nutritional quality of their products at the point where consumers make a choice, i. e., the point of purchase. Nutrition labeling, though more complex than some would desire, has been criticized as not complex enough to meet some special dietary needs. Only experience can tell us whether manufacturers will use it and promote it so that consumers will be aware of it.

From the manufacturer's standpoint, nutrition labeling, though it adds to costs and will require greater attention to the maintenance of quality, provides a way to identify new products that have particularly good nutritional qualities. It can also alert consumers to specific benefits relative to caloric, protein, fat, and/or vitamin and mineral content of traditional foods. It provides a mechanism by which nutritionally distinctive and superior products can be honestly labeled. The manufacturers of many of the major food products have already adopted nutrition labeling, and we anticipate a sizable number of items to be so labeled by the end of 1974.

REGULATORY AGENCIES

The second group with a direct interest in the regulations is the FDA itself and, potentially, other regulatory agencies. Because it is a regulatory agency, some look on FDA as a policeman, solely concerned with forcing people to meet stringent requirements established in regulations. True, the FDA does seek to assure that manufacturers comply with regulations, but the regulations are not designed as part of the game to catch people doing wrong. The new labeling regulations were developed to provide maximum assistance to both consumers and manufacturers—to provide a mechanism by which more information can be provided to consumers. This should allow consumers to make wise choices, not only from the nutritional standpoint but also in relation to cost. The regulations were also designed to assure that the nutritional quality of the foods for sale remains as high as possible, and to stimulate manufacturers to put more effort into nutrition.

EDUCATORS

Educators, those who seek to help the consumer, are the next group considered. The provision of more information on labels offers a mechanism by which consumers can be given specific guidance. Over a period of time, consumers can be alerted to identify products, both new ones and those that are traditional but perhaps which they have not used routinely in relation to nutritional quality. Nutrition labeling, though not designed to meet all special dietary needs, provides significant useful information in terms of modified diets. It has been designed so as to accommodate special labeling—for example, sodium, fatty acid, and cholesterol content of products—which should prove helpful to consumers on modified diets. Caloric content is the first item of information on the nutrition label. With so many people seeking to reduce caloric intake, this could serve as a real stimulus to better selection of a total diet in terms of calories.

With the new regulations, the manufacturer is in a position to identify specific properties of his product that relate to special dietary needs. Those who are trying to help the consumer, for instance, the dietitian, can be a stimulus to manufacturers to place such information on the labels. The FDA sincerely hopes that those who find the presentation of information on the label useful to consumers will tell the manufacturer.

CONSUMERS

The final group we must consider are the consumers—really the most important group in relation to all of our actions. The questions that keep coming back to us are: Will the consumers use nutrition labeling? Can they use it? How will they be assisted so that its use will be appropriate? The FDA knows that nutrition labeling will require the concerted effort of many groups if consumer acceptance and use are to be attained. We do not think it will happen automatically, and we believe that, even with rather comprehensive education information campaigns, it will happen only over a period of time, five to ten years.

Some benefits from nutrition labeling and the other nutritional programs will accrue to the consumer more rapidly and inevitably. One of the most important is the current increased interest in nutrition and the greater concern being expressed by many manufacturers, not only to provide more information but to be sure that their products are produced so that nutritional qualities are maintained. As new products come on the market and displace others, manufacturers will consider the nutritional quality of the new product. Nutrition labeling provides a means by which the consumer can be alerted to the fact that a new product meets certain nutritional requirements or, in some cases, that it is not equal in nutrition to similar products. Though consumer acceptance of foods depends almost always on other attributes—with nutrition being of less importance in selection—it is clear that nutrition labeling, once the consumers become aware of its usefulness, can become a more important tool for selecting the most nutritious product among those that are acceptable.

Increasingly, new food products are being accepted as substitutes for traditional foods, in part because of the high prices, but also because improved technology gives products acceptable qualities. Thus, by including nutritional equivalency as part of the imitation regulations, an important benefit accrues to consumers. Products can be chosen with an assurance that they do provide the nutrients that would be expected from the type of product being purchased.

These are benefits that require little if any consumer input. However, nutrition labeling, if it is to be used to achieve some real nutritional benefits, will require consumer input. Consumers will need to understand what the labeling really means—at least as it relates to their own general nutritional needs. They must be able to make valid comparisons of products.

The various studies carried out by the FDA indicate that consumers who are interested in comparing products *can* do it correctly by using nutrition labeling (4, 5).

For some consumers, identification of special properties within a food is what is most important, i. e., the amount of fat or carbohydrate, the presence or absence of cholesterol, or perhaps the presence of specific vitamins or minerals. Such information will be readily apparent to to those who understand their needs and are concerned with specific dietary modification. Nutrition labeling for such individuals is simply another tool to use in selecting products. If the instructions an individual has received include information on nutrition labeling, selection can be more accurate and appropriate for the diet the patient is trying to achieve.

PROMOTING USE OF NUTRITION LABELING

The more general use of nutrition labeling to select a food or even to identify the most nutritious in a class will require considerable motivation. The FDA will shortly launch a national campaign to sell consumers that nutrition labeling is available and to give some of the basic facts needed to use it. This campaign, we hope, will stimulate others at the state and local levels to provide information to consumers.

The very presence of the label with nutritional information presented in a uniform manner on many products can stimulate action. It also gives writers on consumerism and others a ready opportunity to call consumers' attention to the nutritional value of products and to indicate how to determine which of a group of products provides, for example, the fewest calories, or the most fat, or the broadest array of vitamins. We expect food manufacturers to undertake programs to inform customers, with specific intent to sell their products. Since nutrition labeling appears on all products in a very similar manner, to sell or call attention to the nutritional quality of a product via the label will, in fact, call attention to the labeling for all products.

We do not anticipate that 80, 90, or 100 per cent of the population will use nutrition labeling. We do hope that it will be widely used by the 10 to 15 per cent of the adult population on modified diets, that is, twenty-five to thirty million people.

We also hope that many consumers will use the labeling for some product classes initially to identify products that differ in nutritional quality from others. We sincerely hope that those who provide consumers with information and guidance in selecting more nutritious diets will refer to nutritional labeling and, whenever possible, will use it as a tool to identify products that are the best choice from a nutritional standpoint. This is particularly true when new products are introduced and consumers will be influenced by advertising. The very presence of a new product and the claims of benefits in terms of convenience, appearance, or flavor—all of which are important—will continue to be the most influential factors in food selection. But nutrition is also important, and the nutritional quality of foods eaten plays a role in the overall health of the individual.

Last year, the Department of Health, Education, and Welfare undertook, in cooperation with the Advertising Council, the Department of Agriculture, and the Grocery Manufacturers Association, the development of a national campaign to get across some of the basic facts about food and nutrition. The theme of the campaign is simple: "Food is more than something to eat." The FDA has also initiated a consumer education program for nutrition labeling this spring. It will include: national television public service announcements being developed by a major advertising agency under contract to the FDA; local programs using a film on nutrition labeling and material developed for various aspects of labeling; and special program activities organized by the Consumer Affairs Officers in the FDA regional and district offices.

Nutrition labeling and other labeling information that the FDA has developed over the past three years make it possible for consumers to know more about food. Better identification of new foods, nutritional quality standards for new and traditional foods, and nutrition information on the label all help the consumer to make better food choices.

Finally, another important factor is part of the improved labeling. Those who want to bring about change in the marketplace can do so by calling attention to the specific nutritional qualities—or lack of them—in the products available to consumers. The need for more information or special information can be put in terms of real products. Labeling is a tool that can and should be used to bring about the nutritional improvement of the foods we buy and, thus, the improvement of the nutritional quality of the American diet. Nutrition has a golden opportunity today; there is more interest, more desire on the part of consumers, manufacturers, and educators to make nutrition a meaningful part of the selection of food. It can't be done by any one group; it *can* be done by all groups working together.

REFERENCES

1. Fed. Register 38: 2124 (No. 13, Jan. 19), 1973.
2. Fed. Register 38: 6950 (No. 48, Mar. 14), 1973.
3. Fed. Register 38: 20702 (No. 148, Aug. 2), 1974.
4. Lenahan, R. J., Thomas, J. A., Taylor, D. A., Call, D. L., and Padberg, D. I.: Consumer reaction to nutrition information on food product labels. Search 2, No. 15. Ithaca, N. Y.: Cornell Univ. Agric. Exper. Sta., 1972.
5. Stokes, R. C.: The Consumer Research Institute's nutrition labeling research program. Food Drug Cosmetic Law J. 27: 249, 1972.

9

UPDATE ON NUTRIENT LABELING
consumer awareness, use, and attitudes

Lawrence E. Klinger *

Since the 1969 White House Conference on Food, Nutrition and Health, nutrient labeling has evolved from recommendation to reality. How is it working? Are consumers aware of it? Do they use it?

This article will attempt to describe current consumer awareness, utilization, and attitudes toward nutrition information on food packages by reviewing research reported by Daniel Yankelovich, the Consumer Research Institute, Cornell University, Penn State University, and a survey of food manufacturers, food chains, consumer activist organizations, and the Office of Consumer Affairs. Finally, I will report on a survey conducted in mid-March 1974 in the Chicago metropolitan area to measure consumer awareness, utilization, and attitudes toward the many foods now labeled with nutrient information.

In late 1970, Daniel Yankelovich, Inc., New York City, conducted a study in its simulated super market in Upper Montclair, N. J. to evaluate the effects of nutrient labeling. The results of this study show:

* Consumers feel they have been successful in providing nutritious foods and, therefore, concern over the specific nutritive elements in any

Reprinted from *Food Product Development*, June 1974.

Adapted from a presentation before Food Update XIII, Scottsdale, Ariz., April 23, 1974.

* Director, Public Responsibility, Swift & Co., Chicago.

one category of food is at a very low level. They feel they serve a wide variety of foods and if any one food item is lower in nutritive value than another, it is more than compensated for by other things that the family eats.

- A decision involving the preparation of any one meal or any one course within a meal or any treat or snack does not necessarily have to be based upon the nutritive value of the food.

- There is a general belief among consumers that the well-advertised brands are good products and universally high in nutritive values.

- Women felt they lacked the nutrition knowledge to properly evaluate the information and really didn't have the time while shopping to read the labels of every brand to determine and compare which would be best for their families.

- The dominant brand held its share of purchases even in the face of full disclosure labeling on a secondary brand.

- Store brands do not hold their share in the face of full disclosure labeling on competitive products.

- Full disclosure labeling has its major beneficial effect among secondary brands as long as they are not private label brands. Even in this case, however, the dominant brand does not suffer.

The Consumer Research Institute conducted a series of studies with consumers in 1970, 1971, and 1972 including mail surveys, face-to-face interviews, and a controlled experiment in which food purchases were recorded for a specific period of time. The conclusions which they drew from their research showed:

- Consumers have favorable attitudes toward nutrition.
- They desire more nutrient information on the package.
- They have sufficient knowledge to utilize this information in choosing better nutritional products.
- Some will actually purchase products with superior nutrition when properly motivated.
- The numerical percentage mode of communicating the amount of nutrients is preferred over the verbal or pictorial formats.
- A higher percentage of correct nutrient choices can be made when only those nutrients present are listed as compared to listing all key nutrients.
- A listing of protein, fat, and carbohydrate in per cent composition seems useful to some consumers on some products.

Cornell University has reported on two studies with consumers on this subject. In the first study, personal interviews were conducted with 2,195 men and women, 18 years of age and older, in the spring of 1972. The results of this study showed:

• There was a strong preference for the label stating nutrient content with the per cent of RDA versus test labels containing other means for presenting nutrient information.

• Fifty-eight per cent of the sample indicated they would use the information, but only 44 per cent would be willing to pay for it.

• Labels with nutrient information would be used primarily by those in younger age groups, more highly educated, in the higher income groups, and of the white race.

• Agreement concerning non-use benefits of nutrient labeling was strong.

The second study reported by Cornell was an analysis of consumer reaction to private label products containing different forms of nutrient information which were made available for sale in the stores of Jewel, First National, Kroger, and Giant Food in late 1971 and early 1972. Consumer surveys were conducted between two and four months after the initiation of the program. While there naturally are some differences in the results obtained between the individual super markets, the overall results of this study can be summarized as follows using weighted averages:

• Perception: 26.3% recalled seeing the test products.
• Understanding: 15.6% understood the labels.
• Used the labels to make a purchase decision: 9.2%.
• After the labels were explained:
  a. Thought they were a good idea: 96.5%
  b. Would use: 50.9%
• Non-use benefits: 30.9%.
  a. The consumer has the right to know the nutritional value of food products: 97.5%.
  b. Nutrition information for food products will increase consumer confidence in the food industry: 86.7%
• Willingness to pay something: 35.8%.
• Results over time: perception doesn't change; understanding and use increases, but willingness to pay for the information decreased.
• Promotional activity: perception increases, but willingness to pay and recognition of non-use benefits decreased with higher levels of promotion.

Two comments mentioned in the conclusions of this report are most pertinent:

. . . although experts, particularly nutritionists, tend to see nutrition labels on food products as directly influencing the food purchase decision, consumers tend to see their value in a much more general way.

If, as we surmise, the consumer considers this information nice to have primarily for non-use benefits, then exact accuracy in the presentation is not necessary. . . . The consumer wants to know some information is there, as well as accountability, and seems to desire general information on the relative nutritional quality of various products. . . . Since potential cost is directly related to the degree of accuracy, careful consideration should be given to these views of consumer reaction.

Pennsylvania State University also has conducted several studies which included questions regarding consumer interest in nutrient labeling. Each of these studies was conducted under the direction of Dr. R. O. Herrmann and consisted of telephone surveys among consumers in Pennsylvania in 1969 and 1971. The results of the information in these studies concerning nutrient labeling could be summarized as follows:

- Consumers want more nutrition information.
- Nutritional concerns differ with age and family composition.
- Consumers regard nutrient labels favorably although use rates have been relatively low.

When talking about the interests of consumers regarding the various information programs proposed for food products, the easiest thing to say is that the consumer is interested in nutrient labeling, food ingredient information, open dating, and many other of these issues. In the main, such a statement would be correct. I attempted, however, to find some measure which would quantify the degree of this consumer interest. I contacted a sampling of consumer activist organizations, the Office of Consumer Affairs, food retailers, food manufacturers, and The Nutrition Foundation. I also collected several articles pertaining to this subject from the literature. Our request to these groups was basically the same— would they share the results of any consumer studies which they have conducted to show interest, awareness, and utilization of nutrient labeling? Most of those contacted responded.

The additional information obtained in this survey is summarized as follows:

- The Office of Consumer Affairs reported that nine per cent of the food packaging and labeling complaint cases in a six-month period referred to either the absence of nutrient information on labels or lack of consumer understanding of the information available.

• Of the food retailers contacted, only one had conducted a small, informal survey prior to the Cornell study. One additional chain is planning an evaluation of consumer awareness, understanding, and use of this data in the future. In the interim, they feel it is too early to determine if consumers are changing their buying habits because of the availability of nutrient labeling on some foods. All of the retailers contacted are placing this information on some of their private label brands and are supporting this label change with in-store promotional materials and newspaper ads.

• Only one food manufacturer in this survey reported having conducted any consumer research. This firm found:

a. Interest: strong; would like to see nutrition information on labels.

b. Use: low; do not really understand and feel that they are satisfying the nutritional needs of their families with the variety of foods they serve each day.

c. Would pay more for nutrition information: no.

d. Would switch brands to get nutrition information: no, unless dissatisfied with the quality of their present brand.

e. Which element(s) in the nutrition information table were of most interest: calories.

• For approximately two years, Swift & Company has made available to interested consumers and professionals information concerning the nutrient content of its major branded products. In September 1972, and again in August 1973, we conducted research projects to determine why consumers requested the information from our Nutrition Data Bank, how it was used, was it understandable, etc.? Here are some of the major conclusions from these studies:

a. The consumers motivated to request this information were primarily older, better-educated consumers, most of whom had someone in their family with a dietary or special health need.

b. Forty per cent of those studied felt the average homemaker would not know how to use this information because it was too technical.

c. When asked which nutrients they felt should be placed on food labels, the greatest response was for protein and vitamin content.

• In another study, Swift placed statements on the labels of two of our major, nationally distributed, advertised products, informing consumers that we were willing to supply them with the nutrition information on that product. In the first case, two million packages of product were made available with this statement, and after ten months, we had received 217 requests for this information. In the second case, over thirteen million packages were made available with this offer on the label, and after six months, 34 consumers had requested the data.

• The Canadian Government recently reported the results of the most extensive study ever conducted on the nutritional condition of any nation's population in *Nutrition Canada*. Talking about the Eskimo population the report stated:

> Nutrition labeling so highly regarded as a panacea for malnutrition in most Southern latitudes is lost on the Northern people. Even the few women who can read usually won't bother to do so or to count.

• The Nutrition Foundation is very concerned about the abilities of the average consumer to use this information and the development of effective programs not only to educate the consumer, but also to educate the educators. A comment made by Dr. William Darby in a presentation on this subject in April 1972 fairly well summarizes their feeling: "No label device can possibly give the consumer the nutrition education that he needs in order to understand how to maintain his nutritional health. Nutritional understanding must be developed through a long series of learning experiences to which the individual is exposed from birth (or shortly thereafter)."

• In a presentation before the Chicago Chapter of the American Marketing Association, R. C. Stokes, director of the Consumer Research Institute, described current efforts to communicate more and more information to the consumer as "utter nonesense." As far as nutrient labeling was concerned, he suggested an alternative which would consist of massive education programs directed at the uneducated consumer to acquaint him with the fundamentals of nutrition so that he could make his own decision regarding the nutritional value of particular food products. In addition, producers would be required to provide comprehensive information regarding nutritional value to any consumers who specifically request it. In this presentation, Stokes indicated that nutrient labeling, while helpful to those consumers who understand and would utilize the information, discriminates against the majority of people who presently would not be able to understand or utilize the data.

Preparatory to measuring the awareness, utilization, and attitudes of consumers in the metropolitan Chicago market to food packages containing nutrient information on the label, we measured the availability of such products in this market. The first packages containing this information began appearing in early fall 1973. By early December 1973, there were three lines of products (*Del Monte* canned fruit and vegetable products *Kellogg* breakfast cereals and *Pillsbury* boxed mixes) plus six individual products, four of which were nationally advertised brands. By February 18, 1974, we found this information also on the packages for *Green Giant* frozen vegetables, *Green Giant* canned vegetables, *Hawaiian Punch* products, *Knox* gelatin products, and Jewel Food Company private label products. In addition, there were 24 other national advertised products with this information on their label. By March 18, 1974, the list had grown to include all of the above plus a *Jell-O* instant pudding, an *Armour* canned meat product, a *Pillsbury* frozen roll product, *General Mills Wheaties*, and Food Club (*Topco*) private label items.

With this background, we initiated a market research study involving personal, in-home interviews with 200 homemakers in the metropolitan Chicago area who did most of their grocery shopping and planned the family meals. Because of research which had been conducted by others, we confined this study to middle-class and upper middle-class homemakers. The objectives of the research were to determine:

Consumer awareness, description of nutrient labeling.

Awareness and usage of specific products and brands that contain nutrient labeling.

Extent to which the information was used.

Attitudes toward nutrient labeling.

Research results can be summarized as follows:

* *Awareness*: On an unaided basis, 29 per cent of the consumers contacted were aware and accurately described nutrient labeling, and an additional 57 per cent were aware on an aided basis. Primarily, those who were aware were the younger homemakers (under 35), with at least some college education, and with a family income of $13,000 or more.
* *Brand awareness*: Breakfast cereals were by far the most frequently recalled products having nutrient information. Sixty-two per cent of the responses to this question were for specific brands of breakfast cereals. No other brand or product was mentioned by more than six per cent of the homemakers even with the large number of items presently in the market some of which had been available for approximately six months prior to this study.
* When asked which of the required elements on the nutrient information panel were most useful, no one element was mentioned by even one-half of the homemakers. The average response was for only two elements. Forty-two per cent of the respondents mentioned protein, and 40 per cent mentioned calories.
* Most women agreed there was a need for this information, that it would be helpful, and would be an assurance that they were providing nutritious meals to their families. On the other hand, almost one-half of the homemakers agreed that most women can serve nutritious meals without all the nutrition detail; they don't have time to read labels and they wouldn't pay attention to the information anyway.
* Products with nutrient labeling were not viewed as being better quality and most women were not willing to pay more for a product to get nutrient labeling.

• Only one-third of the respondents said that consumers would switch from their regular brand of product to a competing brand with nutrient labeling.

• Most homemakers do not feel that nutrient labeling is just another gimmick, but feel that it would be more helpful for some products than others.

• Most homemakers agree that by putting this information on the package the manufacturer shows he really cares about the consumer, but he should have a program to explain what the information means.

• Forty-one per cent of the consumers in this study indicated that someone in their household was presently on a diet which would limit or restrict his intake of certain foods. The major program was a low-calorie, weight-loss regimen. Other diet programs included low cholesterol, low fat, and low sodium.

GENERAL CONCLUSIONS

Evaluation of all these data collected from many sources and representing studies conducted over a four-year period of time enables us to reach conclusions regarding the consumer's attitude toward nutrient labeling together with her awareness and utilization.

Three sparate studies have shown that as far as attitude is concerned, housewives feel they are presently doing a sufficient job in preparing nutritious meals for their families, and they depend upon the variety of foods which are served, over time, to satisfy nutritional needs. As far as their attitude regarding nutrient labeling, it would appear from four of these studies that while the housewife reports she would like to have more information concerning the nutritional qualities of the food she is purchasing, the non-use benefits, at least for the foreseeable future will outweigh the direct-use benefits.

With respect to awareness, we see that on an unaided basis, awareness regarding the presence of foods with nutrient labels has not changed too greatly over the past two years. The Cornell study showed an awareness by 26.3 per cent of the consumers interviewed whereas the recent Swift study showed an unaided awareness by 29 per cent. Naturally, when these consumers were shown samples of labels containing nutrient information presently in stores, the Swift study showed a total awareness of 86 per cent. It was interesting to note, however, when asked the brands or products on which they recalled seeing the nutrition information, 62 per cent reported breakfast cereals, a category which has contained this information for over 20 years.

With respect to utilization of the data, a number of conclusions can be drawn:

- In three separate studies, we have seen consumers report that they do not have time to read food labels.
- Two of these studies reported that some nutrient information would be useful to some consumers on some products.
- When asked whether they would use the information, 58 per cent of the consumers responded affirmatively in the initial Cornell national survey, and 51 per cent responded affirmatively after the labels were explained to them following the in-store tests.
- When actual use of the labels was measured, the Cornell in-store study showed only 9.2 per cent of the consumers interviewed used the labels to make a purchase decision. A corollary would be the information obtained in our study wherein we placed an offer on the labels of over 15 million packages of two nationally distributed and advertised brands and after ten months, had received requests for the information from less than 300 consumers.
- There seems to be general agreement among most of the sources that the segment of the population most interested in this information is the younger, higher-educated consumer with a higher income. The one difference was in the Swift study of consumers who requested information from our Nutrition Data Bank wherein the majority of these consumers were over 45 years of age.
- With respect to ability to understand nutrient information on the label, all of the sources studied except the initial Consumer Research Institute study agreed that, in general, consumers lacked knowledge to properly utilize this information. The Cornell study reported a figure of 15.6 per cent of the consumers interviewed who said they understood the information.
- With respect to willingness to pay, the initial Cornell national survey reported a figure of 44 per cent of the consumers who indicated a willingness to pay more for products with nutrient labeling. However, in-store tests evaluated by Cornell showed a figure of 35.8 per cent, with a decrease in willingness to pay, over time, and the recent Swift study showed a figure of only 27 per cent.
- When asked whether or not they were willing to switch brands in order to get nutrient labeling, three sources reported relatively low interest in switching brands in order to get this information.
- Four of the sources asked the consumers which of the elements in the nutrition panel would be most useful to them. Protein content was mentioned by the consumers in three of the studies, calories in two, and vitamin, fat, and carbohydrate content each in one study.

Possibly, the federal agencies issuing regulations on nutrient labeling, and food manufacturers considering the placement of this information on their labels should once again review those two conclusions from the Cornell studies mentioned earlier:

> . . . although experts, particularly nutritionists, tend to see nutrition labels on food products as directly influencing the food purchase decision, consumers tend to see their value in a much more general way.
>
> If, as we surmise, the consumer considers this information nice to have primarily for non-use benefits, then exact accuracy in the presentation is not necessary. . . . The consumer wants to know some information is there, as well as accountability, and seems to desire general information on the relative nutritional quality of various products. . . . Since potential cost is directly related to the degree of accuracy, careful consideration should be given to these views of consumer reaction.

BIBLIOGRAPHY

1. Beaulieu, Andre. 1974. A nutrition surveyor's journal. *Nutr. Today*.
2. Call, D. L., et al. 1972. Consumer reaction to nutrition information on food products labels. *Search Agric. 2*: 15.
3. Campbell Soup Company, personal communication.
4. Darby, W. J. Meaningful consumer education in nutrition. Presentation to the Food Industry Briefing on Nutrient Labeling, Washington, D. C., April 13, 1972.
5. Herrmann, R. O., et al. 1972. Consumer adoption and rejection of imitation food products. Bulletin 779, The Pennsylvania State University, College of Agriculture.
6. Herrmann, R. O., et al. 1972. Consumers' views on their problems—and on what should be done about them. *Farm Economics*. The Pennsylvania State University, Cooperative Extension Service.
7. Herrmann, R. O. Nutrition information: Consumer actions and reactions. Presented at the conference, Nutrition: Marketing and the Law, sponsored by The Nutrition Foundation and the Food and Drug Law Institute, September 1972.
8. How much should the consumer be told? 1973. *Chicago Marketing Scene*, 7: 2.
9. Klinger, L. E. Nutrition labeling: Cost vs. consumer interest. Presentation to the New York Section, Institute of Food Technologists, September 18, 1973.
10. National Consumers League, personal communication.
11. Office of Consumer Affairs, personal communication.
12. Stokes, R. C. 1972. Consumers want nutrition labeling—and can use it. *The National Provisioner, 166*: p. 35.

13. Stokes, R. C. 1972. The Consumer Research Institute's nutrient labeling research program. *Food Drug Cosmetic Law Journal, Vol. 27*: 5. p. 249.

14. Stokes, R. C. 1972. Interim report of the first two phases of the CRI/FDA nutrition labeling research program. Consumer Research Institute, Inc.

15. The Pillsbury Company, personal communication.

16. Yankelovich, D. C. 1971. A consumer experiment to determine the effects of nutrition labeling on food purchases. *Chain Store Age,* p. 55, Jan. 1971.

10 RELATIVE IMPORTANCE OF NUTRITIONAL PROBLEMS IN THE TEN–STATE NUTRITIONAL SURVEY 1968–1970

Low-income-ratio states (Kentucky, Louisiana, South Carolina, Texas, West Virginia)

ETHNIC GROUP	AGE	SEX	Iron	Protein	Vitamin A	Vitamin C	Riboflavin	Thiamine	Iodine	Growth & development	Obesity
BLACK	0–5 years	Both	a	d	b	d	b	d	d	b	e
	6–9 years	Both	a	c	c	d	b	d	d	b	e
		Females	a	c	c	d	b	c	d	c	c
	10–16 years										
		Males	a	d	c	d	b	c	d	c	c
		Females	a	c	d	c	b	d	d	e	a
	17–59 years										
		Males	a	d	d	b	b	d	d	e	d
		Females	a	c	d	d	b	d	d	e	b
	Over 60 years										
		Males	a	c	d	b	b	d	d	e	d
WHITE	0–5 years	Both	b	d	c	d	c	d	d	b	e
	6–9 years	Both	b	d	c	d	c	d	d	b	e
		Females	b	d	c	d	c	c	d	c	c
	10–16 years										
		Males	b	d	c	d	c	c	d	c	b
		Females	b	d	d	d	d	d	d	e	b
	17–59 years										
		Males	b	d	d	b	d	d	d	e	c
		Females	b	d	d	d	d	d	d	e	b
	Over 60 years										
		Males	b	d	d	b	d	d	d	e	d
SPANISH-AMERICAN	0–5 years	Both	b	d	a	d	b	d	d	b	e
	6–9 years	Both	b	d	a	d	b	d	d	b	e
		Females	b	c	a	d	b	d	d	c	e
	10–16 years										
		Males	b	d	a	d	b	d	d	c	e
		Females	b	c	a	d	c	d	d	e	e
	17–59 years										
		Males	b	c	a	d	c	d	d	e	e
		Females	b	c	a	d	c	d	d	e	e
	Over 60 years										
		Males	b	c	a	b	c	d	d	e	e
	Pregnant & lactating women		a	b	e	e	e	e	e	e	e

Legend: a, high prevalence of deficient values; **b,** medium prevalence of deficient values; **c,** low prevalence of deficient values; **d,** minimum deficiences; **e,** figures not available.

High-income-ratio states (California, Massachusetts, Michigan, New York (and New York City), Washington

ETHNIC GROUP	AGE	SEX	Iron	Protein	Vitamin A	Vitamin C	Riboflavin	Thiamine	Iodine	Growth & development	Obesity
BLACK	0–5 years	Both	b	d	c	d	c	d	d	b	e
	6–9 years	Both	b	d	c	d	c	d	d	b	e
		Females	b	d	c	d	c	c	d	c	c
	10–16 years										
		Males	b	d	c	d	c	c	d	c	d
		Females	b	d	d	d	c	d	d	e	a
	17–59 years										
		Males	b	d	d	d	c	d	d	e	d
		Females	b	d	d	d	c	d	d	e	b
	Over 60 years										
		Males	b	d	d	c	c	d	d	e	d
WHITE	0–5 years	Both	c	d	c	d	c	d	d	b	e
	6–9 years	Both	c	d	c	d	d	d	d	b	e
		Females	c	d	c	d	d	d	d	c	c
	10–16 years										
		Males	c	d	c	d	d	d	d	c	c
		Females	c	d	d	d	d	d	d	e	b
	17–59 years										
		Males	c	d	d	d	d	d	d	e	c
		Females	c	d	d	d	d	d	d	e	b
	Over 60 years										
		Males	c	d	d	c	d	d	d	e	d
SPANISH-AMERICAN	0–5 years	Both	b	d	d	d	d	d	d	b	e
	6–9 years	Both	b	d	d	d	d	d	d	b	e
		Females	b	d	d	d	d	d	d	c	e
	10–16 years										
		Males	b	d	d	d	d	d	d	c	e
		Females	b	d	d	d	d	d	d	e	e
	17–59 years										
		Males	b	d	d	d	d	d	d	e	e
		Females	b	d	d	d	d	d	d	e	e
	Over 60 years										
		Males	b	d	d	d	d	d	d	e	e
	Pregnant & lactating women		a	b	e	e	e	e	e	e	e

U. S. Department of Health, Education, and Welfare, Public Health Service. Health Services and Mental Health Administration, Center for Disease Control, Atlanta, Georgia 30333.

11

NUTRITIONAL PROBLEMS GROWING OUT OF NEW PATTERNS OF FOOD CONSUMPTION

L. M. Henderson, Ph.D.*

Foreseeing our future nutritional status is difficult. To begin with the future patterns of food consumption are not at all clear and if they were the nutritional implications of those consumption patterns would not be easily predictable. Obviously our population growth and the health of our economy will influence the patterns of food consumption. If we assume continued concern for population control and a standard of living which continues to require less than 17% of the average total disposable income for food, it seems safe to assume that for most Americans economics will not be the dominant factor in determining the adequacy of the diet. Contrast this value (16.7%) with the 60% of disposable income spent on food in some underdeveloped nations. We should realize, however, that anyone using even 30–40% of his disposable income for food in this country is worse off than the resident of an underdeveloped country because of the much higher price paid here for other necessities. Poverty and ignorance will continue to be the major reasons for inadequate diets.

The lack of certainty in forecasting nutritional status results from the uncertainties regarding our capacity to: 1) eliminate extreme poverty;

Reprinted from the *American Journal of Public Health*, Vol. 62, No. 9, September 1972, pp. 1194–1198.

* Dr. Henderson is Head, Department of Biochemistry, College of Biological Science, University of Minnesota, St. Paul, Minnesota. This paper was presented before the Food and Nutrition Section of the American Public Health Association at the Ninety-Ninth Annual Meeting in Minneapolis, Minnesota, on October 11, 1971.

2) educate the consumer to the point where he is sufficiently nutrition conscious and informed to eat reasonably; and 3) develop realistic guidelines and standards for convenience, prepared foods and snacks whose role in our diets is in a rapid state of change.

On the bright side is the increased awareness of nutrition among the populace and the resulting increased attention to the nutritional value of evolving food patterns and to the programs which are designed to reduce the nutritional impact of low incomes.

Let us examine the trend in food consumption patterns first, then proceed to their nutritional implications. It might be instructive first to look at the changes in consumption levels of the major food groups during the past 50 years. Table 1 shows the trend in food consumption, based upon the food taken off the market for consumer use, that is food that

Table 1: Foods available for consumption per capita per year, retail weight equivalent *

	Meat, fish poultry, eggs and legumes	Dairy products excluding butter	Fats	Vegetables excluding potatoes †	Fruits	Cereals	Sweets
1909–13	225	177	41	14	176	291	89
1925–29	216	191	48	25	189	237	119
1935–39	204	202	49	30	199	204	110
1947–49	240	236	46	31	208	171	110
1957–59	253	240	49	25	183	148	106
1965	258	237	51	24	168	147	112

* From B. Friend, Am. J. Clin. Nutr. 20,907 (1967).
† Potatoes and Sweet Potatoes. 205 lb. in 1909–13 down to 101 lb. in 1965.

disappeared into the civilian consumption channels. This is not a good means of estimating nutrients intake, but it does provide a suitable basis for comparing one time period with another to establish trends. The foods are classified into seven arbitrary groups based upon similarity in nutrient contribution. The most noteworthy changes were the following: 1) a decrease in the potato and sweet potato consumption, and 2) decrease use of flour and cereal products from 291 lbs. in 1909–13 to 147 lbs. in 1965. Both of these changes have been gradual and seem to be leveling off at the present consumption figures. They reflect in part the decreased calorie needs which were about 3,500 calories in 1909–13 and 3,160 cal. in 1965. (Table 2). This 10% decrease in energy resulted from a big decrease in calories from carbohydrate (cereals and potatoes) and a relative increase in calories from fat (32% of calories in 1909–13 and 41% in 1965), while proteins continued to provide about 11–12% of the calories over the 50-year period. It's interesting to note that the vegetable fats increased more than threefold while the animal fat (lard, butter and edible beef fats) declined more than 50%. The linoleic acid contribution to total calories doubled in that 50-year period, most of the change occurring in the last 10–15 years.

Table 2: Food energy available per capita per day and per cent furnished by protein, fat and carbohydrate *

Year	Food energy k cal	Protein	Per cent of calories from Fat	Carbohydrate
1909–13	3490	11.7	32.1	56.2
1925–29	3470	10.9	34.7	54.4
1935–39	3270	10.9	36.9	52.8
1947–49	3230	11.7	38.9	49.4
1957–59	3140	12.0	40.7	47.3
1965	3160	12.1	41.0	47.0

* From B. Friend, Am. J. Clin. Nutr. 20,907 (1967).

The mineral and vitamin content of the food disappearing into the consumption channels is shown in Table 3. The changes are relatively small and probably are of little consequence. Calcium increased, magnesium decreased and largely because of the enrichment of bread starting in 1942, iron, thiamine, riboflavin and niacin increased. Were it not for this remedial practice, thiamine would be lower than in the 1909–13 period when cereal grains were a more important contributor of this vitamin.

Table 3: Minerals and vitamins in foods available per person per year *

	Ca mg	Mg mg	Fe mg	B_1 mg	Riboflavin mg	Niacin mg	Vit. A IU	Vit. C mg
1909–13	816	410	15.2	1.64	1.84	19.0	7600	104
1925–29	859	389	14.4	1.55	1.84	17.8	8000	106
1935–39	894	380	13.8	1.43	1.82	17.1	8300	112
1947–49	994	369	16.7	1.91	2.28	21.0	8700	113
1957–59	978	348	16.1	1.84	2.28	20.6	8000	105
1965	961	340	16.5	1.80	2.26	21.4	7800	102

* From B. Friend, Am. J. Clin, Nutr. 20,907 (1967).

It is reassuring to find that in spite of the changes in life styles that have occurred since the first decade of this century, the nutrient content of the foods we purchase is so similar to that of the diets in the "good old days." This reenforces the oft-repeated counsel that a good mixed diet is the best assurance of nutritional adequacy.

For our purpose more recent trends are of great concern. 1970 figures would be useful. Since these are not available, we might look at the 1955 and the 1965 reports of the USDA on Food Consumption of Households. These reports indicate that in that 10-year period food group consumption (Table 4) had the following changes: milk –10%, fats and oils –10%, flour and cereals –20%, bakery products +14%, meat +10%, poultry and fish +9%, eggs –4%, sweets –11%, potatoes and sweet potatoes –14%, fresh vegetables –17%, fresh fruit –13%, canned vegetables and fruits +11%, frozen vegetables and fruits +18%, juice (vegetables and fruits) +13%, and dried vegetables and fruits −22%. The decreased levels of calcium, vitamins A and vitamin C in diets in 1965 compared to 1955 provided some cause for concern. The decreases in milk and carotene-containing vegetables were the most noteworthy changes in that 10-year period.

Table 4: Comparison of 1955 and 1965 household consumption survey figures for food used at home. (per household per week) *

Food group	Quantity (pounds) 1955	1965
Milk	31.86	28.78
Fats, oils	2.97	2.70
Flour, cereal	5.87	4.69
Bakery products	6.70	7.63
Meat	10.10	11.05
Poultry, fish	3.68	4.03
Eggs	2.81	2.69
Sugar, sweets	4.15	3.70
Potatoes, sweet potatoes	6.23	5.37
Fresh vegetables	8.86	7.33
Fresh fruit	9.52	8.20
Commercially canned		
Vegetables	2.58	2.93
Fruits	1.51	1.59
Commercially frozen		
Vegetables	.46	.62
Fruits	.10	.05
Juice vegetables and fruits	3.50	3.97
Dried vegetables and fruits	.61	.47
Beverages		
Coffee	.80	.74
Soft drinks	2.89	5.09
Fruitade, punch, nectar	.12	1.02
Soup and other mixtures	1.53	1.95
Peanut butter	.19	.30

* USDA, ARS. Report No. 1. 1968 (ARS–34).

A review of surveys done by nongovernmental agencies between 1950 and 1965 was prepared by Davis, Gershoff and Gamble (J. Nutr. Educ. 1, 41, 1969). These surveys which covered over 30,000 subjects in 25 studies were primarily the dietary types, but limited biochemical and clinical examinations were reported also. The conclusions of these reviewers was that the nutritional value of the diet had slipped perceptibly in the period since 1950–55. In view of the greater variety of foods available now, one wonders if the deterioration detected by these and the household surveys doesn't reflect the greater opportunity to make selection errors.

Assessing nutritional status requires more than data from household surveys of food intake. These provide average, not individual, intakes and our estimates of requirements remain rough approximations. The best figures we have are the Recommended Dietary Allowances, (RDA), revised and published periodically by the Food and Nutrition Board. They are recognized as and promulgated as target values at which to aim in planning diets in homes and institutions, but in the absence of something better they have become the standard for most dietary surveys with ⅔ RDA or ½ RDA connoting a certain nutritional risk described as low, deficient levels, etc.

A number of events occurred about the same time that the 1965 household consumption figures were published. A Citizen's Board of Inquiry Report, "Hunger USA" was published, the Senate Select Committee on Nutrition and Human Needs held extended hearings in 1969, a White House Conference on Food, Nutrition and Health was held and a comprehensive National Nutrition Survey was launched to determine the degree of malnutrition in low-income families. All of these placed nutrition in the national spotlight.

What did the results of the National Nutrition Survey have to say about the extent of concern and the nutrients of concern? This matter is important because this survey dealt with nutritional status on a more precise plane, using biochemical and clinical methods. The laboratory analysis of blood and urine samples is particularly useful because it deals with individuals on an objective basis. Clinical examination provides unique advantages in detecting residual signs of past malnutrition, but the lack of reliable signs limits its usefulness. The National Survey combined all three methods and if it continues as an ongoing program, we may project trends in nutritional status with much greater confidence in the next decade.

The National Nutrition Survey is familiar to most of you. It's purpose was to: 1) Study the nutritional status of low income families; 2) obtain data on other than those at the lowest economic levels, as they reside in the low income enumeration districts; 3) to identify nutritional problems including information needed to provide a sound basis for action at federal, state and local levels; and 4) create interest in and establish ongoing programs in nutrition.

It was conceived as a collaborative effort involving local, state, and federal groups and it was sponsored by local or state health departments and involved personnel from academic and health services in the states. The methodology was that tested extensively in this country and in 33 foreign surveys and was carefully standardized.

The results of the ten state surveys are not yet available in other than preliminary form, released to the Congress in April 1971 by H.E.W.[1] Table 5 is an attempt to summarize the biochemical findings for the lowest

[1] Complete report has appeared: Ten State Nutrition Survey 1968–1970. USDHEW Health Service and Mental Health Administration, Center for Disease Control, Atlanta, Ga. DHEW Public, No. (HSM) 72–8130–8133.

Table 5: Biochemical findings national nutrition survey of 8 or 10 states, poverty level and below, all ages

	No. of subjects	% deficient	% deficient and low	Age of greatest concern	Correlates with poverty index
Hemoglobin	10,629	5.0	25.1	—	yes
Plasma vit. A	4,455	1.5	8.5	1–9	no
Plasma vit. C	6,693	1.5	7.2	—	yes
Urinary riboflavin	6,896	2.9	17.8	1–16	yes
Two or more	5,776	0.4	7.7	not reported	yes

income group. The standards adopted for the metabolites measured are shown in Table 6. Low hemoglobin levels were observed in all of the surveys. While the causation is related to iron deficiency, possible other deficiencies complicate the anemia. The low hemoglobin values in adult males was an unexpected result. The calculated iron intakes based on food consumption data were also low. While the exact percentage of the population affected and the severity and cause may be in doubt, it is clear that the hemoglobin findings reflect a widespread health problem.

The vitamin A serum levels were deficient or low in 8.5% of the poverty group. The age group most seriously low were the children, ages 1–9. Follicular hyperkeratosis, suggestive of vitamin A deficiency was observed in 1% of all children examined in the first five states surveyed.

Table 6: Deficient, low and acceptable standards of biochemical values. National nutrition survey

Measurement	Age	Deficient	Low	Acceptable
Hemoglobin gm/100 ml	6–23 mos.	< 9.0	9.0–9.9	⩾10.0
	2–5 years	<10.0	10.0–10.9	⩾11.0
	6–12 years	<10.0	10.0–4.4	⩾11.5
	13–16 male	<12.0	12.0–12.9	⩾13.0
	13–16 female	<10.0	10.0–4.4	⩾11.5
	>16 male	<12.0	12.0–13.9	⩾14.0
	>16 female	<10.0	10.0–11.9	⩾12.0
	Preg. 3rd trimester	< 9.5	9.5–10.9	⩾11.0
Plasma vit. A μ/100 ml	all ages	<10	10–19	⩾20
Serum vit. C mg/100 ml	all ages	< 0.1	0.1–0.19	⩾ 0.20
Urinary riboflavin μ/gm creatinine	1–3	<150	150–499	⩾500
	4–6	<100	100–299	⩾300
	7–9	< 85	85–269	⩾270
	10–15	< 70	70–199	⩾200
	Adult	< 27	27–79	⩾ 80
	Preg. 3rd trimester	< 30	30–89	⩾ 90

Thiamine, riboflavin and niacin did not appear to be of major concern, based upon clinical examinations. The preliminary report of the biochemical findings dealt only with riboflavin, whose urinary levels showed that a rather large percentage (17.8%) of those in the poverty group were excreting riboflavin in smaller amounts than is considered acceptable. The per cent in the deficient category was 2.9% and the excretion was lower in the children and youth than in adults. The excretion varied directly with the income of the subjects.

The ten state results indicated 1.5% deficient and 7.2% deficient or low in ascorbic acid based upon the plasma vitamin C levels. The percentage of subjects with deficient and low excretion values varied from none in one state to 15% in another. Bleeding gums which is suggestive of vitamin C deficiency was observed in 1.1% of the population in all states.

Some past vitamin D deficiency in the form of residual skeletal changes was observed. These were in the range of a few tenths per cent to 5% in different states, suggesting that too little attention is being devoted to the availability and cost of vitamin D fortified milk in some localities.

Dental findings, while not complete, suggest that in these low-income families, dental caries largely go untreated until age 18 and thereafter are treated by extraction. The extent to which nutrition is responsible for the poor dental health will be difficult to determine because of the widespread neglect of dental hygiene and routine dental care.

As in foreign surveys the height-weight measurements indicated that the welfare of the preschool age child should be of greatest concern. The poverty-level children were shorter in stature and lighter in weight than the above-poverty group.

The per cent of subjects who had unacceptable biochemical levels for two or more nutrients was 7.7% in 5,776 subjects in the poverty level and below, but only 0.4 were in the deficient range. The corresponding values ran as high as 16.4% and 0.5 in one state and down to 2.0% and 0.0% in another state. This important index was highly correlated with economic status.

In dealing with the nutritional deficiencies of this country we should obviously concentrate on low-income groups. The degree to which we will alleviate the nutritional crunch for them depends upon how effectively the food stamp and other such programs function, how successful we are in establishing realistic guidelines and standards for the nutritional improvement of low cost foods and how successful we are in nutritional education of all segments of our population. The lack of strong correlation between income and the per cent who were deficient or low in two or more nutrients at poverty levels, above the very poor, suggests that only at the very bottom of the economic scale is lack of funds the dominant factor in determining nutritional status. More studies with a broader spectrum of economic levels will be needed to establish this lack of correlation with certainty.

Some say that nutritional education has failed to solve our nutritional problems. Certainly up to now nutritional value of the diet has not been the primary basis for selecting what the average citizen eats. On the other hand, the current concern has made some more teachable than they have ever been before. Nevertheless, sensory rewards seem to be the basis for most food selection. If food researchers succeed in improving on nature in pleasing our senses we must indeed take care to see that the nutritional value is assured.

The prediction regarding the nutrient intake and nutritional health of our people, on the basis of the trends in recent years would have to be somewhat pessimistic. We should ask, can the trend be reversed and do we see present programs as successful in doing this? A number of circumstances place the very poor in a relatively unfavorable position today. Greater urbanization reduces the opportunity for the family to produce its own food. There are fewer opportunities for family labor to be used to enhance the food supply, e. g., picking and canning of fruits and vegetables and the seasonal depression of the price of foods has largely disappeared. If we assume that the nutritional problems will arise from selection errors by our more affluent consumers and from economic pressure on the very poor, how can we cope with the potential undernutrition?

A hasty consideration leads us to say "fortify." Fortify an inexpensive widely accepted staple in the diet, or fortify the major items for all, to insure adequate intake of micronutrients. The cost of nutrients would not be excessive, but what of the technical problems in such a process? What of the cost of controlling this process so that the composition matches the label? What do you do about Zn and Mn, what about folacin and vitamin B_{12}, where the requirements are not known and the analysis a problem?

The opposing philosophy would say that we don't know enough about men's requirements to tamper with the food consumption patterns of the past. Let's depend upon good quality, standard foods and educate and otherwise foster wise selection. As we approach the period when greater manipulation of man's food is a certainty, where greater control of sensory acceptability will make substitutes for traditional foods feasible, we will be obliged to find practical solutions.

These are difficult problems with far-reaching implications. At the present time bread and flour enrichment is accepted as a sound practice. I recall how in 1941 C. A. Elvehjem brought the debate on bread and flour enrichment to the classroom. There were many pros and cons, some of which concern marketing and advertising policies which grow out of attempts to enhance nutritive quality of any product. Many of these problems are as real today as they were 30 years ago. Many still feel that we should go slow in tampering with natural foods. Should substitutes for traditional foods duplicate the item it replaces in nutrient content? If vitamins and minerals are added thereby making less expensive substitutes, should they be advertised as equivalent to the food they simulate? This gets us into the area of regulation, labeling and food standards with all of the inherent thorny problems. We want an inducement for food processors and manufacturers to improve the nutritional value of their products, but we are sometimes not willing to see them take marketing advantage of a nutritional edge obtained by adding nutrients. This view is understandable but it is inconsistent with our system and it leads to a de-emphasis of nutritional considerations in product development. If it tastes better, you can tell people so, and be excused for some slight exaggeration and sell more of it. Extravagant and inaccurate claims regarding taste appeal are not questioned, because we know that the eating public will pass judgment. Nutritional claims are always questioned because we have no jury and no foolproof basis of judgment. Let me illustrate with a problem now being discussed in connection with the FDA's attempt to establish nutritional guidelines for frozen convenience dinners. Several of those now on the market fall short in one or two nutrients; some fall short in 4 or 5 nutrients and some contain ample nutrients for their caloric value. Should those who market a nutritionally inferior product be allowed to add 4 or 5 nutrients to that product, thereby bringing it up to guideline values? If this is allowed, they then can use a label indicating that the product meets the guidelines and sell it in competition with products whose basic composition is so good that they require addition of none or one vitamin to meet the guidelines. What of the many nutrients not included in the guidelines, either because we don't have good enough information on their distribution or on the amounts man requires? Thus enrichment or fortification provides a means for giving an inferior product a seal of approval and an unfair marketing advantage over the better product. These kinds of questions are being asked by FDA now and the Food and Nutrition Board has a committee working hard on this and related questions.

More informative labeling of all foods is needed and several schemes are being examined by FDA for testing in the market place. Some of these guidelines may be discussed by Dr. Forbes in greater detail.

What is the nutritional significance of the increase in meals taken outside of the home? If I were to judge from my own experience, the only nutritional problem associated with eating out is obesity. Perhaps there are others, but professional or semiprofessional dietitians are involved in many food-away-from-home institutions. Meals in restaurants, air lines, school cafeterias, etc. are likely to be very nutritious.

The magnitude of this change in eating patterns is great, 35 billion dollars annually with predictions of $75 billion by 1980. At present about 23% of the food dollar is spent for meals outside the home. In the period from 1947 to 1965 there was 131% increase in working mothers. The working mother's family eats out more and often eats restaurant-prepared meals carried home. Many office and factory workers, particularly the younger ones, are now eating breakfasts away from home. One report indicates that less than 10% of Americans eat a midday meal at home on weekdays. Food service is now the third largest industry in the nation. The nutritional impact of this, except for the overindulgence it encourages, is probably not a negative one. Its influence on what we consume at home has not been determined.

The spiraling use of snack foods is the other major change in consumption patterns which will influence nutrition in the immediate future. Snacks vary widely in nutrient content. I'm inclined to feel that those items which survive will not be washouts nutritionally. Potato chips of various kinds are up to 6.5 lbs. per person per year or $600 million projected to 1 billion for this year. Some have estimated that in unusual circumstances snack foods could account for 30% of the caloric intake. Should they be fortified in any way? They are not intended as meals and normally would provide less than 10% of the caloric intake, therefore should be exempted. On the other hand, if they become sufficiently varied with enough taste appeal to replace meals, they might threaten adequate nutrition of the user. Soft and hard drinks plus snacks might provide a substandard substitute to a few meals a month but probably they pose no great threat to our nutritional well-being, except in the fringe consumers.

In conclusion let me reiterate that short supply of nutrients in our society stem from inability to *pay* or to *choose* and, for most, it is *choose*. As long as we eat, public health agencies must continue to be involved in what we eat and what it provides. Hopefully, we will remain cognizant of our responsibility to monitor the nutritional well-being of those for whom we have responsibility.

Some elementary lessons have come from the national survey. Goiter and its cause is being rediscovered by the grandchildren of those who suffered from it. Rickets occurs in children whose parents do not see the need to pay the extra cost of vitamin D fortified milk. Increasing numbers of our young people have turned to "natural foods" and "health foods" on the basis of unwarranted fear of chemicals added to food or on the basis of misinformation regarding elementary biology and agriculture, but chiefly on the basis of an emotional appeal by some who do not want to be bothered with the facts. Phil White, of the Council on Foods of the American Medical Association, recently made the telling point that food additives presented a less serious threat to health than does overeating. In the decision to add or not to add a chemical to foods we are choosing between the slight risk and the alternative of stale or otherwise inferior food. Overeating is far more dangerous with the attendant obesity and in this case there are no benefits to weigh against the risk. The person who wishes to get involved in a cause related to food and its effect on health might more properly turn his attention to finding a means of preventing our most serious malnutrition, overconsumption of calories.

12

THE PARADOX OF TEEN–AGE NUTRITION

Ruth M. Leverton, Ph.D.*

It is common practice today to believe that many teen-agers have atrocious food habits and are on the brink of nutritional disaster. The basis for such a generalization is questionable. We point with pride to our youth—their size, their attainments, and their vitality, even though we view with alarm their food habits. Are we implying that food has no relation to fitness, or do we have a distorted picture of their food choices and eating patterns?

Surveys show that some teen-agers do have food intakes that fail to supply the Recommended Dietary Allowance for each of the nutrients. Some diets fail to supply even two-thirds of the recommended amounts, and these we rate as inadequate or poor. The number of teen-agers classified as having inadequate nutrient intakes, however, depends on which revision of the Recommended Dietary Allowances has been used as the basis for evaluation.

EFFECT OF CHANGED ALLOWANCES

Since the first edition in 1941 (1), the Allowances have been reviewed and revised as needed to reflect the best available scientific evidence. In

Reprinted from *Journal of The American Dietetic Association*, Vol. 53, No. 1, July, 1968. © The American Dietetic Association. Printed in U. S. A.

Presented at the Golden Anniversary Meeting of The American Dietetic Association in Chicago, on August 16, 1967.

* Former Assistant Deputy Administrator, Agricultural Research Service, U. S. Department of Agriculture, Washington, D. C.

the 1963 revision (2), the allowances for teen-agers for several nutrients were significantly reduced. For instance, the allowance for protein for the thirteen-to-fifteen-year-old girl was 80 gm. in the 1941 edition (1). It continued to be 80 gm. in the revisions through 1958 (3–7). But, in the latest 1963 revision, it was reduced to 62 gm. for the twelve-to-fifteen-year-old girl. Many of the dietary evaluations we "view with alarm" are from studies made prior to 1963, using comparisons with the earlier and higher Allowances.

A few figures will illustrate the differences in the assessment of adequacy that occur when an allowance is revised. In the late 1940's, the dietary intakes of 281 girls thirteen to fifteen years old in three northeastern states were evaluated (8). Only 45 per cent had protein intakes that equalled the allowance which was then 80 gm. However, when the intakes are compared with the 1963 allowance of 62 gm., instead of 45 per cent, 74 per cent of the girls had protein intakes that met or exceeded the allowance (assuming a distribution which is normal in the area of the mean, plus or minus one standard deviation). The figures are similar for thiamine—the percentage of intakes that met or exceeded that allowance rose from 46 when judged by the 1948 allowance to 73 when judged by the 1963 allowance.

When I reviewed a Nebraska study made in 1949–50 (9), I found that certain conclusions were no longer justified. Using the 1953 Allowances, we had reported that half of the thirteen-to-fifteen-year-old girls had thiamine intakes that were less than 70 per cent of the allowance. By the present standard, however, there would have been no intake of thiamine that rated this low. Instead of reporting that only half of the girls met the allowance for riboflavin, we would now report that 92 per cent had intakes that met or exceeded the allowance.

There has been no downward revision, however, in the allowances for calcium and iron for the teen years. In fact, in the 1953 edition, the calcium allowance for the sixteen-to-twenty-year-old girl was increased from 1.0 to 1.3 gm. Thus, if these two nutrients were in short supply when compared with the Allowances of the 1940's, they would still be in short supply when compared with later revisions. We might ask the reason for such steadfastness in recommendation. Has the research on which the 1941 recommendations were based withstood the impact of newer findings, or have normal human requirements for these nutrients been neglected in the competitive research arena?

ALLOWANCES FOR IRON

For an answer, I studied the table and the text of each of the seven editions of the Allowances from 1941 through 1963. I was particularly interested in the iron allowance which has remained at 15 mg. for both boys and girls in the teen years. There was no text explaining the basis for the figures for the individual nutrients in the Allowances in 1941 and 1943. When discussing their scientific basis, however, Roberts wrote (10): "No data were available for the [iron] requirements of adolescents. The allowances were set empirically on the assumption that the needs would be actually greater than those of the adult during these years and increases [over the allowances for younger children] of the order used would probably be justified."

The text accompanying the 1945 revision, states: "No data are available for the [iron] requirement during adolescence. The allowances recommended were estimated on the assumption that needs are greater than those of the adult." Similar statements were made in the 1948 and 1953 revisions. In the 1958 revision, there are no references to new metabolic studies but the statement was changed to: "Iron requirements during adolescence are enhanced because of the growth spurt which occurs at this age. Allowances of 15 milligrams have therefore been proposed for age groups from 13 to 15 years." In the 1963 revision, no new studies were cited and the statement was made that "iron requirements during adolescence are enhanced because of the growth spurt which occurs and are probably equal to or exceed the adult requirement, particularly in the case of adolescent girls who have passed the menarche."

THE CALCIUM ALLOWANCE

A review of the texts on calcium allowances for adolescents indicates concern over the scarcity of data. Studies made in 1922 (11), 1930 (12), and 1936 (13) are the chief sources of the figures which have been evaluated and recalculated in light of newer findings on younger and older age groups.

In reading a journal recently, I saw that the Chairman of the Subcommittee on Calcium of the Food and Nutrition Board had reported "that the committee was not prepared to make specific recommendations concerning the calcium allowance, but that the problem was beginning to emerge." There is nothing unusual about this report, except that it was made in May of 1952—fifteen years ago.

APPLYING THE ALLOWANCES

We are deeply indebted to the Food and Nutrition Board for its leadership in developing and keeping current the Recommended Dietary Allowances. Without these, the evaluation of diets of groups and of individuals as a basis for educational and action programs could not have progressed as it has. The scientists on the Board have documented carefully the limits of knowledge on these requirements and thus on the allowances for adolescents, but sometimes we, as practitioners, have tended to ignore the "fine print." The relationship between the scarcity of data on which to base a nutrient allowance and the prevalence of dietary inadequacies in that nutrient is indeed food for thought.

We tend to use the Recommended Dietary Allowances in a most rigid way for measuring the adequacy of diets and the prevalence of poor diets. We classify a diet as "poor" if it supplies less than two-thirds of the allowance for any one nutrient. Using this criterion, a teen-ager's diet that provides at least two-thirds of the allowance for every nutrient except one bears the same stigma, "a poor diet," as one that fails to supply two-thirds of the allowance for all nine nutrients. Granted, nutrients are not interchangeable in their usefulness to the body—an over supply of one cannot make up for a shortage of another. It seems a distortion, however, to throw into the category of "poor," diets of every degree of inadequacy from one to nine nutrients.

Teen-ager's diets studied to date are most likely to fall short of the allowances in calcium, iron, and ascorbic acid. I have mentioned the limited basis for the allowances for calcium and iron. Opinions about the allowances for ascorbic acid differ widely. Many scientists view them as unnecessarily high.

It should be of great concern to us that so little research is being done on nutrient requirements of normal people of all ages. Fantastic advances have been made in the science orientation of every segment of our world with funds made available for scientific searching in fields from cells to the whole arena of outer space, and in the precision of instrumentation and techniques. Why, then, has an area as urgent as nutrient requirements of people been so neglected?

I think that the specialization involved in these advances has reduced the interest and concern of scientists in the heterogeneous, baffling collection of cells, tissues, systems, and processes that make up the human body. Yet our responsibility is to understand and serve the entire organism in its functioning as a whole person.

The limited knowledge of the precise quantitative requirements for the nutrients does not relieve us of responsibility for helping the adolescent to be well fed. We must give support to good food habits so they will be continued and work to improve habits that need improvement.

Despite our efforts to date, we have not always done enough of the right things. As professional "people feeders," we must take more responsibility and find more opportunities to provide teen-agers with the food they need and like at the times they need and like it.

Perhaps we need to try harder to recognize and respect the complexity of the needs and problems that characterizes the teen-ager's world today. Even if we think that we had some of the same problems when we were teen-agers, we must realize how different it is to be a teen-ager and to look back on having been one.

The period of transition from childhood to adulthood has been progressively telescoped into fewer and fewer years. "Instant adulthood" seems to be the current demand.

THE LIABILITIES AND ASSETS

Under such stress, what chance is there of today's adolescent following the guidelines for good nutrition? There are several counts against it:

(a) Too often teen-agers have been given the idea that nutrition means "eating what you don't like because it's good for you," rather than "eating well because it will help you in what you want to do and become."

(b) Adolescents are not experiencing the nutritional disaster that adults are telling them will result from poor food habits.

(c) Food is only one component of the busy lives of teen-agers and can receive only a fraction of their attention. What they need and will eat is not always available to them at places and times when they do eat.

(d) Many persons who are in strategic positions to help them are not knowledgeable about practical nutrition. Some are actually misinformed.

Fortunately, there is a plus side to the ledger, i. e., reasons why there is a good chance for teen-agers to be well fed:

(a) Adolescents get hungry.

(b) They like to eat.

(c) They want energy, vigor, and the means to compete and excel in whatever they do.

(d) Many have good food habits established in childhood. "Habits are hard to break," applies to *good* habits as much as it does to bad habits.

We have not always appreciated these assets and the opportunities they offer for effective nutrition education.

DETERMINING "ACCESS POINTS"

I suggest that our greatest responsibility now is to identify "access points" to our teen-agers—points in time and place when we can make available for them food they like and that will contribute to meeting their physical and social needs. Access points means doing things *for* the teen-ager, not *to* him, and they should be serviced without adult prejudice and mores. Their major purpose should be to offer the adolescent food he will enjoy. Examples of such access points are: (a) the home refrigerator and the kitchen cupboard with foods easily available in a permissive, pleasant atmosphere, at any time of day, but especially in the morning; (b) school lunches that recognize that teen-agers want some choice, even within the framework of the Type A lunch—choice that permits variation in the caloric value and allows for favorite foods, and (c) dispensing machines that offer foods with more than empty calories.

Basic to the success of access points is a schedule that permits time for eating and snacking. Some school schedules are so packed with activities that there is scarcely time for mid-day eating and even less time for refueling before the after-school activities. Such schedules practically force teen-agers into a distorted pattern of grabbing any food they can during the school hours and using the hours late in the day for catching up on their food intake.

SPACING OF MEALS AND EATING

We know little about what is desirable in the spacing and the size of meals. We do know that it is undesirable to crowd a large proportion of the day's food intake into a small time space or a single meal. Such quantities not only tax physiologic processes at the time but mean that during much of the day the body's needs for nourishment are likely to have been neglected. Also, omission of "food in the morning" can adversely affect the total nutrient intake for the day. So it should be reason for concern and action when teen-agers eat much of their total food for the day after school hours and before bedtime.

Little relationship has been found between frequency of teen-age eating and overall nutritive quality of their diet except that when they ate fewer than three times a day, the nutritive intake usually suffered (14).

The teen-ager is a snacker and there is no research evidence to indicate that frequent eating *per se* is detrimental to health. We have talked a good deal about planning balanced meals with a caloric value low enough to permit "snacks in addition." We have moved on to a concept of food on a daily basis—servings of all the kinds of food that are needed for good nutrition during the day. Thus we have admitted snacks into the inner circle of the foods that can contribute to good nutrition and be enjoyed at the same time. We no longer regard them as being limited to empty calories or to carrot sticks and raisins. Such permissiveness, however, must carry with it responsibility for developing a sense of orderliness and organization about meals and about snacking. Acceptance of snacking does not give a license for overeating or for ignoring total daily nutrient needs.

THE SCHOOL LUNCH

The school lunch is an access point that has not always been used to advantage. Programs as extensive as the School Lunch must aim to do the greatest good for the greatest number. Teen-agers represent a relatively small portion of that "greatest number" but their participation is relatively high in programs managed by directors who are alert to their needs and preferences. The Type A pattern is flexible enough to be interpreted with foods that are appealing to the teen-age population. Usually teen-agers like many kinds of foods but they do like choice. They also like fast service. If some low-calorie choices are available, the lunch is more acceptable, especially to the girls, even if they do not take these choices.

This always raises the question of skim milk vs. whole milk as a choice in the lunch. Any school can offer the children the choice of skim or whole milk. Reimbursement for the lunches of those who choose skim milk, however, is given for the cost of the lunch excluding the cost of the skim milk. The school that offers skim milk as a choice has an obligation to teach the marginally nourished child to select whole milk. Whole milk with its vitamin A and calories is one of the safeguards that has been built into the Type A pattern.

The school lunch as an access point is strengthened when there is understanding and cooperation of administrators, parents, and other community members. School lunch operations that have good communication and good working relationships with these groups also have good participation.

Nutrition education to undergird and accompany whatever access points we identify is an art and science in itself. There are as many approaches as people have time and training to develop. In the total health picture, as much attention needs to be given to rest and exercise as to food selection. Whatever methods and materials we use in our nutrition programs, we must not be tempted to judge the individual teen-ager by generalizations about the group. Even if half the teen-agers *are* poorly fed, this means that there is still the other half that is well fed. It is just as much our responsibility and privilege to help them remain so as it is to help others attain the well-fed status.

REFERENCES

1. Comm. on Food and Nutr.: Recommended Daily Allowances for Specific Nutrients. Washington, D. C.: Natl. Research Council, 1941.

2. Food and Nutr. Bd.: Recommended Dietary Allowances, Sixth Revised Edition, 1964. Natl. Acad. Sci.—Natl. Research Council Pub. 1146, 1964.

3. Food and Nutr. Bd.: Recommended Dietary Allowances. Natl. Research Council Repr. & Circ. Series No. 115, Jan. 1943.

4. Food and Nutr. Bd.: Recommended Dietary Allowances, Revised. Natl. Research Council Repr. & Circ. Series No. 122, 1945.

5. Food and Nutr. Bd.: Recommended Dietary Allowances, Revised. Natl. Research Council Repr. & Circ. Series No. 129, Oct. 1948.

6. Food and Nutr. Bd.: Recommended Dietary Allowances, Revised 1953. Natl. Acad. Sci.—Natl. Research Council Pub. 302, 1953.

7. Food and Nutr. Bd.: Recommended Dietary Allowances, Revised 1958. Natl. Acad. Sci.—Natl. Research Council Pub. 589, 1958.

8. Cooperative Nutritional Status Studies in the Northeast Region. IV. Dietary Findings. R. I. Agric. Exper. Sta. Bull. 319, Contribution 802 (Northeast Regional Pub. No. 11), 1952.

9. Leverton, R. M., and Pazur, J.: Food Practices and Nutritional Status of Typical Nebraska Families. Neb. Agric. Exper. Sta. Misc. Pub. 5, 1957.

10. Roberts, L. J.: Scientific basis for the Recommended Dietary Allowances. New York J. Med. 44: 59, 1944.

11. Sherman, H. C., and Hawley, E.: Calcium and phosphorus metabolism in childhood. J. Biol. Chem. 53: 375, 1922.

12. Wang, C. C., Kern, R., and Kaucher, M.: Minimum requirement of calcium and phosphorus in children. Amer. J. Dis. Child. 39: 768, 1930.

13. Wang, C. C., Kaucher, M., and Wing, M.: Metabolism of adolescent girls. 4. Mineral metabolism. Amer. J. Dis. Child. 52: 41, 1936.

14. Hampton, M. C., Huenemann, R. L., Shapiro, L. R., and Mitchell, B. W.: Caloric and nutrient intakes of teen-agers. J. Am. Dietet. A. 50: 385, 1967.

13

EATING BETWEEN MEALS

a nutrition problem among teenagers?

Jean A. Thomas and David L. Call *

Much concern has been voiced in recent years over the nutritional quality of the American diet. In the USDA's 1965 Household Food Consumption Survey, food consumption data indicated decreased intakes of calcium, vitamin A, thiamine, riboflavin and ascorbic acid when compared with the findings of the 1955 Survey. When a 24-hour dietary recall was carried out as part of the 1965 Survey, groups with average diets below the Recommended Dietary Allowance (RDA) for more than one mineral or vitamin included all females of age nine years and older and boys 12 through 17.

The adolescent period has been pointed out by many as a cause for nutritional concern. Females of ages 12 through 17 were found in the 1965 Household Food Consumption Survey to have average intakes of calcium and of iron about 30 percent below the RDA for each of these nutrients, while intakes of thiamine and vitamin A were also below the RDAs for this age group. Nutrient intakes of adolescent males were about 10 to 20 percent below the RDA for calcium, 20 to 30 percent below the RDA for iron, and the thiamine intake also fell below the RDA.

Reprinted from *Nutrition Reviews*, Vol. 31, No. 5, May, 1973. Printed in U. S. A.

* Jean Thomas is Research Assistant, Graduate School of Nutrition, Cornell University; Dr. Call is Professor of Food Economics, Graduate School of Nutrition, Cornell University, Ithaca, New York, 14850.

In the Ten-State Nutrition Survey it was reported that adolescents between the ages of ten and 16 years had the highest evidence of unsatistory nutritional status of any of the age groups surveyed.

A knowledge of adolescent eating habits has resulted in a great deal of the attention given to the quality of the teenage diet being focused on the habit of eating between meals, a frequent practice among this group. One often finds reference to the practice of eating between meals as being undesirable—an examination of several basic nutrition textbooks, for example, revealed that many writers consider that eating between meals spoils the adolescent's appetite for "regular" meals and that foods eaten between meals provide the teenager with a substantial proportion of his daily calorie requirements, but little else in the way of nutrients.

The feeling that the calories provided by foods consumed between meals are "empty" is reinforced by the prominent advertising and large sales of volume of potato chips, pretzels, soft drinks, candy and other items which many persons associate with between-meal eating. Some nutritionists have called for the development of foods specifically intended for consumption between meals which are low in calories but provide significant amounts of various nutrients. Others suggest "balanced" snack foods where nutrients are included in some prescribed relationship to the caloric content.

The problem with the statements made by many nutritionists concerning the nutritive quality of foods eaten between meals is that they have been derived largely from sales figures for certain foods and personal opinion based on informal observations. In an effort to obtain an objective estimate of the nutritional quality of foods eaten by teenagers between meals, we examined data from the Ten-State Nutrition Survey.

We combined the data on mean intake per person and percent supplied by between-meal foods for white males and black males, ages 12 to 14 and 15 to 16 years, in low and high income-ratio states and for females of corresponding groups for calories, protein, calcium, iron, vitamin A, thiamine, riboflavin and ascorbic acid. The data included *only* those teenagers in the Ten-State Survey who reported eating between meals on the day of the 24-hour recall—about 78 percent.

The actual amount of each nutrient supplied by the between-meal foods was calculated and then combined into one group for each sex to show the nutrient intake from between-meal foods for persons 12 to 16 years of age. The resulting figures represented the weighted mean intake per person for the combined group. Conversion to a per 100 Kcal. basis was accomplished by dividing the mean calorie intake per person in the aggregate by 100, and dividing the mean intake per person for the other nutrients by the resulting number. Intake of nutrients per person for the entire period covered by the dietary recall was converted to a per 100 Kcal. basis in a similar fashion. The resulting figures were compared to the appropriate RDAs, also converted to a per 100 Kcal. basis.

Calculation of the amount of each nutrient in this way indicates how well the actual nutrient intake compares to a standard distribution of nutrients in the diet.

Results are shown in the table, based on a calorie intake from between-meal foods of 634 Kcal. for males and 495 Kcal. for females, and a total calorie intake of 2,770 Kcal. for males and 2,157 Kcal. for females. Since the RDAs for calories for these groups are 2,800 and 2,350 respectively, it is readily seen that of the teenagers who reported eating between meals, both males and females obtained a substantial proportion of their recommended caloric intake—about 23 percent—from foods eaten between meals.

Mean nutrient intake per 100 calories from between-meal foods and total nutrient intake per 100 calories for males and females ages 12 to 16 years, based on data from ten-state nutrition survey, 24-hour recalls

| | Males [1] | | | Females [1] | | |
| | RDA per 100 Kcal [2] | Mean Intake per 100 Kcal [3] | | RDA per 100 Kcal [2] | Mean Intake per 100 Kcal [3] | |
		Between-meal foods	24-hour total		Between-meal foods	24-hour total
Protein (g.)	2.0	2.3	3.8	2.2	2.2	3.7
Calcium (mg.)	50.0	39.1	44.6	55.3	34.3	41.0
Iron (mg.)	0.64	0.33	0.55	0.77	0.34	0.53
Vitamin A (IU)	178.0	128.0	193.5	212.0	117.4	196.0
Thiamine (mg.)	0.05	0.03	0.05	0.05	0.03	0.06
Riboflavin (mg.)	0.05	0.07	0.09	0.06	0.06	0.09
Ascorbic acid (mg.)	1.7	2.6	2.8	2.0	3.9	2.9

[1] Number of teenagers reporting snacking on day covered by recall: 1,351 males, 1,460 females.

[2] Based on RDA for calories of 2,800 for males and 2,350 for females.

[3] Based on calorie intake from between-meal foods of 634 Kcal for males and 495 Kcal for females, and total intake of 2,770 Kcal for males and 2,157 Kcal for females.

Source of data: Tables 4–7, pp. V–312–V–314, Ten-State Nutrition Survey, Vol. V. Dietary, Atlanta, U. S. Department of Health, Education, and Welfare, 1972.

For both sexes the mean nutrient intake per 100 Kcal. from between-meal foods met or exceeded the RDA for protein, riboflavin and ascorbic acid, while the intake of thiamine was slightly below standard. When data for the entire period covered by the 24-hour recall are considered, however, RDAs per 100 Kcal. were met or exceeded by both males and females for all four of these nutrients.

Both males and females had vitamin A intakes from foods eaten between meals which were below the RDAs. For the entire period of the recall, the mean vitamin A intake per 100 Kcal. among males exceeded the RDA. Among the females, however, the mean vitamin A intake per 100 Kcal. during the 24-hour period was 196 IU, which represents about 92 percent of the RDA of 212 IU per 100 Kcal.

Calcium and iron presented the most serious problems relative to adequacy of intake. For the males, foods eaten between meals provided 39.1 mg. of calcium and those eaten at meals supplied 46.2 mg. of calcium per 100 Kcal., resulting in a 24-hour total of 44.6 mg. of calcium, about 89 percent of the RDA per 100 Kcal. of 50 mg. Foods eaten between meals provided females with 34.3 mg. of calcium per 100 Kcal., while 43.1 mg. of calcium were obtained from foods eaten at meals, the resulting total for the period covered by the recall being 41.0 mg. of calcium, about 74 percent of the RDA per 100 Kcal. of 55.3 mg.

Males obtained 0.55 mg. of iron per 100 Kcal. during the day of the recall, about 86 percent of the RDA per 100 Kcal. of 0.64 mg. Of this, 0.33 mg. per 100 Kcal. came from foods eaten between meals and 0.61 mg. per 100 Kcal. from foods eaten at meals. Although the RDA per 100 Kcal. for iron is 0.77 mg. for females of this age, the mean intake per 100 Kcal. over the 24-hour period was 0.53 mg. of iron, about 69 percent of the RDA. Between-meal foods supplied 0.34 mg. per 100 Kcal. and foods eaten at meals provided 0.59 mg. of iron per 100 Kcal.

Based on the foregoing analysis, one can conclude that on the basis of the nutrients examined, the calories supplied to teenagers by between-meal foods are far from empty. On the other hand, there are indications of some dietary problems, especially with regard to calcium and iron. On a per 100 Kcal. basis the mean intake of these nutrients both from meals and foods eaten between meals was just too low. The between-meal foods contributed to the problem but even if all the calories had come from the regular meals, the problem of dietary inadequacy would remain. Unfortunately, the data as presented do not allow an assessment of the potential impact of the proposed change in the cereal enrichment formula which should help on the iron problem. Although the use of average data can be misleading, it seems clear that several conclusions can be drawn from the data. Certainly there is no evidence that more protein should be added to so-called "empty calorie foods." Not only is protein enchancement a relatively expensive process but its inclusion would imply a definite dietary need which runs counter to the available facts. Calcium presents another interesting problem since it is seldom included in enrichment or fortification efforts for technical reasons. Inclusion of more dairy products in the diet either at meals or between meals is still a valid suggestion. The evidence would indicate little need for widespread fortification with the B vitamins or vitamin C leaving vitamin A and iron as candidates for serious study. A major problem with any program of encouraging the fortification of "empty calorie foods" is the lack of control over the amount consumed by an individual. The policy of fortifying foods that are consumed by most people in relatively controlled amounts, for example bread and milk, is still sound.

The dietary problem of iron and calcium in teenage diets should be approached with specific group oriented efforts. A surgeon's scalpel is often more appropriate than a meat ax.

In conclusion, although large quantities of the empty calorie foods which many persons associate with between-meal eating are consumed annually, it seems on the basis of the existing data that the place which such foods occupy in the teenage diet has been exaggerated, since foods eaten between meals provided a relatively good balance of nutrients. Instead of simply attempting to break the teenager of the habit of eating between meals or providing more nutrients in foods that are often eaten between meals, it seems more reasonable to give special attention in nutrition education efforts to helping the teenager to link up food with various nutrients and give special emphasis to those foods which supply calcium and iron in his diet. The potential beneficial effect of the proposed change in the iron enrichment formula on teenage diets should be examined in more detail.

14

SUPPLEMENTATION OF FOODS vs NUTRITION EDUCATION

nutritional improvement debate

in favor of nutrition education

Henry A. Dymsza

I challenge the concept that an expanded program of fortification and supplementation—including nutrification (Lachance, 1972)—other than in specific foods where there is sound evidence of possible benefit, is a better way to achieve nutritional status improvements in the United States than is nutrition education.

ADEQUATE NUTRIENTS ARE AVAILABLE

The first premise which supports the education position is that adequate nutrients are available in the food supply. Friend (1972a) com-

Reprinted from *Food Technology*, July 1974, pp. 55–63.

This debate is based on papers presented at the 33rd Annual Meeting of the Institute of Food Technologists, Miami Beach, Fla., June 10–13, 1973. Co-sponsored by the National Dairy Council, the debate was chaired by Bernard S. Schweigert, University of California, Davis, CA 95616.

The authors of the papers are: Benjamin Borenstein, Manager, Food Industry Technical Services Dept., Roche Chemical Div., Hoffman-La Roche Inc., Nutley, NJ 07110; Henry A. Dymsza, Professor and Chairman, Dept. of Food & Nutritional Science, College of Home Economics, University of Rhode Island, Kingston, RI 02881; Helen Kiesel, 141 W. Gravers Ln., Philadelphia, PA 19118; Paul A. Lachance, Professor of Nutritional Physiology, Dept. of Food Science, Rutgers University, P. O. Box 231, New Brunswick, NJ 08903; Donald McAfee, Director of Nutrition Education, National Dairy Council, 111 N. Canal St., Chicago, IL 60606; Elwood W. Speckmann, Director of Nutrition Research, National Dairy Council, 111 N. Canal St., Chicago, IL 60606.

puted that the levels for food energy and 11 major nutrients available for U. S. civilian consumption per capita per day in 1972 were sufficient; and Murphy et al. (1969) reported that the content of seven vitamins in Type A lunches served to children in the sixth grade in 300 schools was generally satisfactory.

The Ten-State Nutrition Survey (HEW, 1972), which included, dietary, clinical, and biochemical evaluations of nutritional status, provides no evidence supporting the need for greatly increased fortification with several nutrients, except iron, the level of which the Food and Drug Administration has proposed increasing in enriched bread and flour (FDA, 1973); recently, however, enactment has been postponed pending the outcome of another hearing and reconsideration.

I support the present enrichment and fortification programs regulated by the FDA and endorsed by the Food and Nutrition Board of the National Academy of Sciences and the Council on Foods and Nutrition of the American Medical Association.   However, the contribution of enrichment and fortification to available nutrient levels is already greater than most people realize.   Friend (1972b) reported that in the 1970 food supply, fortification added the following amounts of nutrients: thiamine 40%, iron 25%, niacin 20%, riboflavin 15%, vitamin A value 10%, ascorbic acid 10%, vitamin B_6 4%, and vitamin B_{12} 2%.   With the trend to fortify beverages, breakfast products, and desserts, I suspect that the ascorbic acid levels provided by fortification are now greater than 10%.

KNOWLEDGE OF REQUIREMENTS INADEQUATE

Fortification of such products as snack items, cakes, desserts, and beverages on the basis that they contribute a significant portion of the caloric intake may be nutritionally defeating.   If consumption is increased at the expense of staple foods because of greater consumer acceptance of these fortified foods, a cycle may be triggered where inadequate and unbalanced nutrient intakes will need to be constantly compensated for by adjustments in fortification.

The problem of adjustment would not be so serious if we had a sufficient bank of knowledge on nutrient requirements, food composition, and appetite control.   These we do not have.   Our present knowledge of nutritional requirements or allowances is, in my opinion, inadequate to support extensive expansions in food fortification.   The USDA's Agriculture Research Service is reviewing the world literature (Irwin and Hegsted, 1971a; b) and finding wide gaps in the state of knowledge of nutritional requirements, particularly in regard to infants, adolescents, the aged, and pregnant and lactating women.   .   .   .

Knowledge, in many instances, is also limited on factors which may be related to fortification, such as food composition; loss of nutrients during processing, handling, storage, heating, and reheating; and preservation of nutrient value.

It is apparent that much more research is needed on human nutritional requirements and on the nutrient content of foods subjected to various treatments. Without an improved data base, I do not see how we can proceed much further with any form of fortification, especially of fabricated or engineered foods.

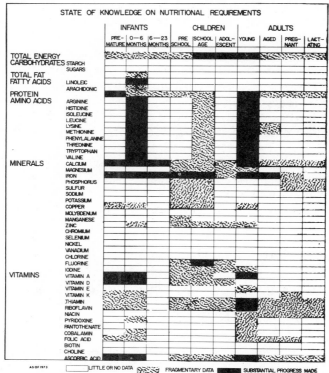

STATE OF KNOWLEDGE ON NUTRITIONAL REQUIREMENTS

Nutrition Institute
Agriculture Research Service
United States Department of Agriculture
Beltsville, Md. 20705

REGULATIONS NOT ENOUGH

While it is of value to the consumer, nutrition labeling (FDA, 1973) is not a substitute for nutrition education. If nutrients are added, nutrition claims made, or nutrition information voluntarily provided, the label must list only calories, protein, fat, carbohydrate, vitamin A, vitamin C, thiamine, riboflavin, niacin, calcium, and iron. The regulations do not require the listing of the remaining 12 nutrients for which U. S. RDAs have been established or the many other nutrients essential to man.   Under the present labeling regulations, therefore, nutrification or fortification can give consumers a false sense of nutritional security.

Malnutrition can be associated with an excess of specific nutrients. In spite of FDA regulations, it is possible for consumers to obtain excessive levels of vitamins, and unnecessary fortification increases the chances of hypervitaminosis.   Our work on excessive intake of polyvitamins and iron in rats (Dymsza et al., 1972) clearly indicates that such hypernutrition is undesirable.   A few reports are now appearing on vitamin or mineral overnutrition (Thompson et al., 1973), but in general, data are lacking on the health risks which may result from excessive intakes of many vitamins and minerals.

EDUCATION OFFERS MORE POTENTIAL

The AMA's Council on Foods and Nutrition has stated (AMA, 1961) that:

> the requirements which should be met for the addition of a particular nutrient to a given food include (a) acceptable evidence that the supplemented food be physiologically or economically advantageous for a significant segment of the consumer population, (b) assurance that the food item concerned would be an effective vehicle of distribution for the nutrient to be added, and (c) evidence that such addition would not be prejudicial to the achievement of a diet good in other respects.

It is of interest that the recent policy statement of the Food and Nutrition Board (NAS/NRC, 1974) on enrichment, fortification, and formulation of new foods recognizes that nutritional understanding is needed by the consumer; that enhanced levels of nutrients should not be harmfully excessive and not likely to create a dietary imbalance; and that a product designated primarily as a meal replacer should provide for those essential nutrients for which allowances have and have not been established.

I would be less than candid if I did not affirm my support for the development of new foods and admit that there is a place for both fortification and nutrition.   It is a matter of priority.

I maintain, however, that the fortification case has not been adequately supported on the basis of need or social or scientific merit.   There is also an inadequate base of knowledge to support an increased fortification program, especially with fabricated or engineered foods.   Other problems may include hidden costs, more regulations, and increased chance of excessive nutrient intake.

It is apparent that much of the malnutrition (over and undernutrition) found today is due to a lack of nutrition knowledge or motivation to apply existing knowledge. While research is needed on making nutrition education more effective, the education approach offers, I believe, more potential at less cost and risk than does fortification or any form of food modification.

REFERENCES

1. AMA. 1961. General policy on addition of specific nutrients to food. Am. Med. Assn. Council on Foods and Nutrition. J. Am. Med. Assoc. 178: 1024.

2. HEW. 1972. "Ten-State Nutrition Survey 1968–1970." Pub. No. (1) 72–8130 to 8134. Dept. of Health, Education and Welfare, Center Disease Control, Atlanta, Ga.

3. Dymsza, H. A., Reddi, A. K., Constantinides, S. M., and Bergan, 1972. Adverse effects of excess dietary vitamins and iron in growing rats. Abstracts of Short Communications. IX Int. Cong. of Nutr., Mexico.

4. Friend, B. 1972a. Nutrition review. National Food Situation. USDA/ARS, Consumer and Food Economics Inst., Hyattsville, Md.

5. Friend, B. 1972b. Enrichment and fortification of foods, 1966–70. National Food Situation. USDA/ARS, Consumer and Food Economics Inst. Hyattsville, Md.

6. Irwin, M. I. and Hegsted, D. M. 1971a. A conspectus of research on protein requirements of man. J. Nutr. 101: 387.

7. Irwin, M. I. and Hegsted, D. M. 1971b. A conspectus of research on animo acid requirements of man. J. Nutr. 101: 541.

8. Lachance, P. A., Moskowitz, R. B., and Winawer, H. H. 1972. Balanced nutrition through food process or practice of nutrification: Model experience in school food service. Food Technol. 26(6): 30.

9. Murphy, E. W., Koons, P. C., and Page, L. 1969. Vitamin content of type A school lunches. J. Am. Dietetic Assn. 55: 372.

10. NAS/NRC. 1974. How far shall we go in the enrichment, fortification and formulation of new foods? Food and Nutrition Board, National Academy of Sciences-National Research Council. J. Am. Dietetic Assn. 64: 255.

11. Thompson, M. F., Morse, E. H., and Merrow, S. B. 1973. Evaluation of vitamin-mineral supplements taken by pregnant women. Federation Proc. 32: 926 abs.

in favor of supplementation

Benjamin Borenstein

There is no dichotomy between well-planned fortification and well-planned nutrition education. Well-planned fortification, by its very concept, means the addition of micronutrients to appropriate foods at conservative levels. It does not mean fortification of everything or at high levels.

There are legal restrictions on fortification of foods which have either FDA Standards of Identity or USDA Standards, and we frequently forget that most staple foods cannot legally be fortified or can only be fortified under specific restrictive conditions. In addition, the FDA regulations on nutrition labeling further control the maximum inputs of micronutrients into foods.

EDUCATION CAN'T SOLVE ALL PROBLEMS

The failure of nutrition education is possibly best shown by the enormous success of "health foods"—which may indeed be nutritionally good, but for which fantastic claims and profits are made. Nutrition education is important, but it can never be a panacea because of specific problems. These include strong food likes and dislikes, ethnic habits, and poverty.

Education also cannot solve the problem of poor distribution of some nutrients in the dietary. For example, since dairy foods supply 76% of the available calcium in the U. S. diet (Hodgson, 1973), it is almost impossible to obtain the Recommended Dietary Allowance for calcium without being at least a moderate consumer of dairy products. And it is almost impossible to obtain the RDA for iron and vitamin B_{12} without consuming moderate quantities of meats, particularly red meats: the RDA for iron is 18 mg/day—muscle meats contain 2–4 mg/100 g, and organ meats contain 7–20 mg/100 g; milk (0.1 mg/100 g) and other important foods have low iron levels; most fruits have only 0.2–0.5 mg/100 g; spinach, traditionally thought of as a good source of iron (2–3 mg/100 g), was recently reported to have a bioavailability of only 2% (Layrisse, 1970).

Other nutrients with distribution imbalances include vitamins C and E. The major vitamin C sources in the diet are citrus products, and the vitamin C content of these products may be more variable than we think. The major source of vitamin E in the diet is vegetable oils, the vitamin E content of which varies extremely from oil to oil, as well as within a specific type. Davis (1972) studied the range of vitamin E in baby menus, using commercial infant formulas, made with vegetable oils to replace the milk fat, as the major food source of vitamin E. These formulas supplied 0.42–12.4 IU/day; this 30-fold variation among commercial formulas designed for the same use is quite surprising. The range of vitamin E in the total baby menus was 0.94–17 IU/day.

ASSUMES KNOWLEDGE OF NUTRIENTS

Education of the consumer assumes that we actually know the nutritional value of key foods as eaten. Not only are there weaknesses in this assumption, as already discussed, but we must add nutrient changes caused by food technologists, plant geneticists, and, our changing food supply:

Food technology. A major product change has been the packaging of reconstituted orange juice in paper milk cartons for sale in dairy cases. The vitamin C content of this product depends on the oxygen permeability of the package as well as losses during reconstitution of the concentrate. Samples purchased from retail stores have been found to contain as little as 25% of the USDA Handbook No. 8 value for vitamin C in orange juice.

Plant genetics. Although plant geneticists may not have changed the vitamin C content of tomato juice when they developed new varieties in order to enable mechanical harvesting of tomatoes, the vitamin C content of canned tomato juice reported by Farrow et al. (1973) varied from 1 to 25 mg/100 g, compared to the handbook value of 16 mg/100 g.

Changing food supply. The rapid change in our food supply is shown by the commercial success of processed potatoes. Only 16% of the total U. S. food potato supply in 1956 was processed; by 1969, it was up to 47%. Dehydrated potatoes have little, if any, residual vitamin C in the finished, ready-to-serve, reconstituted product, yet nutritionists traditionally think of potatoes as a major dietary source of ascorbic acid in the U. S.

RESTORATION RATHER THAN FORTIFICATION

Perhaps in discussing nutritional improvement of processed juices, potatoes, and other products which sustain losses in processing, we should use the term standardization or restoration rather than fortification to indicate our objectives. It is ironic that processing procedures that degrade vitamin E in vegetable oils or vitamin C in orange juice are not discouraged, but restoration of these nutrients is. For example, in 1966, the FDA proposed legislation which would have made it illegal to restore vitamin C to tomato juice cocktail (and other foods) without preclearance by FDA.

New foods are competitive with, not additive to, the food supply since they vie essentially for the same consumers and for the same number of calories consumed. They cannot be included in the diet without either increasing the amount of food we eat or reducing the consumption of more classical foods.

The high cost of meat has resulted in a new retail product which is a combination of 25–30% reconstituted textured soy protein and 70–75% ground beef. Since the substitute ingredient has no native vitamin B_{12}, this product tends to lower the vitamin B_{12} supply in the dietary. It seems to me that a processor making such a change has the nutritional obligation to replace or add back nutrients which are in effect being reduced in the dietary supply.

OVERFORTIFICATION DISCOURAGED

A major concern of some nutritionists is the potential toxicity of fortification. It is interesting to note that Filer (1973) rated protein more toxic for infants than vitamins A and D and iron, the three micronutrients which are normally thought of as having the highest potential toxicity.

We should note that there are technological difficulties which do tend to discourage overfortification: It is difficult to fortify most foods with iron except at modest levels. Vitamin A has an odor and flavor which are noticeable in some foods, particularly at higher levels. Vitamin B_2 has an intense color at 3–6 ppm in solution, prohibiting its use in some applications. Vitamin B_1 produces off-odors and -flavors which are not noticeable in baked goods but which can be very severe in most foods.

The argument has been made that food fortification is not necessary because a vitamin pill is the cheapest way to obtain micronutrients. This is not so. Assuming an average overage of 50% above label claim in both industries and similar quality control costs, the food industry can deliver 100% of the U. S. RDA of nine vitamins (A, D_2 E, B_1, B_2 niacin, B_6, B_{12} and C) for a total cost (including overages) of 0.30–0.35¢, whereas the vitamin-pill-producer has these same costs plus the cost of tablet excipients, the bottle, label, and transportation (food delivery costs already include the container, label, transportation, etc., which are not affected by fortification).

A long-range consideration which has not received adequate attention is the possibility that a significant shift may occur in the international distribution of food to produce more equitable distribution among nations, since the increase in food production in underdeveloped nations is barely keeping up with the population increase (Harris, 1973). This could conceivably result in much less freedom of choice of foods in this country and, hence, the need for more standardized, inexpensive, designed foods.

SAFE, CONSERVATIVE APPROACHES

There are several very conservative and safe approaches to the fortification of foods. Leading among these are Lachance's nutrification procedure (Lachance, 1972), which titrates the micronutrient content of foods to the protein content and cannot result in overfortification from a nutrition, cost, waste, or toxicity viewpoint; and Borenstein's caloric density approach (Borenstein, 1971), which may be appropriate for snack foods. These conservative rationales for fortification should not discourage the applied or basic nutritionist from improving the nutritional quality of foods.

REFERENCES

1. Borenstein, B. 1971. Rationale and technology of food fortification with vitamins, minerals and amino acids. Crit. Rev. in Food Technol. 2(2): 171.

2. Davis, K. C. 1972. Vitamin E: Adequacy of infant diets. Am. J. Clin. Nutr. 25: 933.

3. Farrow, R. P., Lamb, F. C., Elkins, E. R., Jr., Low, N., Humphrey, J., and Kemper, K. 1973. Nutritive content of canned tomato juice and whole kernel corn. J. Food Sci. 38: 595.

4. Filer, J. J., Jr. 1973. U. S. RDA doesn't meet population needs. Food Prod. Dev. 7(4): 103.

5. Harris, M. 1973. The withering green revolution. Natural Hist. 82 (March): 20.

6. Hodgson, R. E. 1973. That fluid called milk. J. Dairy Sci. 56: 500.

7. Lachance, P. A. 1972. Nutrification: A concept for assuring nutritional quality by primary intervention in feeding systems. J. Agr. Food Chem. 20: 522.

8. Layrisse, M. 1970. Informal meeting on Bioavailability of Supplemental Iron. Assn. Offic. Anal. Chem., Washington, D. C., Oct. 14.

in favor of nutrition education

Elwood W. Speckmann and Donald McAfee

It is difficult to debate nutrition education vs nutrient supplementation, because there is little room for argument. Nutrition education is a fact of life and is on the increase. So, too, is supplementation a fact of life, with fortification of natural foods on the increase and a trend toward fabricated foods that will contain whatever nutrients we wish them to have. Rather, we wish to debate the merits of *effective* nutrition education vs *unlimited* nutrient supplementation.

SUPPLEMENTATION IS NOT THE ANSWER

We must recognize that a major cause of poor diet and malnutrition in the United States is lack of knowledge and skill in choosing and preparing foods. Most of us generally consider the majority of people in the U. S. to be well nourished. However, as many as 100 million persons in the U. S. have been said to show some signs of being malnourished. Among "malnourished" people, we include those who exhibit evidence of overconsumption of calories (leading to obesity) or specific nutrients (such as sucrose, leading to tooth decay), as well as those who do not eat sufficient amounts of needed nutrients and therefore exhibit some clinical manifestation. In addition, there may be many more persons in subclinical situations wherein no specific nutrient deficiency can be identified but who are growing at a reduced rate and/or are performing below their biological capacity.

Unlimited nutrient supplementation of common foods is not the answer to this problem. At best, it might help selected groups of citizens with specific dietary problems or habits over critical periods of nutritional need, but in order for it to truly be of value for the general population, *all* foods would have to be supplemented with *all* nutrients so as to establish a common desirable nutritional profile. Otherwise, we run the risk of supplementing certain foods that are popular with certain consumer groups but never eaten by others. Such a concept has many inherent pitfalls:

• The theory behind the addition of nutrients is to alleviate nutritional deficiencies. Thus, the food industry through widespread supplementation would place itself in the position of practicing medicine. And there is real danger of overconsumption of certain nutrients when all major foods are supplemented.

• Do we really know enough about nutrition to make all foods nutritionally complete? Supplementation generally adds to foods only those major nutrients which we know something about. Addition of trace nutrients to foods is rarely done for nutritional purposes, yet these nutrients are just as essential as the well-known vitamins and minerals generally added to food. In addition, laboratory experiments reveal that ordinary foods contain unidentified nutrients necessary for optimal growth and development. It is thus desirable to eat a wide variety of traditional foods in order to ensure the intake of all essential nutrients, as well as fiber.

• While there may be merit in fortifying certain foods (such as flour with vitamins and iron, milk with vitamin D, and salt with iodine) to satisfy carefully established needs and to minimize specific diseases that may otherwise be epidemic (such as anemia, rickets, and goiter), there are both legal and moral issues to be considered in supplementing *all* foods with nutrients for *all* people.

• How would supplementation help reduce tooth decay, diabetes, and other nutritionally related disorders, including obesity? We believe that generalized supplementation leads people to be non-discriminating and would therefore contribute to the problem of overconsumption of calories. It is not unreasonable to suppose that many obese individuals would go on an all-pastry diet, since theoretically all the essential nutrients would be found in cream puffs, cup cakes, pies, and donuts. Why should the overweight consumer consider the addition of low-calorie foods such as vegetables and fruits to his diet if he is promised his nutrients in foods more attractive to him?

THE ANSWER IS EDUCATION

The answer to the problem lies in nutrition education—education that stresses individual responsibility and relies upon an intelligent, informed population being able to make decisions that are compatible with their ethnic, religious, and economic backgrounds and habits. We concede that nutrition education has not been an overwhelming success, but we reject the accusation that it has been a complete failure.

There are many reasons why nutrition education has not been as effective as we would like it to be. One major reason is that it has not really had much of a chance. Nutrition education in elementary schools is scanty and inadequate, and nutrition is seldom taught in high schools outside of home economics classes where emphasis is frequently more on food preparation than on health and only a small number of students are reached. And, to the best of our knowledge, there presently is not one state in this nation that requires elementary teachers to take a course in nutrition in order to qualify for a teaching license.

But things are changing. Many state departments of education and state legislatures are considering nutrition education as a basic responsibility of the schools. Health education is now being mandated in many states, with a strong nutrition component.

Not only are curricula and requirements changing, but how teachers teach and how students are expected to learn are also changing. Techniques learned from industry, principles of management, and the psychology of learning are being blended into usable formator packages, sometimes known as learning modules. These modules carefully spell out what is expected of the student, how he is to learn, and how we will know if he has learned, and can be applied to nutrition education by a wide variety of educators with a minimum of preparation and training.

The National Dairy Council has designed, piloted and transmitted newer approaches to nutrition education that utilize conceptual modules based upon behavioral objectives and is teaching teachers how to design objectives in nutrition education and how to measure student achievement of these objectives. Our Big Ideas Program and our Washington State Model are designed to teach teachers how to teach nutrition, and our University of Tennessee Curriculum Model is designed to develop a high school health education curriculum with a strong nutrition education component. We have combined basic concepts of nutrition with innovative and sound educational techniques to achieve effective nutritional education of tomorrow's consumer through today's teachers.

In addition, the federal government has intensified its programs in nutrition education; the USDA has given grants to six states to develop model programs in nutrition education; the Department of Health, Education and Welfare has awarded grants to develop a nutrition education curriculum for elementary and secondary schools; legislation has been introduced to provide greater funding of nutrition education in medical and dental schools and to establish a program of nutrition education for children as part of the National School Lunch and Child Nutrition Programs; and the Society for Nutrition Education is providing impetus to the role of nutrition in education.

WHAT THE FOOD INDUSTRY CAN DO

And now, with the advent of more extensive food labeling, the food industry has an excellent opportunity to educate the consumer about its foods and the nutrients they contain. The food industry can show people that we have an excellent food and nutrient supply, that they do not have to rely to a major extent upon supplementation to obtain a nutritionally adequate diet.

We feel that a broad supplementation program by the food industry removes consumer option in selecting a nutritionally adequate diet from a variety of foods and may not improve the major nutrition-health problems confronting Americans today. We are convinced that most people, especially teachers and children, are eager to learn and practice good nutrition. We feel that if nutrition education is given a chance under the best teacher-learning situation and specific methodology is carefully and consistently evaluated using the best-known educational research criteria, consumers can be guided to achieve a better nutritional status through the selection of a variety of foods.

We therefore urge government, the food industry, and the educational community to join together to develop and implement an expanded and coordinated program of nutrition education.

in favor of supplementation

Paul A. Lachance and Helen Kiesel

We believe that the consumer, irrespective of his or her lifestyle, has a right to a balanced dietary and that the food industry has a responsibility (Lachance, 1971b) to provide nutritive food value in addition to organoleptic value.

Nutrification (Lachance, 1972a) is a technological concept for assuring balanced nutriture. It is based on the RDA (now, the U. S. RDA) and the presence in a product, as manufactured or used, of significant utilizable protein. Although some may have falsely interpreted the concept to advocate the promotion of "supernutrition" which could lead to possible imbalances due to excess micronutrient intakes, a critical analysis of the concept and the products which have adopted the concept (Lachance et al., 1972) reveals that the result is a better-balanced nutritive profile and an increase in the likelihood that the consumer realize a more balanced dietary than his food choices currently provide.

NOT MUTUALLY EXCLUSIVE

Nutrification and nutrition education are not mutually exclusive: they are complementary. Both enhance the nutritive value of food as ingested by the consumer, but nutrification is a technological practice, whereas nutrition education is a teaching/learning practice. The issue, then, is whether nutrification is justified, in addition to nutrition education, in light of existing knowledge about nutrient requirements, nutrient intakes, nutritive status, food habits, and food technology.

Nutrient requirements. Our knowledge of nutrient requirements, although not complete, has substantially improved in the last 20 years. This is reflected in the changes which have occurred with each revision since

1943 of the NAS/NRC Recommended Dietary Allowances: The number of nutrients recognized as essential has increased, as has the number of nutrients for which an RDA has been established, and some of the RDA values have decreased, including those for protein, calories, and vitamins C, B_{12}, and E (Harper, 1974).

One could argue that there are nutrients yet to be discovered (Murphy, 1972), but it is interesting to note that animals fed semi-purified rations have been known to have longer than usual life expectancy (Ross, 1959) and that man has been satisfactorily sustained for extended periods on completely chemical diets (Stephens and Randall, 1969; Winitz et al., 1970).

Nutrient intake and nutritive status.   The nutritive status of individuals is related to their intake of essential nutrients.   The nutritive status of Americans with respect to some key nutrients leaves something to be desired (HEW, 1972; Babcock, 1972), and this is probably also true for other micronutrients as well (Schroeder, 1971; Pennington, 1973).   In fact, the U. S. dietary is stated to have deteriorated by 10% from 1955 to 1965 (USDA, 1968), and meals such as school lunches have been shown to not provide a profile of even the RDA nutrients (Miskimin et al., 1974).
Food habits.   McLinton et al. (1971) reported that the Basic Seven and Basic Four were not the pattern of eating for a total sample of 4,529 food records, including those with satisfactory nutrient intakes, and that only 34% of those with satisfactory food intakes met the food guide criterion.

It should be evident that if food habits could be changed, the dietary might be improved.   However, food habits are continually changing (Lachance, 1973) and are more responsive to social, cultural, and economic influences than to the invisible changes in nutritive value of foods per se. Compared to the 1940s, Americans today consume less bread, less fluid milk, and fewer vegetables—bread has lost out to the erroneous awareness that it is fattening; milk has lost out to the very questionable awareness that it is related to heart disease and is fattening; and vegetables have apparently been forced aside by a combination of higher cost and unrecognized nutritive value.   The vegetarian stands as evidence of the fallacy of the latter, but few Americans are willing to trade-off the acceptance, status, and apparent nutrient significance of meat and protein foods for that of cereals and vegetables.

Food technology.   The most significant advancement of the food industry in the same 20-year period has been in providing convenience to meet the demands of the marketplace.   Whereas 10% of foods in the marketplace in 1940 were convenience foods, today fully 55% are convenience foods (Trager, 1972).   Moreover, the fabrication of "analogous" foods at lower economic cost is a rapidly growing factor in food product development.

The food industry has been slow to recognize that as it shifted from the business of simple preservation to the business of preservation and convenience, its responsibility for nutritive value had to increase. Not only must nutrient retention in the preservation of a commodity be of concern, but nutritive value as various convenience foods are formulated, fabricated, and merged into convenience meals by the food service industry and the public must also be of concern.

The consumer has become increasingly dependent upon the nutritive value decisions that are made *for* him rather than *by* him—it has become increasingly difficult to interpret convenience foods in terms of food guides (Lachance, 1972b). However, we now have a very significant stepping-stone in nutritional labeling (Lachance, 1973a), not so much because it is a nutrition education tool but because it • establishes a reference nutrient standard, the U. S. RDA • makes industry think about the nutritive component of the definition of food • permits the consumer to associate certain foods as sources of particular nutrients and to compare otherwise analogous products on nutritive grounds.

IMPORTANT IN SCHOOL FEEDING

Children need to be educated about nutrition—there is a lack of nutrition knowledge at all school levels—yet the paucity of adequate programs and time to inculcate desirable results is almost overwhelming, especially when the population, as in inner-city school situations, is very mobile. Children's food preferences are diverse, and the unfamiliarity of many foods requires systematic education. Because this is lacking, much nutritious food is wasted.

In addition, from the food service viewpoint, there is uncertainty about the nutritional content of many products, including raw products, and there are variances in otherwise similar products. Furthermore, there are differences in preparation practices and satelliting procedures, which need to be corrected so that the nutrient value of meals as served is assured.

These concerns lead us to the conclusion that nutrification must be given priority along with nutrition education.

NUTRIFICATION LOGICAL AND FEASIBLE

Nutrification is not a new practice, but is a logical extension or coupling of existing restoration and public health enrichment practices (Sebrell, 1972) with the longer-range implications that a balanced profile of RDA nutrients in formulated convenience foods and fabricated convenience foods can mean to the public health. Nutrification is very compatible with both a new and systematic nutrition education (Lachance,

1971a)—extending from labeling to nutrient standard menu planning—and actual consumer practice of menu assembly from commodity foods, formulated convenience foods, and fabricated convenience foods.

We submit that nutrification's feasibility and suitability (commercial application) have been demonstrated. What has not occurred is a new and needed nutrition education compatible with nutrification, nutrition labeling, and consumer needs.

REFERENCES

1. Babcock, M. J. 1972. The status of nutrition in the United States. Food Prod. Dev. 6(4): 56.

2. Harper, A. E. 1973. Recommended Dietary Allowances (Revised 1973). Nutr. Reviews 31(12): 393.

3. HEW. 1972. "Ten-State Nutrition Survey, 1968–1970." Pub. No. (HSM) 72–8134. U. S. Dept. of Health, Education and Welfare, Washington, D. C.

4. Lachance, P. A. 1971a. Point of view: Nutrition education. J. Nutr. Educ. 3(2): 52.

5. Lachance, P. A. 1971b. Innovation vs nutrition as the criterion for product development. Food Technol. 25: 615.

6. Lachance, P. A. 1972a. Nutrification: A concept for assuring nutritional quality by primary intervention in feeding systems. J. Agr. Food Chem. 20: 522.

7. Lachance, P. A. 1972b. Point of view: Food guides. J. Nutr. Educ. 4(2): 44.

8. Lachance, P. A. 1973a. A commentary on the new FDA nutrition labeling regulations. Nutrition Today 8(1): 18.

9. Lachance, P. A. 1973b. The vanishing American meal. Food Prod. Dev. 7(9): 36.

10. Lachance, P. A., Moskowitz, R. B., and Winawer, H. H. 1972. Balanced nutrition through food processor practice of nutrification. Food Technol. 26(6): 30.

11. Miskimin, D., Bowers, J., and Lachance, P. A. 1974. Nutrification of frozen preplated school lunches is needed. Food Technol. 28(2): 52.

12. McLinton, P., Milne, H., and Beaton, G. H. 1971. An evaluation of food habits and nutrient intakes in Canada: Design of effective food guides. Can. J. Public Health 62: 139.

13. Murphy, W. B. 1972. Some things you might not know about the foods served to children. Nutrition Today 7(5): 34.

14. Pennington, J. T. 1973. Unpublished Ph.D. dissertation, Dept. of Nutritional Sciences, Univ. of California, Berkeley.

15. Ross, M. H. 1959. Protein, calories and life expectancy. Federation Proc. 18: 1190.

16. Schroeder, H. A. 1971. Losses of vitamins and trace minerals resulting from processing and preservation of foods. Am. J. Clin. Nutr. 24: 562.

17. Sebrell, W. H. 1972. Chemical aspects of updating diet quality. J. Agr. Food Chem. 20: 518.

18. Stephens, R. V. and Randall, H. T. 1969. Use of a concentrated, balanced, liquid elemental diet for nutritional management of catabolic states. Am. Surg. 170: 642.

19. Trager, J. 1972. "The Bellybook," p. 171. Grossman Publishers, New York.

20. USDA. 1968. Dietary levels of households in the U. S., 1965–66. USDA/ARS, Washington, D. C.

21. Winitz, M., Seedman, D. A., and Graff, J. 1970. Studies in metabolic nutrition employing chemically defined diets. 1. Extended feeding of normal human adult males. Am. J. Clin. Nutr. 23: 525.

C

Nutrients in the diet

the controversy and crisis

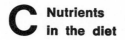

C **Nutrients
in the diet**

THE FOOD WE EAT, besides supplying us with our basic need for calories, also supplies many nutrients needed on a much smaller scale—vitamins and minerals. Much controversy exists over requirements for these nutrients. This chapter presents some of the arguments that have appeared recently in the scientific literature.

Jane Heenan of the FDA discusses vitamin needs and abuses in the first article. She examines the vitamin pill syndrome, or the habit of popping a pill every day "just to be sure." This syndrome was given further credence when Bobby Riggs was seen taking 300 to 400 vitamin pills a day, certainly not needed and of little help.

Literature on vitamin C, the subject of recent controversy, illustrates the crisis; the major questions center around whether over-consumption of this vitamin is harmful or beneficial. Dr. A. K. Sim reviews the history and biochemistry of ascorbic acid (vitamin C). He then reviews the relationship of vitamin C to smoking, an area which seldom is publicized but which has definite potential for helping the heavy smoker. Sim believes that vitamin C's usefulness in curing colds is unproven, and draws a similar conclusion about the vitamin's affect on other ailments.

The next article reviews the research publications that Dr. Linus Pauling used to prove that vitamin C cures colds. The author believes Pauling's evidence is inconclusive since the experiments were either uncontrolled or based on too few subjects.

Vitamin E also has been in the spotlight recently. The next article, from *Consumers Union*, concludes that the intake of extra vitamin E is, at best a waste of money and could delay needed medical treatment—a far greater danger.

In the following article, Dr. Reuben Bitensky presents an interesting thesis on why people take high doses of vitamins. He states: "By ingesting vitamins one could fight the establishment with the kind of activism that required no more effort than swallowing." The vitamin intake controversy has intensified since the FDA's recent ruling that no food or over-the-counter pill which contains more than 150 percent of the RDA could be sold.   Many Senators have introduced bills to overrule the FDA's action, in order to protect the rights of whose who wish to take high doses.

Another issue is the nutritional value of synthetic versus natural vitamins.   Pelletier and Keith show in the next article that synthetic vitamin C is slightly superior to the natural vitamin C from orange juice. This refutes the claim that natural bioflavonoids and rutin in orange juice increase vitamin C absorption.

In the area of minerals, calcium has been the subject of controversy. Dr. Leo Lutwak supports the claim that the cause of bone weakening in older age is low calcium intake or the imbalance of calcium with other minerals especially phosphorus.   But he blames not so much low calcium intake as high phosphorus intake from ingestion of processed meats and canned beverages.

Whenever a processor creates a substitute food, such as the new soy analogs which partially replace meat in the diet, a common question arises: are there trace elements present in the original food which will not be present in the substitute, and will this lead to nutritional deficiencies?   Dr. F. Nielsen covers a number of the "newer" trace elements that have been found to be essential.   He points out that our knowledge about them is minimal, and concludes by warning of the possible crisis that could erupt if we don't obtain more knowledge about them.

15

MYTHS OF VITAMINS

Jane Heenan

Once a day, "just to be sure," millions of Americans take a multivitamin pill. Then, when cold season comes around, some stock up on vitamin C.

Others whose sex lives seem to be lagging may reach for vitamin E, with the added hope that it will stave off heart disease. And if all these vitamins don't prevent that "rundown feeling," they might try a little—or a lot—of all the vitamins, with an added boost of vitamin B_{12}.

According to some of the latest "literature" appearing in books by nutrition "experts" and in magazine articles, this sort of therapy should do the trick. But as millions of Americans now know, it doesn't necessarily mean you can even win a tennis match.

And as a 4-year-old boy in Kansas will never forget, taking a whole bottle of 40 children's vitamins at once won't help him grow stronger, faster. He spent the following 2 days in intensive care with vitamin A and iron poisoning. His experience was added to the statistics compiled by FDA's National Clearinghouse for Poison Control Centers which reveal that 4,000 cases of vitamin poisonings are reported each year, with some 3,200 involving children.

Other Americans, with rashes, diarrhea, or headaches, may also be unwary victims of the belief that since vitamins are good for them, the more the better.

Of course, this is just one of the many myths about vitamins that is accepted by many health-conscious Americans. Some of the myths have been with us so long they're difficult to distinguish from fact. For instance, many people will tell you that vitamins provide extra energy. False.

Reprinted from *FDA Consumer*, March 1974, by permission of the publisher.

Some of the B vitamins do aid in the conversion of food to usable energy, but in amounts greater than the U. S. Recommended Daily Allowance (U. S. RDA), they provide nothing of value.   Only people with a relatively rare medically diagnosed deficiency of a vitamin would benefit from an amount greater than the U. S. RDA levels.

FDA has promulgated regulations which are designed to prohibit false and misleading promotional and labeling claims about vitamins and minerals, and to distinguish between vitamins and minerals that are dietary supplements, and those that should be sold as drugs.   Still, educational efforts are required for the public to be able to know what vitamins can, and cannot, accomplish.

THE DAILY MULTI-MYTH

An advertisement on television shows a person explaining how he stays healthy and looking "great."   He says he watches his diet, gets plenty of exercise, and, "just to be sure," takes a vitamin-mineral supplement every day.

This is the way we have come to expect the marketing of dietary supplements.   They are promoted as an "insurance" policy to guarantee good health.   The implication of such advertising has contributed to the myth that even a balanced diet cannot provide adequate nutrients.

Some people have gone further and maintain that modern farming methods have depleted the soil and that food itself no longer contains adequate nutrients.

This is untrue.   More is known about the nutrient content of food today than ever before.   And more is done, through modern farm practices, to protect and enrich the soil than was even known about in the good old days.   Crop rotation, soil tests, and routine enrichment of crop soil were developed because the oft-revered "natural" way of farming was quantitatively and qualitatively unreliable.

In addition, the protein, carbohydrate, fat, fiber, and vitamins are controlled primarily by the plant's genetic structure, not by the soil.   Excess mineral elements in soil beyond the plant's requirements may be reflected in the plants, but these differences are usually small.   Both desirable (magnesium, zinc, iron, etc.) and undesirable (lead, cadmium, selenium, etc.) elements are similarly accumulated.

A balanced diet which generally meets the U. S. RDA requirements for vitamins A, B₁, B₂, C, and D will nearly always provide the needed amounts of other vitamins, despite the claims of some people that these other vitamins are hard to find and therefore must be eaten in special foods or taken by pill.   Even though eating is a personal thing and the acceptability of foods varies from person to person, it is possible to obtain the U. S. Recommended Daily Allowance (U. S. RDA) in many different diet patterns because of the wide variety of foods containing similar nutrients. But the simplest, surest guide to follow for a good daily balance of nutrients is still the selection of foods from each of four larger groups—milk, meat, vegetable/fruit, and bread/cereal.

There are substances in food which some "experts" glibly term vitamins although they are of no importance in the diet for human nutrition. Examples are inositol, PABA (para-aminobenzoic acid), citrus bioflavonoid complex, hesperidin, and rutin. Many companies have marketed these substances individually or in combination with essential vitamins, but consumers should not be misled by claims for them that ignore the fact that their absence from the diet does not cause a disease or any form of illness.

Foods can and do supply most Americans with adequate nutrients, and consumers should not expect any major physical benefits from multivitamin pills, contrary to the myth.

MUCH ADO ABOUT E

Vitamin E supplements have been found useful in only two conditions —in premature babies who because of poor placental transfer may have received too little of the vitamin before birth, and in persons with intestinal disorders in which fats are poorly absorbed.

This view by the National Academy of Sciences Committee on Nutritional Misinformation is vastly different from claims that have more than doubled the sales of vitamin E in the last 5 years.

Among the latter claims are assertions that the vitamin can promote physical endurance, enhance sexual potency, prevent heart attacks, protect against air pollution, and slow the aging process. But there is virtually no scientific proof for the majority of these claims.

In fact, the new interest in E has been based on misinterpretations of animal research studies: Male rats that deliberately had been deprived of dietary sources of vitamin E became sterile, but the use of large doses in treating human sterility or impotence has not been successful. Similarly, it is known that E is essential to maintain pregnancy, but it has not been found to be a factor in fertility.

One reason so little is known about vitamin E is that E deficiency is almost impossible to produce in human subjects. To withdraw all sources of vitamin E is almost to withdraw food itself, since the vitamin is present to some extent in most foods and in large amounts in vegetable fats and oils.

Discovered about 50 years ago, the vitamin has also been described as a cure, preventive, or treatment of cancer, muscular dystrophy, ulcers, burns, and skin disorders. Again, science does not back this up. In muscular dystrophy patients for example, no deficiency of vitamin E has been found and large-dosage treatments have been ineffective.

The vitamin has been used in some cosmetics for its antioxidant properties, but one popular new deodorant containing E was recalled last year when widespread incidence of severe rashes were reported after use.

C FOR COLDS?

James Lind, surgeon's mate on the H.M.S. *Salisbury*, and "the father of nautical medicine," conducted the first properly controlled clinical therapeutic trial on record in 1747. Aboard ship, his experiment determined the value of citrus fruit in the prevention and cure of scurvy.

Forty-two years later, the Royal Navy adopted the administration of 1 ounce of lemon juice to each man each day. It wiped out scurvy in the Royal Navy and preserved its numbers to the extent that vitamin C is credited with having done as much as Lord Nelson to break the power of Napoleon.

So began the recorded and gradual recognition of vitamin C, which was isolated and so named in 1933.

Today, these things are known about C: It helps hold body cells together and strengthens blood vessels; it helps heal wounds; it helps tooth and bone formation; and it helps in resistance to infection.

It is also known that C does not cure or prevent colds. The claims that C lessens the number and severity of colds remains controversial, for in several clinical studies, subjects who believed they were being given C but who were actually receiving inert tablets reported fewer colds than they expected to have, and, in some cases, those taking C reported no change.

Some research has indicated difficulties associated with large doses of C, including kidney stones, severe diarrhea, and possible harm to diabetics. Also, because the body does pass off excesses of vitamin C, its presence in the urine makes accurate testing for diabetes impossible, since it gives a false indication of sugar levels. At this point, unless a physician has diagnosed vitamin C deficiency, the safe, practical course is to get the U. S. Recommended Daily Allowance of 60 milligrams per day (see table).

B VITAMINS

A common belief about B vitamins is that the old "rundown feeling" can easily be overcome by vitamin B_{12} supplements. But unless there is actually a deficiency—which is extremely rare—amounts beyond the U. S. RDA will not be of any benefit to the body, and any apparent effect has been shown to be psychological. In the case where vitamin B_{12} treatment is

U. S. RDA's for vitamins

	Unit of measurement	Infants	Children under 4 years of age	Adults and children 4 or more years of age	Pregnant or lactating women
Vitamin A	International units	1,500	2,500	5,000	8,000
Vitamin D	"	400	400	400	400
Vitamin E	"	5	10	30	30
Vitamin C	Milligrams	35	40	60	60
Folic acid	"	0.1	0.2	0.4	0.8
Thiamine	"	0.5	0.7	1.5	1.7
Riboflavin	"	0.6	0.8	1.7	2.0
Niacin	"	8	9	20	20
Vitamin B_6	"	0.4	0.7	2.0	2.5
Vitamin B_{12}	Micrograms	2	3	6	8
Biotin	Milligrams	0.15	0.15	0.30	0.30
Pantothenic acid	"	3	5	10	10

recommended, when a person actually cannot absorb the vitamin properly, the treatment must be carried out through injections, and it is relatively ineffective when administered orally.

Another exotic claim for vitamins involves pantothenic acid and is also based on misinterpretation of animal experiments. When a severe deficiency was produced deliberately in male rats, their hair turned grey, and when the process was reversed, the color was restored. From this, some "experts" have deduced that deficiencies of pantothenic acid are responsible for greying hair in humans. Although greying hair may occur because of severe deficiency, grey hair per se does not mean a deficiency, since there are many other reasons for the condition. Clinical deficiencies in man are truly rare. There has been no discovery so far to prevent grey hair.

Skimping on protein and overcooking vegetables in water will cut back on the amount of B vitamins in a diet. But a rush for vitamin pills or expensive brewer's yeast does more damage to the budget and offers far fewer benefits to health than consuming a proper selection of foods carefully prepared.

NATURAL vs. SYNTHETIC

"Getting back to nature" can sometimes be an expensive trip—especially when you wind up where you started. Such is the case for persons paying close to $5 for 100 tablets of vitamin C "from pure rose hips," from acerola cherries, or for a host of combinations with natural but ungermane ingredients, such as honey, when the same amount of pure ascorbic acid can be bought for under $1.

Two major fallacies lie behind the rush for so-called "natural" vitamins: (1) Natural vitamins are superior to those synthesized by man; (2) vitamin products sold as "natural" don't contain synthetic ingredients.

In truth, each vitamin has a particular molecular structure that remains the same whether it's synthesized in a laboratory or extracted from an animal or plant or consumed as part of an animal or plant. To be called "vitamin A," for example, there has to be a specific molecular arrangement that is identical no matter where it is found or how it is derived. The body cannot distinguish in any way between a vitamin from a plant or animal and the same vitamin from a laboratory. Only the pocketbook "knows for sure."

Perhaps even more revealing is that some synthetic ingredients many persons are trying to avoid today are also present in the "natural" products. In processing tablets and capsules, vitamin manufacturers must use excipients and binders, such as ethyl cellulose, Polysorbate 80 (a synthetic emulsifier), as well as gum acacia, etc.

So it comes back down to some basic rules about eating. Your body not only needs vitamins and other nutrients, it needs the bulk and textures of real food. And it needs a *balance* of those foods, a balance that may not be provided in fad dieting or in an endless array of tablets and capsules.

VITAMINS A AND D TOXICITY

Vitamins A and D were the first to explode the myth that vitamins are not toxic when administered in doses beyond body requirements.

Excessive amounts of vitamin A taken over long periods can increase pressure within the human skull and may mimic a brain tumor. In fact, one teenager actually was hospitalized and prepared for brain surgery only to find out the trouble was simply an overdose of vitamin A. Large doses of this vitamin taken over extended periods have also been known to retard growth in children and cause dry and cracked skin, headaches, bone pain, and other symptoms—in fact, almost the same symptoms as for a severe deficiency.

Excessive doses of vitamin D have been known to retard mental as well as physical growth in children. It can also cause nausea, weakness, stiffness, constipation, hypertension, and even death.

Because of this, FDA prohibits, except by prescription, any daily recommended intake of a tablet or capsule of more than 10,000 International Units (IU) of vitamin A and 400 of vitamin D. While this in no way prevents the consumer from taking as much as he chooses at any one time, it does control the strength and labeling for each package.

From this regulatory action a new myth may have arisen: That all vitamins are nontoxic except for A and D. In fact, the correct interpretation of this action is that the only conclusive, actionable proof of toxicity so far is with excessive A and D. Medical libraries contain numerous refences to adverse side effects from ingestion of high levels of niacin or vitamin C. In addition, the interaction of nutrients within the body is affected by high intakes of certain vitamins and minerals.

Other problems, involving vitamins E, C, and folic acid, have also been reported recently. For instance, there is evidence of a possible antagonistic effect of high intake levels of vitamin C on the nutritional status of A.

As research continues, there will be more answers as to how much is too much of a vitamin, what the entire scope of usefulness of each vitamin is, and which medical conditions may respond well to vitamin therapy. In the meantime, consumers should know that elaborate testimonials, miraculous claims, and vitamins supposedly derived from exotic sources result from mere guesswork, confusion, and, often, outright fraud.

BEST SOURCES

Vitamin A—Fish-liver oils, liver, butter, cream, whole milk, whole-milk cheeses, egg yolk, dark green leafy vegetables, yellow vegetables, yellow fruits, fortified products.

Vitamin D—Fish-liver oils, fortified milk, activated sterols, exposure to sunlight.

Vitamin E—Plant tissues—Wheat germ oil, vegetables oils (such as soybean, corn, and cottonseed), nuts, legumes.

Vitamin K—Green leaves such as spinach, cabbage; cauliflower, and liver.

Vitamin C—Citrus fruits, tomatoes, strawberries, cantaloupe, cabbage, broccoli, kale, potatoes.

Folic acid—Widespread in foods. Liver, kidney, yeast, deep green leafy vegetables are highest sources.

Thiamine—Pork, liver, and other organs, brewer's yeast, wheat germ, whole-grain cereals and breads, enriched cereals and breads, soybeans, peanuts, and other legumes, milk.

Riboflavin—Milk, powdered whey, liver, kidney, heart, meats, eggs, green leafy vegetables, dried yeast, enriched foods.

Niacin—Lean meat, fish, poultry, liver, kidney, whole-grain and enriched cereals and breads, green vegetables, peanuts, brewer's yeast.

Vitamin B_6—Wheat germ, meat, liver, kidney, whole-grain cereals, soybeans, peanuts, corn.

Vitamin B$_{12}$—Amply provided by small daily intakes of animal protein.

Biotin—Liver, sweetbreads, yeast, eggs, legumes.

Pantothenic acid—Almost universally present in plant and animal tissue.   Liver, kidney, yeast, eggs, peanuts, whole-grain cereals, beef, tomatoes, broccoli, salmon.

Choline—Egg yolk is best source.   Liver, heart, sweetbreads, milk, meats, nuts, cereals, vegetables, soybeans.

16

ASCORBIC ACID
a survey, past and present

A. K. Sim *

This survey summarises investigations of the role of ascorbic acid, principally in human nutrition, carried out over the past thirty years. Beneficial effects and untoward side effects are documented and methods of analysis discussed since these have changed over this period and doubt still remains of the relevance of most recent methodology.

ROLE OF ASCORBIC ACID

The role of ascorbic acid in particular circumstances has been well documented (1) and the general metabolism and physiology of the vitamin has been reviewed. The latter needs only a brief mention here.

It has been recognised for some considerable time that most sources of life, with the exception of man, most primates (2) and the guinea pig, are capable of synthesising ascorbic acid. The exceptions are dependent on a regular exogenous supply of the vitamin, the optimum levels of which are described below. It is obvious from even a brief review of the litera-

Reprinted from *Chemistry and Industry*, 1972, pp. 160–165.

* A. K. Sim is head of the Biochemical Section of the Biological Sciences Division at Inveresk Research International, Inveresk Gate, Musselburgh, Scotland.

This survey formed part of a study of ascorbic acid utilisation in health and disease, sponsored at Inveresk Research International by Roche Products Ltd, Welwyn Garden City. The financial support and encouragement by members of this company is gratefully acknowledged by the author, as well as the cooperation and assistance of Dr. W. Lumsden, General Practitioner, Edinburgh, and Ann P. McCraw of this organisation.

ture that ascorbic acid is multifunctional and is involved in many aspects of human physiology, some of which are still poorly understood. It is involved in the tricarboxylic acid and Krebs' cycles involving body minerals, carbohydrates, fats and other vitamins. It is involved in cell function, enzyme action and protein metabolism.

Harris has classified the action of ascorbic acid in terms of:

1.   Its considerable reducing activity, which may contribute to many biochemical reactions
2.   Its contribution in the regeneration of tissue, collagen formation and bone deposition
3.   Its participation in the conversion of folic acid to folinic acid and the metabolism of aromatic amino acids
4.   Its involvement in other biological systems such as blood lipids/cholesterol levels, many of which are discussed in more detail below.

It is also considered to be intimately involved in the absorption and transport of iron from blood to tissue, in the synthesis of steroids, leucocyte activity, the function of the reticuloendothelium and in antibody formation.

DIETARY REQUIREMENTS

The optimum daily requirements of ascorbic acid recommended by the BMA Committee on Nutrition (1950) is 20–30mg/d. In America 70mg/d is advised rising to 130mg for example during lactation (3, 4). The protective daily dose against scurvy is 10mg, although Srikantia *et al*, (5, 6), have reported that this is sufficient to maintain a maximum leucocyte level in many individuals (in India) with 22mg/d or less as a maximum overall requirement.

The clinical signs of scurvy are very slow to develop and were only observed after six months on a diet containing 1mg/d ascorbic acid. For this reason, diagnostic signs of deficiency probably reflect many years of deprivation. Moreover, the author and other investigators (7–10), have shown that there is a considerable variation in the mean leucocyteascorbic acid level between January and May and this may even extend as far as August. Allen's report (7) also reflects this in terms of dietary intake and the availability of foods rich in the vitamin during these months. The annual average intake per person therefore may conceal an intake below the mean for up to six months of the year. In addition, it has been shown (11) that Scottish households consume more starch and less vitamin C than any other region of the UK, and current figures indicate that this imbalance is continuing.

MEASUREMENT OF ASCORBIC ACID

Many chemical methods have been described for the measurement of ascorbic acid including that in tissue, whole blood, plasma, serum, leucocytes, platelets and urine. These methods have been described on the macro scale, micro scale (12) and more recently, utilising automated procedures (13).

The relevance of various measurements to the nutritional status for ascorbic acid in humans has been the subject of much controversy, and now it is generally accepted that the level of ascorbic acid in leucocytes (and platelets) of the buffy layer provides the most reliable index of vitamin C nutrition and of tissue saturation.

One of the most traditional methods for the assessment of vitamin C deficiency is the measurement of urinary excretion levels at relatively high doses of the vitamin. This 'saturation' test is fraught with difficulties, not least, that supplemented individuals excrete, in the urine, a substance which reacts chemically as ascorbic acid, but which has not yet been identified. The two compounds have been separated by thin-layer chromatography (14).

Urinary measurements may also be complicated by a variable renal threshold or an increase in requirement and utilisation (15). Large oral doses tend to be reflected rapidly in the plasma and subsequently in the urine without necessarily reflecting leucocyte or tissue saturation. Conversely, low-dose supplementation may be carried out over a long period with a gradual but persistent increase in leucocyte (and tissue) level without significant urinary excretion. Indeed, there are reports of individuals who appear to be impossible to saturate (16). Burch (17) and others have shown the 'threshold' phenomenon to be clearly related to plasma ascorbic acid level while many have shown that the latter does not give a good indication of tissue saturation (14, 17–19).

It is generally agreed that one of the best methods of assessing the tissue level and nutritional status of the individual with respect to vitamin C is by measuring the level in blood leucocytes or in the leucocyte/platelet buffy layer (5, 19–21). This would seem to correlate well with the level of ascorbic acid in the issues which is obviously of greatest significance but difficult to measure. Most leucocyte methods are adaptations of the original procedure described by Bessey and Lowry (12, 22) for serum and leucocytes. In their communications, the ascorbic acid level was related to the acid-insoluble phosphorus of the sample, but more recently, this has been expressed as $\mu g/10^8$ white blood cells (WBCs) in the buffy layer (23, 24). The leucocyte count is usually carried out manually although some recent work has been reported using automated methods (25). The measurement of ascorbic acid in the sample is based on the reaction of dehydroascorbic acid and diketogulonic acid with 2, 4-dinitrophenyl-hydrazine.

Using this method, the leucocyte (and platelet) ascorbic acid has been shown to be directly proportional to the intake of ascorbic acid (17, 26), but this is in contrast to the findings of Disselduff and Murphy (27). This remains a major point of dispute and may not indeed be resolved until controlled trials take into account the past and present nutritional status and vitamin C level of the individual, as well as the widely reported variation in individual requirements and therefore marked variation in response to dietary supplementation (9). A direct proportionality between leucocyte and total body ascorbic acid has been shown in the guinea pig (17), and it is claimed that there is indirect evidence that this also holds for humans. It is not usually found to be necessary to use the conversion factor advocated by Gibson *et al* (28), in normal, thrombocytopenic, thrombocythaemic and cases of high leucocyte to platelet ratio. Cohen and Duncan (29) and others (10, 27, 30) have found this factor unnecessary and indeed, its use may indicate very abnormal results.

Alternative methods described for ascorbic acid measurement include the use of *C*-labelled material (14), fluorimetric (31) and other chemical and/or colorimetric methods (32, 33), some of which have also been automated (13, 34). Very many factors may be reflected in this measurement and these must be accounted for before the relevance of the data can be appreciated. Some of the more important parameters which may influence these results are discussed in detail below.

DEFICIENCY STATES

Effect of Age on Ascorbic Acid Level

The initial aim of the present survey was to examine the effect of age on leucocyte ascorbic acid level, with particular reference to those over 65 years old. It soon became obvious, however, that in the main, they were not significantly deficient and it was subsequently shown that they were not significantly different from those under 65. Instances were found of considerable deficiency among the 18–25 age group which is probably accounted for by bad dietary habits or in some instances through 'diseased' states and/or a general malabsorption. This has been confirmed by the work of Brook and Grimshaw (25).

In general, men have been reported to be more deficient in ascorbic acid than women (25, 35–37), with a significant decline with age. This decline has not been observed in women by most workers (38). This survey found some tendency for lower levels in elderly men although these are not significantly different from the data on females. Morgan *et al* (35) have claimed, however, that men have a higher vitamin requirement than women, but this remains very speculative.

Many reports are to be found in the literature which would appear to substantiate the theory of deficiency in the elderly (39). Some examples of such reports are given in Table 1.

Table 1

		Leucocyte ascorbic acid level (μg/10^8 WBCs)	
		Mean	Range
Denson and Bowers [23]	50 elderly at home (in the London area)	13·7	2–36
	Controls (working adults)	35·0	21–53
Bowers and Kubik [40]	50 elderly (mean age 76·2 years) in Industrial Midlands	12·3	2–27
Kataria et al [41]	25 elderly in London (at home)	26·0	
	15 elderly (hospitalised)	14·0	5–22
	16 elderly (institutionalised)	8·0	4–16

Griffiths *et al* (42) in a geriatric survey of patients admitted to hospital, indicated chemical evidence of deficiency in 41 per cent. However, in the elderly at home, the figure was 27 per cent. Brocklehurst *et al* (43) studied 80 geriatric hospital patients for one year and concluded that there was definite evidence of deficiency in many elderly people in hospital for long periods.

Andrews *et al* (44) reported a significant fall in the leucocyte ascorbic acid level in the elderly in winter. This is not surprising in view of the variation in dietary habits throughout the year. Apart from social and dietary habits and certain diseased states, it is likely that control values will depend particularly on the geographical site of the study.

Taylor (45) originally suggested that there may be a connexion between 'senile purpura' and sublingual petechial haemorrhages and chronic vitamin C deficiency (43). This, at first sight, seems very reasonable, since these clinical manifestations are well recognised in scorbutic states. Andrews and Brook (46), however, confirmed the earlier work of Tattersall and Seville (47) which indicated that 'senile purpura' and hypovitaminosis were not related. The classical signs of deficiency, e. g. the caviare tongue [Mendes da Costa and Cremer (48), Bean (49)] and petechial haemorrhages were indeed common in the elderly, but were shown by Andrews (9) on histological examination to be aneurysmal dilatations of the venules and mostly unrelated to the vitamin status.

Andrews and Brook (46) originally described these lesions as manifestations of deficiency, but later failed to produce any improvement by vitamin C supplementation, although they did achieve an obvious improvement in the leucocyte ascorbic acid level. There is, however, no doubt that the true petechiae of scurvy readily respond to ascorbic acid supplementation [cf Arthur *et al* (50)]. Similarly, conjunctival lesions in deficiency respond rapidly to supplementation (51).

Other authors have reported multiple vitamin deficiencies in the elderly, particularly in serum folic acid, B_{12} and ascorbic acid [Batata *et al* (52)

Read *et al* (53)]. These may well be interrelated and are worth evaluation in any future survey. Batata *et al* (52) have reported that while reduced food intake and malabsorption are the most likely causes of these deficiencies, they did not all respond similarly, or occur to the same degree in one individual.

Smoking

Many reports have recently indicated a possible association between cigarette smoking, related diseases and ascorbic acid deficiency (20, 54–62). Brook *et al* (25) have reported a significant reduction in plasma ascorbic acid for non-smokers with increasing age in men and women, but leucocyte levels did not change with age. Cigarette smoking, however, significantly lowered both plasma and leucocyte levels.

Indeed, it has been suggested that smoking tended to increase the 'apparent' age of an individual by 40 years with respect to leucocyte ascorbic acid level (35). This must, however, be regarded with some suspicion and moreover serves to illustrate the difference in opinion between authors on the true effect of ageing, smoking and other parameters on different blood components. Typical figures quoted for the effect of smoking are shown in Table 2 (25).

Table 2

Smoking habits	No. males	Mean ascorbic acid	No. females	Mean ascorbic acid
None	32	24.6±1.3	50	30.7±1.4
Moderate	14	19.6±1.7	28	25.6±1.6
Heavy	8	17.4±3.5	6	27.8±1.4
Moderate plus heavy	22	18.4±1.6	34	26.0±1.3

MacCormack (63) has claimed that smoking one cigarette destroys 25mg ascorbic acid in the body. Calder *et al* (64) have confirmed by *in vitro* tests that tobacco smoke actually destroys vitamin C in solution, but were unable to show that the plasma level was reduced in smokers or non-smokers who smoked one cigarette every half hour over a period of 6h or in smokers who smoked 19–25 cigarettes in 6h.

While the real relevance of such an *in vitro* test is not clear, it is not surprising, in view of the considerable data on short and long-term supplementation and depletion, that a 6h test period should indicate nothing conclusive. In most studies the reports of deficiency states associated with smoking habits fail to take into account the many other parameters which may also be involved. In other instances, there are too few subjects per group [e. g. five smokers versus five non-smokers (62)].

Bailey *et al* (65) have found no difference in the response of smokers and non-smokers in relation to ascorbic acid supplementation and exercise performance. Pelletier (54, 62, 66) attempted to control the diet of his patients rigorously and confirmed the results of Brook and Grimshaw (25). By saturation tests carried out in conjunction with carefully con-controlled dose schedules and blood measurements, he concluded that in smokers, less ascorbic acid is effectively available for utilisation or that this group utilises the vitamin differently from non-smokers.

Ascorbic acid is involved in the synthesis of neuro-transmitters such as noradrenalin and 5-hydroxytryptamine (67) and in the function of the adrenal gland. This organ contains the highest concentration of the vitamin of any tissue in the body and this must therefore have some influence on catecholamine and steroid production.

Smoking is well known to induce increased adrenalin secretion via nicotinic stimulation by nicotine and hence in smokers there is probably an abnormal demand on the adrenals and an increased utilisation of ascorbic acid at this site. Moreover, Lipscomb and Nelson (68) have shown that *in vivo*, the release of ascorbic acid precedes corticoid output with no detectable release in the absence of steroid secretion. It is also postulated by Kitabuchi (69) that a high concentration of ascorbate in the adrenal prevents steroidogenesis and therefore during stress or stimulation with ACTH (or smoking?), the adrenal must first release the bulk of its ascorbate before stimulation can commence. The effect of smoking and adrenal function could thereby represent one consistent source of ascorbic acid depletion.

It has also been shown here and elsewhere that after a prolonged period of smoking (six months or more), there is a significant proliferation of goblet cells of the epithelium of the trachea, which in turn results in an excessive secretion of mucus. Such induced cell turnover and proliferation may also represent a source of ascorbic acid depletion in smokers. The possibility of secretion of the vitamin in mucus has not been investigated, but may be of interest.

Depending on the significance of these effects, there may be a good case for the prophylactic and possibly therapeutic use of ascorbic acid in combating some of the untoward effects of heavy smoking.

Tissue damage and regeneration

While many diseased states could be classed under this heading, we are particularly concerned here with the levels of ascorbic acid in such cases as gastric/duodenal ulceration, accidental tissue damage, and the effects of post-operative surgery.

Attention has recently been drawn to the low leucocyte levels of ascorbic acid in many surgical patients (70) and particularly in patients with peptic disorders (29). The fundamental importance of vitamin C in the healing process has been demonstrated in guinea pigs (71) and in humans (29, 72). There is also a consistently low level in patients with peptic ulcer and since these may, by necessity, be subjected to surgery, supplementation may be of considerable importance.

Cohen and Duncan (29) found that patients with gastro-duodenal disorders had significantly lower leucocyte ascorbic acid levels than normal healthy adults. The mean levels quoted were $11.0\mu g/10^8$WBCs and 22.9 $\mu g/10^8$WBCs respectively. Dymock *et al* (73) confirmed these results but also found that the depletion was more severe in ulcer patients with stenosis. Patients with previous gastric surgery and in good health were also nearer the normal level than those similarly treated but with symptoms. They suggest, as Williamson and others (74) that this indicates inadequate absorption or increased utilisation and not, as has been claimed, malabsorption induced by antacid administration.

Russell *et al* (20) has shown that in cases of peptic ulcer with gastro-intestinal haemorrhage, the leucocyte ascorbic acid is even lower and this is more exaggerated if the haemorrhage may be attributed to aspirin or alcohol induction. Similarly, Russell and Goldberg (75) reported that with aspirin-induced lesions in guinea pigs, the mucosal haemorrhage which often followed, was significantly more severe when subclinical scurvy was present. These observations have been supported by Croft (76) who suggested that increased haemorrhage in elderly people may be due to a low turnover of gastric epithelial cells which rendered the mucosa particularly susceptible to aspirin. The effects of aspirin in subscorbutic states may also, however, be explained as a direct effect of platelet adhesiveness and the inhibition of aggregation (77).

Typical signs of clinical scurvy have been described by Williamson *et al* (72, 74) in patients who had previously undergone gastric surgery and this was also associated with low levels of leucocyte ascorbic acid (12.7 $\mu g/10^8$WBCs versus $20.8\mu/10^8$WBCs control). Collins *et al* (71) have shown a significant improvement in the rate of gingival wound healing in guinea pigs and suggest that the therapeutic supplementation with ascorbic acid, at least following surgical procedures, is indicated.

Atherosclerosis

One of the most common features of cardiovascular disease is the presence of an abnormal blood lipid pattern. This is usually manifested in raised cholesterol and triglyceride fractions, although other lipids, e. g. cholesterol esters and phospholipids are also known to be altered.

It is not yet clear what role cholesterol plays in the etiology of the disease and indeed there is considerable divided opinion whether it is causitive or merely indicative of a high risk situation. There is some indication that atherosclerotic plaques—certainly an important feature in thrombus formation—may be initiated by cholesterol deposition on the endothelial wall. A type of cholesterol-induced atherosclerosis may be induced by feeding a diet rich in the sterol, but because of the short time factor involved, some doubt the relevance of this lesion to the naturally-occurring intimal deposit.

Sokoloff *et al* (78, 79) have shown that long-term administration of ascorbic acid is effective in the prevention of this experimentally induced atherosclerosis in rats, rabbits and guinea pigs, and indeed, appears to act successfully as a therapeutic agent in clinical atherosclerosis. Changes in blood triglyceride levels and lipoprotein lipase activity were observed as well as a lowering of blood cholesterol. Incorporation of ascorbic acid in a high cholesterol diet in animals effectively reduced the blood lipid levels compared with controls which were only fed the cholesterol-rich diet. Similarly, the vitamin appeared to have significant protective effect in the fatty infiltrations of liver and kidney. Similar observations were reported in coronary patients with hyperlipaemic conditions.

Myasnikov (80) and others (81) have claimed that ascorbic acid markedly influenced the development of experimental atherosclerosis in the aorta of rabbits as well as alimentary cholesterolaemia. The mechanism of action proposed for the vitamin is the augmenting of ketone bodies in blood which stimulates the metabolism of fat. By increasing the functional capacity of the liver, ascorbic acid stimulates the secretion of cholesterol with bile.

The introvenous administration of ascorbic acid to patients with atherosclerosis and hypertensive disease and a high blood cholesterol level leads, according to the Soviet scientists, to a markedly lowered cholesterol and a simultaneous increase in the duodenal and faecal cholesterol levels. The antioxidant effect of the vitamin may also play an important role in fat metabolism.

In contrast, the influence of ascorbic acid deficiency in cholesterol metabolism and atherogenesis has been reported by Ginter *et al* (82, 83). This group studied the effect of chronic hypovitaminosis (C) on these parameters in cholesterol-supplemented guinea pigs and found that, while brain and blood cholesterol levels were not significantly altered in the deficient state, significantly more vascular atheromatous lesions were found in these animals. A role involving ascorbic acid in the hydroxylation of cholesterol and the formation of bile acids is proposed. Willis (84, 85) has reported atheromatous changes in the aortae of scorbutic guinea pigs even without an atherogenic diet.

Chronic ascorbic acid deficiency (two weeks scorbutic regime) in guinea pigs was also reported by Ginter *et al* (82, 83) to produce hypercholesterolaemia and an increased accumulation of liver cholesterol. The vitamin deficiency also increased significantly the content of saturated fatty acids (up to C_{16}) and decreased the amount of mono and polyunsaturated fatty acids and cholesterol esters of liver. In blood, the cholesterol esters contained an increased amount of linoleic acid and a decreased amount of palmitic and oleic acids. The fatty acids and triglycerides were, however, not significantly altered. A possible sex difference was also noted. These observations were thought to be due to a disturbance of cholesterol metabolism induced by the vitamin deficiency.

Shaffer (86, 87) has reviewed the role of ascorbic acid in atherosclerosis and points out that local ground lesions which may be readily induced by ascorbic acid deficiency could readily be the sites of atherosclerotic/thrombotic deposits, particularly cholesterolaemic. The guinea pigs and primates, which are unable to synthesise ascorbic acid, therefore provide acceptable experimental animals for this study.

If the development of atherosclerosis via cholesterol deposition in the intima is to be accepted as relevant to human atherosclerosis, then the use of these experimental animals through the medium of induced ascorbic acid deficiency provides an ideal model system for studying the reversibility of atherosclerosis.

In a recent article Dunnigan *et al* (88) reported a seasonal variation in the incidence of myocardial infarction, which Spittle (89) has since attributed to the seasonal variation in the intake of ascorbic acid. While there may be some involvement between ascorbic acid intake, lipogenesis and cardiovascular disease, such sweeping claims are hardly justified.

Folic acid deficiency

Some workers believe that ascorbic acid deficiency alters folate metabolism (7, 90, 91), while others claim that the dual deficiency which often exists is a result of a diet deficient in ascorbic acid and folate (92). Folic acid and ascorbate deficiencies have been reported in several geriatric surveys (52, 53, 91) and while this could not be ascribed to dietary factors in all cases, it seems unlikely that the two are inter-related in any way other than in intake.

Malabsorption

Ascorbic acid deficiency is a frequent occurrence in malabsorption states, although this seldom reaches the level of clinical scurvy. Badenoch (93), for example, has noted many instances of deficiency in steatorrhea, but only one case of clinical scurvy.

Williamson *et al* (74) have described an investigation of surgical cases (already discussed) and cases of malabsorption including pancreatic steatorrhea, reticulum cell sarcoma, intestinal diverticulosis, and idiopathic steatorrhea, all of which were significantly lower than normal in leucocyte ascorbic acid level ($10.7\mu g/10^8$ WBCs versus $20.8\mu g/10^8$ WBCs).

Many studies of malabsorption states have indicated that the low ascorbic acid levels are not due to impaired absorption of the vitamin, but rather by way of an abnormal utilisation of requirement (73, 94). The pathogenesis of ascorbic acid malabsorption is, however, still obscure and each situation requires separate consideration (95).

EFFECTS OF ASCORBIC ACID

Common cold

It is generally believed that ascorbic acid supplementation may offer some protective effect against the common cold, either therapeutically or prophylactically. There is, however, very little clinical evidence to substantiate this claim and, indeed, most trials have indicated a marked beneficial effect from placebos. Under these circumstances, the claim is therefore equally difficult to disprove (96, 97).

There is evidence, however, of the therapeutic and prophylactic effects of the vitamin in certain infections (98–104), although again it may be argued that the infection itself may be a direct result of the deficiency, or at least the latter is a contributing factor towards its development.

Ritzel (105) has claimed an improvement in upper respiratory tract infections of skiers on supplementation, while Barnes (106) has noted a reduction in the number of colds in children and basketball players with additional vitamin C.

It is tempting to suggest that, in view of the well-documented individual variation in ascorbic acid requirements, there may be a norm for each individual, above which he is less prone to infections and below which these occur more readily. Leucocytes respond rapidly to ascorbic acid supplementation and multiply equally rapidly during infection.

Mental health

Recently Pauling reiterated in the popular press the claims that ascorbic acid supplementation improves mental alertness, performance and efficiency. These claims, like the therapeutic effectiveness of the vitamin, are without adequate supporting data and must await verification. Indeed, Chatelier has found the vitamin in his experience a panacea in psychotic illness (16).

Rheumatoid arthritis

Many years ago, Rinehart *et al* (107) reported that patients with rheumatoid arthritis were deficient in ascorbic acid. This observation has been verified since then by many workers and more recently, Abrams and Sandson (108, 109) showed that the serum and synovial fluid ascorbic acid concentration in patients with rheumatoid synovitis were the same and significantly lower than in normal individuals.

Duthie (110) has confirmed the need for supplementation in rheumatoid patients and a detailed investigation of these cases has revealed essentially three groups in which the severity of the disease varies and on which ascorbic acid utilisation/deficiency appears to be dependent. These groups have, as yet, not been studied in terms of their utilisation of the vitamin but are well worth further investigation.

Bone growth

The role of ascorbic acid in collagen synthesis is frequently quoted, but its direct influence on calcium mobilisation and bone growth has received less attention. The extent of the physiological function of the vitamin is unclear, but it is thought to be concerned chiefly with matrix formation (111, 112). There is evidence that the vitamin may affect the mobilisation of calcium from bone to plasma and thus it may have a more profound effect on skeletal physiology than currently believed. There is good evidence that ascorbic acid supplementation/depletion markedly affects serum alkaline phosphatase levels (113), and this effect would explain grossly elevated enzyme levels in undernourished primates in our own colony immediately after supplementation of their diet with fresh fruit and ascorbic acid. Alkaline phosphatase levels are of course higher in immature animals, but we have noted an inexplicable rise immediately after inclusion in the colony, which gradually returns to normal when the condition of the animal is nutritionally adequate.

MISCELLANEOUS EFFECTS

Large doses of vitamin C are said to have a beneficial effect on muscular exercise (114), but this still remains somewhat speculative. It was believed that large quantities of the vitamin were excreted in perspiration and supplementation may be required, for example, in tropical climates (101, 102, 115). Further investigation disproved this theory.

The effect of vitamin C on the rate of ethanol metabolism has been investigated (116) and appears to be without effect.

The use of ascorbic acid in conjunction with iron in anaemia has been described by many (117–122). We have also found that the vitamin effectively increases the rate of iron absorption possibly even to the extent of dependence of dietary iron without supplementation. The response to ascorbic acid supplementation was more rapid in males than females although the effect seemed to be more long-lasting in the latter. Its effectiveness on iron absorption appears to follow a similar pattern.

Loh and Wilson (123) have recently shown a close relationship between ascorbic acid excretion and the excretion of luteinising hormone at the time of human ovulation.

REFERENCES

1. 'Todays drugs', *B.M.J.*, 1969, 1, 493.
2. Lehner, N. D. M., Bullock, B. C. & Clarkson, T. B., *Proc. Soc. exp. Biol. Med.*, 1968, 128, 512.
3. Food and Nutrition Board, 'Recommended dietary allowances', 1964, 6 ed., *Natural Academy of Sciences.*
4. King, C. G., *Nutr. Rev.*, 1968, 26, 33.
5. Srikantia, S. G. *et al.*, *Am. J. clin. Nutr.*, 1970, 23, 59.
6. Mohanran, M., *Indian J. med. Res.*, 1965, 53, 891.
7. Allen, R. J. L., Brook M. & Broadbent, S. R., *Br. J. Nutr.*, 1968, 22, 555.
8. Medical Research Council, *Lancet*, 1948, i, 853.
9. Andrews, J., Letcher, M. & Brook, M., *B.M.J.*, 1969, 2, 416.
10. Griffiths, L. L., in 'Vitamins in the elderly', ed. A. N. Exton-Smith & D. L. Scott, p. 34, 1968, *Bristol: J. Wright & Sons Ltd.*
11. National Food Survey Committee Report, 1967, *London: HMSO.*
12. Bessey, O. A., in 'Vitamin methods', ed. P. Gyorgy, 1, 1950, *New York: Acad. Press Inc.*
13. Nesset, B. L. *et al.*, *Analyt. Biochem.*, 1967, 19, 89.
14. Hodges, R. E., Baker, E. M., Hood, J., Sauberlich, H. E. & March, S. C., *Am. J. clin. Nutr.*, 1969, 22, 535.
15. Andrews, J. & Brook, M., *B.M.J.*, 1969, 3, 176.
16. Chatelier, A., personal communication, 1969.
17. Burch, H. B., *Ann. N. Y. Acad. Sci.*, 1961, 92, 268.
18. Cutforth, R. H., *Lancet*, 1958, i, 454.
19. Bartley, N. H. Krebs, A. & O'Brien, J. R. P., *Spec. Rep. Ser. med. Res. Coun.*, 1953, No 280, *London: HMSO.*
20. Russel, R. I., Goldberg, A., Williamson, J. M. & Wares, E., *Lancet*, 1968, 2, 608.
21. Lloyd, B. B. & Sinclair, H. M., *cit.* Bourne, G. H. & Kidder, G. W., 'Biochemistry and physiology of nutrition', 1, 369, 1953, *New York: Acad. Press.*
22. Bessey, O. A., Lowry, O. H. & Brock, M. J., *J. biol. Chem.*, 1947, 168, 197.
23. Denson, K. W. & Bowers, E. F., *Clin. Sci.*, 1961, 21, 157.
24. McCraw, A. & Sim, A. K., *Clinica chim. Acta*, 1969, 25, 286.
25. Brook, M. & Grimshaw, J. J., *Am. J. clin. Nutr.*, 1968, 21, 1254.
26. Davey, B. L., Wu, M. L. & Storvick, C. A., *J. Nutr.*, 1952, 47, 341.
27. Disselduff, M. M. & Murphy, E. LaC., in 'Vitamins in the elderly', ed. A. N. Exton-Smith & D. L. Scott, p. 60, 1968, *Bristol: J. Wright & Sons Ltd.*
28. Gibson, S. L. M., Moore, F. M. L. & Goldberg, A., *B.M.J.*, 1966, 1, 1152.
29. Cohen, M. M. & Duncan, A. M., *ibid.*, 1967, 4, 516.

30. Williamson, J., personal communication, 1970.

31. Deutsch, M. J. & Weeks, C. E., *J. of the A.O.A.C.*, 1965, 48, No 6, 1248.

32. Murty, C. N. & Bapat, M. G., *Z. analyt. Chem.*, 1964, 199, 368.

33. Beckman Ultra-Micro Method Sheet, Ascorbic Acid, No UAS-TB-21-E.

34. Wilsson, S. S. *et al.*, *Clin. Chem.*, 1969, 15, 282.

35. Morgan, A. F., Gillum, H. I. & Williams, R. I., *J. Nutr.*, 1955, 55, 431.

36. Spathis, G. S. & Hallpike, J. F., *Guy's Hosp. Rep.*, 1967, 110, 148.

37. Brin, M., Dibble, M. V., Peel, A., McMullen, E., Bourquin, A. & Chen, N., *Am. J. clin. Nutr.*, 1965, 17, 240.

38. Brocklehurst, J. C. *et al.*, *B.M.J.*, 1969, 2, 824.

39. Patnaik, B. K., *Nature, Lond.*, 1968, 218, 393.

40. Bowers, E. F. & Kubik, *Br. J. clin. Pract.*, 1965, 19, 141.

41. Katatia, M. S., Rao, D. B. & Curtis, R. C., *Geront. clin.*, 1965, 7, 189.

42. Griffiths, L. L., Brocklehurst, J. C., MacLean, R. & Fry, J., *B.M.J.*, 1966, 1, 739.

43. Brocklehurst, J. C., Griffiths, L. L., Taylor, G. F., Marks, J., Scott, D. L. & Blackley, J., *Geront. clin.*, 1968, 10, 309.

44. Andrews, J., Brook, M. & Allen, M. A., *ibid.*, 1966, 8, 257.

45. Taylor, G., *Lancet*, 1966, i, 926.

46. Andrews, J. & Brook, M., *ibid.*, 1966, i, 1350.

47. Tattersall, R. N. & Seville, R., *Q. Jl. Med.*, 1950, 19, 151.

48. Mendes da Costa, S. & Cremer, G., *Derm. Wschr.*, 1930, 91, 1206.

49. Bean, W. B., *Trans. Am. clin. clim. Ass.*, 1952, 64, 40.

50. Arthur, G. *et al.*, *B.M.J.*, 1967, 1, 732.

51. Hood, J. & Hodges, R. E., *Am. J. clin. Nutr.*, 1969, 22, 559.

52. Batata, M., Spray, G. H., Bolton, F. G., Higgins, G. & Wallner, L., *B.M.J.*, 1967, 2, 667.

53. Read, A. E., Gough, K. R., Pardoe, J. L. & Nicholas, A., *ibid.*, 1965, 2, 843.

54. Pelletier, O., *Am. J. clin. Nutr.*, 1970, 23, 520.

55. US Public Health Service Review, 'The health consequence of smoking', 1967, 1696.

56. Kershbaum, A. & Bellet, S., *Geriatrics*, 1966, 21, 155.

57. Solomon, H. A., Priori, R. L. & Bross, I., *J. Am. dent. Ass.*, 1968, 77, 1081.

58. Bodansky, O., Wroblewski, F. & Markardt, B., *Cancer Res.*, 1951, 11, 238.

59. Esposito, R. & Valentini, R., *B.M.J.*, 1968, 2, 118.

60. Willis, G. C. & Fishman, S., *Can. med. Ass. J.*, 1955, 72, 500.

61. Hoffer, A. & Osmond, H., *Dis. nerv. Syst.*, 1963, 24, 1.

62. Pelletier, O., *Am. J. clin. Nutr.*, 1968, 21, 1259.

63. MacCormack, W. J., *Archs. Pediat.*, 1952, 69, 151.

64. Calder, J. H., Curtis, R. C. & Fore, H., *Lancet*, 1963, March 9, 556.

65. Bailey, D. A., Carron, A. V., Teece, R. G. & Wehner, H. J., *Am. J. clin. Nutr.*, 1970, 23, 905.

66. Pelletier, O., *J. Lab. clin. Med.*, 1968, 72, 674.

67. Franchimont, P. & Delwaide, P. J., *Revue fr. Etud. clin. biol.*, 1966, 11, 876.

68. Lipscomb, H. S. & Nelson, D. H., Endocrinology, 1960, 66, 144.

69. Kitabuchi, A. E., *Nature, Lond.*, 1967, 215, 1385.

70. Cohen, M. M., *B.M.J.*, 1967, 2, 243.

71. Collins, C. K. *et al.*, *Int. Z. VitamForsch.*, 1967, 37, 492.

72. 'Useful vitamins', *Nature, Lond.*, 1968, 220, 329.

73. Dymock, I. W., Turck, W. P. G., Brown, P. W., Sircus, W., Small, W. P. & Thomson, C., *B.M.J.*, 1968, 1, 179.

74. Williamson, J. M. *et al.*, *ibid.*, 1967, 2, 23.

75. Russell, R. I. & Goldberg, A., *Lancet*, 1968, ii, 606.

76. Croft, D. N., *ibid.*, 1968, ii, 831.

77. Macmillan, D. C. & Sim, A. K., *Thromb. Diath. haemorrh.*, 1970, 24, 385.

78. Sokoloff, B., Hori, M., Saelhof, C. C., Wrzolek, T. & Imai, T., *J. Am. Geriat. Soc.*, 1966, 14, 1239.

79. Sokoloff, B., Hori, M., Saelhof, C. C., McConnell, B. & Imai, T., *J. Nutr.*, 1967, 91, 107.

80. Myasinikov, A. L., *Circulation*, 1958, 17, 99.

81. *Nutr. Rev.*, 1967, 25, No 6, 183.

82. Ginter, E., Babala, J. & Cerven, J., *J. Atheroscler. Res.*, 1969, 10, 341.

83. Ginter, E., Ondreicka, R., Bobek, P. & Sinko, V., *J. Nutr.*, 1969, 99, 261.

84. Willis, G. C. & Fishman, S., *Can. med. Ass. J.*, 1955, 72, 500.

85. Willis, G. C., *ibid.*, 1957, 77, 106.

86. Shaffer, C. F., *Am. J. clin. Nutr.*, 1970, 23, No 1, 27.

87. Taylor, C. B. *et al.*, *Illinois med. J.*, 1961, 119, 80.

88. Dunnigan, M. G., Harland, W. A. & Fyfe, T., *Lancet*, 1970, ii, 793.

89. Spittle, C. R., *ibid.*, 1970, October 31, 931.

90. Fleming, A. F. *et al.*, *Am. J. clin. Nutr.*, 1969, 22, 642.

91. *Nutr. Rev.*, 1967, 25, No 8, 237.

92. *Ibid.*, 1969, 27, 139.

93. Badenoch, J., *B.M.J.*, 1960, 2, 879, 963.

94. Aterman, K., Boscott, R. J. & Cooke, W. T., 1953, *Nutr. Rev.*, 1967, 25, 239.

95. Laikakos, D., Matsaniotis, N., Karpouzas, J., Morphis, L. & Agathopoulis, A., *Clinica chim. Acta*, 1969, 26, 197.

96. *Nutr. Rev.*, 1967, 25, 228.

97. Regnier, E., *Rev. Allergy appl. Immun.*, 1968, 22, 835.

98. Fletcher, J. M. & Fletcher, I. C., *B.M.J.*, 1951, 1, 887.

99. Dey, P. K., *Naturwissenschaften*, 1966, 53, 310.

100. Hindson, T. C., *Lancet*, 1968, i, 1347.

101. Hindson, T. C. *et al.*, *Br. J. Derm.*, 1969, 81, 226.

102. Reiss, F., *J. Lab. clin. Med.*, 1943, 28, 1082.

103. Fiedoruk, T., *Wiad. parazyt.*, 1968, 14, 69.

104. Hoffman, B. *et al.*, *ibid.*, 1969, 15, 343.

105. Ritzel, G., *Helv. med. Acta*, 1961, 28, 63.

106. Barnes, F. E., *N. Carol. med. J.*, 1961, 22, 22.

107. Rinehart, J. F., Greenberg, L. D. & Baker, F., *Proc. Soc. exp. Biol. Med.*, 1936, 35, 347.

108. Abrams, E. & Sandson, J., *Ann. rheum. Dis.*, 1964, 23, 295.

109. Sandson, J. & Hamerman, D., *J. clin. Invest.*, 1962, 41, 1817.

110. Duthie, J. J. R., personal communication, 1970.

111. Thornton, P. A., *Proc. Soc. exp. Biol. Med.*, 1968, 127, 1096.

112. Follis, R. H., *Bull. Johns Hopkins Hosp.*, 1951, 89, 9.

113. Bourne, G. H., in 'The biochemistry and physiology of bone', 1956, *New York: Acad. Press.*

114. Bourne, G. H., *Br. J. Nutr.*, 1948, 2, 261.

115. Ellis, F. B., *Lancet*, 1968, ii, 173.

116. Pawan, G. L. S., *Nature, Lond.*, 1968, 220, 374.

117. McCurdy, P. R. *et al.*, *Am. J. clin. Nutr.*, 1968, 21, 284.

118. Asquith, P. *et al.*, *B.M.J.*, 1967, 4, 402.

119. Bryson, D. D., *Practitioner*, 1968, 200, 694.

120. Schleicher, E. M., *Minn. Med.*, 1970, 53, 135.

121. Wapnik, A. A. *et al.*, *Br. J. Haemat.*, 1969, 17, 563.

122. Gomez, G. *et al.*, *Br. J. clin. Pract.*, 1969, 23, 421.

123. Loh, H. S. & Wilson, C. W., *Lancet*, 1971, January 16, 110.

17

ASCORBIC ACID AND THE COMMON COLD

It is widely believed that ascorbic acid may have some protective effect against the common cold, lessening the incidence of infection, and that it can also exert a beneficial therapeutic effect, shortening the course of the common cold. Ascorbic acid is commonly taken as a preventive measure, and large doses are frequently consumed at the onset of symptoms. There is, however, little or no factual evidence that, given to healthy individuals not depleted of ascorbic acid, it has any such prophylactic or therapeutic effect.

Assessment of any beneficial effect of ascorbic acid on the natural course of the common cold is made difficult by the usual self-limited and short duration of the disease, and by the fact that evaluation of any possible therapeutic effect is often determined on purely subjective and clinical grounds. In addition, the placebo effect of any agent in the treatment of the common cold is marked. H. E. Tebrock, J. J. Arminio, and J. H. Johnston (*J. Am. Med. Assn.* 162, *1227* (*1956*)), in their large series of over 1,900 subjects, noted a high percentage of reactors to placebos, and in a recent study by G. H. Walker, M. L. Bynoe, and D. A. J. Tyrrell (*Brit. Med. J.* 1, *603* (*1967*)) it was observed in two series where the volunteers were told before their colds were finished whether or not they were receiving ascorbic acid, that the duration of colds in the treated group was shorter than in the control subjects. In a third trial in which no information was given, the colds lasted the same length of time in the ascorbic acid and placebo recipients.

Many trials claiming a beneficial effect of ascorbic acid in colds have been completely uncontrolled studies, and in many instances conclusions have been based solely on clinical impressions. In some studies, ascorbic

Reprinted from *Nutrition Reviews*, Vol. 25, No. 6, August, 1967. Printed in U. S. A.

acid has been given together with other active agents, thereby making evaluation of effect difficult or impossible.

In an experimental study of vitamin C deprivation in man (W. Bartley, H. A. Krebs, and J. R. P. O'Brien, *Medical Research Council Special Report Series No. 280. Her Majesty's Stationery Office, London, 1953*), the mean length of colds in deprived subjects was 6.4 days as compared with 3.3 days in non-deprived controls. The authors stated that their data supported the hypothesis that the colds of subjects deprived of ascorbic acid lasted longer, but did not establish it.

In observations of a group of 1,500 adolescents, none of whom showed clinical evidence of scurvy, in an institution which provided a diet containing only 10 to 15 mg. ascorbic acid daily, A. J. Glazebrook and S. Thomson (*J. Hyg.* 42, 1 (*1942*)) noted that supplements of 50 to 200 mg. ascorbic acid daily had no effect on the incidence of colds and tonsillitis. The duration of tonsillitis was shorter in the supplemented groups, but the duration of colds was completely unaffected. Sixteen cases of rheumatic fever and 17 of pneumonia occurred in the unsupplemented group of 1,100, but none occurred in the youths receiving the supplements.

N. W. Maxwell (*Med. J. Aust.* 2, 777 (*1947*)) enthusiastically advocated ascorbic acid therapy for the common cold, claiming on the basis of his experience in over 100 cases that there was a better than one in two chance of stopping a cold if a large enough dose of ascorbic acid was taken early. This report is an example of a completely uncontrolled study where conclusions were based solely on clinical hunches. Maxwell stated that 0.5 g. ascorbic acid taken at the first sign of a cold was inadequate to arrest development of the infection and recommended a dosage schedule with an initial 0.75 g. followed by 0.5 g. in 3 to 4 hours if unimproved, with 1 g. on the second and third days if symptoms persisted. J. M. Fletcher and I. C. Fletcher (*Brit. Med. J.* 1, 887 (*1951*)) though 50 to 100 mg. supplements of ascorbic acid increased resistance to infection in children, but added that their experience was limited and suggested the necessity for control studies.

G. Ritzel (*Helv. Med. Acta* 28, 63 (*1961*)) in a study of 279 skiers, allocated by alternate numbers to groups receiving either 1,000 mg. ascorbic acid daily or identical inert placebo, reported a reduction of 39 per cent in the number of days ill from upper respiratory tract infections and a reduction of 35 per cent in the incidence of individual symptoms in the supplemented group as compared with the placebo group. A slight reduction in the mean duration of illness from 2.6 in the control series to 1.8 days in the treated series was noted. In this study, the assessment was largely based on subjective reports from the participants and only limited clinical observations were made.

A study sometimes quoted as evidence of a beneficial protective effect of ascorbic acid in reducing the number of colds is that of F. E. Barnes, Jr. (*N. Carolina Med. J.* 22, 22 (*1961*)). He studied two groups of school children, a group of basketball players receiving therapy and a control group of nonplayers receiving no therapy. There was a marked reduction in the number of days on which colds were reported in those receiving daily supplements which, however, contained many other vitamins in addition to 200 mg. of ascorbic acid. Apparent improvement on the second day of medication was noted by W. L. Macon (*Indust. Med. Surg.* 25, *525* (*1956*)) in subjects receiving a mixture of bioflavinoids, ascorbic acid, and aspirin, the control group receiving aspirin, phenacetin, and caffeine. It is again difficult to conclude from the results of this study that ascorbic acid had any definite effect.

Tebrock *et al.* (*loc. cit.*) studied in a series of over 1,900 workers the effect of 1 g. bioflavinoids, 200 mg. ascorbic acid, or 1 g. bioflavinoids plus 200 mg. ascorbic acid daily given at the onset of a cold and noted "a singular lack of effect" of therapy in aborting or curing the common cold. The members of this large group, apart from an initial examination, were examined once only on the third day and the control group given placebos and three supplemented groups all received a cold therapeutic mixture of salicylamide, acetophenetidin, caffeine, and an antihistaminic thonzylamine. No evidence of subjective or objective improvement was noted and no decrease in time lost from work occurred in the three groups treated with bioflavinoid and ascorbic acid as compared with the group receiving the cold therapy alone.

H. Banks (*Lancet* 2, *790* (*1965*)) reported the results of three double blind controlled trials comparing the effect of antibiotics and ascorbic acid on the common cold, using as a criterion of assessment, during ten days of observation, whether the nasal discharge remained clear, or stopped, or became mucopurulent. In the first trial, the ascorbic acid was intended as a placebo, but similar results were obtained in those patients receiving antibiotics and those getting ascorbic acid. The nasal discharge remained mucoid or stopped in 62 per cent of 101 cases on tetracycline, 75 per cent of 84 cases on spiramycin. and 70 per cent of 90 cases on ascorbic acid.

In the second trial the nasal discharge remained clear or dried up in 70 per cent of 37 cases on tetracycline, 73 per cent of 34 cases on spiramycin, 51 per cent of 37 cases on ascorbic acid, and in 30 per cent of 30 controls on inert kaolin. In a third study good results were obtained in 68 per cent of 71 cases on spiramycin, 56 per cent of 71 cases on ascorbic acid, and 80 per cent of 41 cases on spiramycin and ascorbic acid. A combination of spiramycin and ascorbic acid was claimed to be statistically (at 5 per cent level) more effective than ascorbic acid alone only when given within 12 hours of the onset of symptoms. Ascorbic acid within the first 12 hours was also stated to be more effective than ascorbic acid given later. The dose of ascorbic acid employed in these studies was not stated.

In view of the differing and often unwarranted conclusions drawn by many previous investigators, the recent report by Walker *et al.* (*loc. cit.*) of a carefully planned controlled study with objective measurements of assessment of infection is welcome. They found, in *in vitro* studies and observations of both animals and human beings, that ascorbic acid had no effect on viruses producing the common cold.

In their *in vitro* studies, exposure of tissue culture cells to ascorbic acid did not increase resistance to infection with viruses. Using strains of viruses chosen from biological groups known to cause colds and representative of the picornavirus, myxovirus, adenovirus, enterovirus, and herpesvirus families, Walker *et al.* noted no antiviral effects of ascorbic acid added in nontoxic doses (10 mg. per 100 ml.) to the tissue culture medium before use.

In the studies, except for the myxovirus which was tested after several days of hemadsorption, the cytopathic effect of the various viruses in tissue cultures was studied daily. The minimum infectious dose of virus was the same in cultures treated with ascorbic acid as in untreated cultures. Since with the passage of time, a marked decrease in the ascorbic acid content of the culture medium was noted whether or not the medium was in contact with cultures, an experiment was conducted with adenovirus 5 in which the medium was changed every 12 hours for four days in order to maintain ascorbic acid levels, but here again no antiviral effect of vitamin C was noted.

In animals studies, a strain of influenza A was given to mice by intranasal instillation under light ether anesthesia. The treated group received daily intraperitoneal injections of 4 mg. ascorbic acid in saline for six days before and nine days after instillation and the control group received only saline injections. No difference in mortality or in the extent of the lung lesions was noted between the group receiving daily approximately 300 mg. per kilogram ascorbic acid and the control group getting saline.

These investigators state that the colds induced under their experimental conditions by artificial inoculation of human beings are very similar to those occurring naturally in clinical practice where there is a possibility of developing secondary bacterial infection. The 91 volunteers used in this study were aged between 18 and 50 (mean 30.2) years of age and received a generous mixed diet, the vitamin C content of which was unknown but which contained fresh fruit and cooked vegetables. The trials were conducted between January and May when the dietary intake of vitamin C was expected to be low, so any effect of the ascorbic acid supplements would be maximal.

Inoculations were made in the volunteers with virus propagated by man-to-man passage, and all the viruses used are known to be frequent causes of colds. Influenza B was used as a typical representative myxovirus, a family that includes the influenza and parainfluenza viruses which cause an appreciable proportion of colds, especially in young children. Also studied were three strains of rhinovirus and the B814 virus, which is morphologically similar to that of avian bronchitis, and at least one other virus causing human colds.

Forty-seven volunteers received 1 g. ascorbic acid thrice daily (approximately 75 mg. per kilogram) for three days prior to challenge with virus and for six days after inoculation. Absorption of the ascorbic acid was proven by urinary excretion studies. Forty-four controls received identical but chemically inert placebo tablets. No evidence of a general prophylactic effect on colds was noted, and with these massive doses of ascorbic acid no difference was noted in the number and severity of colds as compared with the placebo group. The mean length of the incubation period and the duration of symptoms were the same in both groups, and the incidence of sore throat and muco-purulent nasal discharge was also similar.

In the volunteers who received influenza B and two of the three strains of rhinovirus used, two serum specimens were tested for antibodies against the inoculated virus before and two weeks after inoculation. In these subjects nasal washings were collected daily from the first day after virus inoculation and the representative viruses isolated and typed by neutralization tests with specific antiserum. No laboratory evidence for any protective effect of ascorbic acid against viral infection was found. The results of these *in vitro* animal and human studies show that ascorbic acid has no effect against viruses frequently causing the common cold.

There is no conclusive evidence that ascorbic acid has any protective effect against, or any therapeutic effect on, the course of the common cold in healthy people not depleted of ascorbic acid. There is also no evidence for a general, antiviral, or symptomatic prophylactic effect of ascorbic acid.

18

THE VITAMIN E CURE–ALL

The overpromotion of vitamins is by now a familiar story, but in recent years one vitamin in particular has been selected by its proponents to be the savior of humanity. Vitamin E is widely promoted as a preventive, a treatment, or a cure for literally scores of human ailments—ranging from diabetes and heart disease to infertility, ulcers, and warts. It is even touted as an antidote for air pollution.

Millions of patients, it is alleged, are currently suffering from painful, crippling, life-threatening diseases because their misguided physicians refuse to recommend vitamin E supplements to them. And we are said to be rearing a new generation of children destined in turn to suffer and to die prematurely because they are not receiving daily preventive doses of vitamin E. Such claims as these have appeared in magazine articles, and in widely circulated paperback books bearing such titles as *Vitamin E for Ailing and Healthy Hearts*, *Vitamin E: Your Key to a Healthy Heart*, and *Vitamin E: Key to Sexual Satisfaction*.

Are any of these allegations justified? What is vitamin E really good for?

It was more than fifty years ago that scientists isolated a group of six or more substances called tocopherols (designated as alpha, beta, gamma, and so on). The alpha form of tocopherol was found to be the most biologically potent. In 1938 tocopherol was synthesized. However, although early research had shown alpha-tocopherol—now called vitamin E —to be a dietary essential for many animal species, no human disorder could be found for which vitamin E offered benefits. For years it remained "a vitamin in search of a disease." In 1953 Dr. M. K. Horwitt, head of the Biochemical Research Laboratory at Elgin State Hospital in Elgin, Illinois, made the first study of what happens when humans are maintained for protracted periods on low-E diets. The project spanned more than eight years—making it one of the longest as well as one of the most thorough studies of human metabolism under controlled conditions. A total of thirty-eight subjects participated in the study.

The outcome of the project can be simply stated: *There was no apparent physical or mental impairment caused by the restricted intake of vitamin E.* Low-E patients remained in satisfactory health, despite the lowering of alpha-tocopherol in their blood by 80 percent. Their red blood cells had somewhat shorter survival times—on the average, about 110 days instead of 123—than those of the two comparison groups (those on a low-E diet who received vitamin E supplements, and those on a standard diet). But the cells remained adequate for their function. Nevertheless, the shorter survival time was considered sufficient reason for terminating the experiment. In earlier studies, monkeys maintained on diets severely deficient in vitamin E had developed anemia, and Dr. Horwitt did not want to risk that possibility with the Elgin patients. In short, the study showed that humans apparently need *some* vitamin E, but that the requirement is a modest one and can be satisfied by typical, everyday diets.

Nine patients in the project developed peptic ulcers, which showed up in X-ray examinations although not in patient symptoms. After an extensive study, experts in peptic ulcer disease concluded that the ailment was caused by factors other than vitamin E deficiency. Significantly, the incidence of ulcers was no higher among low-E patients than among those who received the same diet plus vitamin E supplements. The ulcers healed with standard therapy without complications. (Despite this experience, vitamin E is still being touted as a treatment for ulcers.)

In 1973 the National Research Council (NRC) announced a new much lower recommended daily allowance of vitamin E. The former figure for adults of 25 to 30 international units (IU) was cut by half to 12 to 15 IU (equivalent to approximately 8 to 10 milligrams of natural vitamin E in foods).

Vitamin E enthusiasts point out that millions of Americans whose intake of polyunsaturated fats is low obtain less than that amount in their diets. The deficit, they insist, should be made up by vitamin E supplements.

The fact is, however, as the NRC made clear in a June 1973 statement, that vitamin E is available in adequate quantities in the ordinary diet: "Dietary vitamin E is supplied in substantial amounts by most vegetable oils as well as by margarine and shortening made from these oils, and significant inputs are made by many vegetables and by whole-grain cereals. Meats, fish, poultry, milk, eggs, legumes, fruits, and nuts also contribute to the dietary supply."

Margarine has at least thirteen times more vitamin E than butter. A salmon steak contains ten times the vitamin E of a beefsteak, pound for pound. And most vegetable oils, which are relatively high in polyunsaturated fats, are also adequate sources of vitamin E, despite refining procedures used in processing. In short, when we eat more polyunsaturated fats, our intake of vitamin E is concomitantly increased. Even though there is an increased requirement for vitamin E in a diet high in polyunsaturated fats, that requirement is automatically met. In contrast, when the intake of polyunsaturated fats is low, the need for vitamin E is also low. "The apparent absence of vitamin E deficiency in the general population suggests that the amount of vitamin E in foods is adequate," the NRC has stated.

Vitamin E enthusiasts sometimes allege that, while ordinary diets may be good enough for ordinary good health, vitamin E supplements may lead to even better health—with greater physical vigor, strength, and endurance.

Three researchers in Britain, Drs. I. M. Sharman, M. G. Down, and R. N. Sen, subjected that possibility to a test. Thirteen boys in a boarding school swimming club were given 400 milligrams of vitamin E daily during a six-week program of intensive physical training. Before and after the six-week period, they were subjected to a variety of tests—including pull-ups, push-ups, sit-ups, breathholding, running, and swimming endurance. Significant improvement was shown at the end of the six weeks— which might lead some vitamin E enthusiasts to call out "Aha!" But thirteen other boys, matched to the thirteen test subjects in age, weight, and other criteria, were put through the same training program and evaluation. They were given a placebo similar in appearance to the vitamin E capsule taken by the test subjects. And guess what? The placebo group also improved! "No significant differences were found between the group given vitamin E and that given placebo tablets," the British researchers reported.

In addition to the claims made for alpha-tocopherol as a *vitamin*, the same chemical has for more than a quarter of a century also been touted, when used in far larger amounts, as a *medicine*. The doses specified in medicinal use commonly range from 300 to 600 milligrams a day or even higher—from thirty to seventy-five times the recommended daily allowance of the NRC.

The news magazine *Time* first broke the story of vitamin E as a medicine in its issue of June 10, 1946:

"Out of Canada last week came news of a startling scientific discovery: a treatment for heart disease (the nation's No. 1 killer) which so far has succeeded against all common forms of the ailment. . . . Large, concentrated doses of vitamin E . . . benefited four types of heart ailment (95 per cent of the total): arteriosclerotic, hypertensive, rheumatic, old and new coronary heart disease. The vitamin helps a failing heart. It eliminates anginal pain. It is non-toxic."

The clinical trials that *Time* thus enthusiastically recounted were conducted by three Canadian physicians—Dr. Evan Shute, a fellow of the American College of Obstetricians and Gynecologists and of the Royal College of Surgeons (Canada); his brother, Dr. Wilfrid E. Shute, a specialist in heart disease; and Dr. Albert Vogelsang. They based their enthusiasm for vitamin E on their personal experiences with patients. An example, reported by Dr. Wilfrid E. Shute, involved a fifteen-year-old boy who had suffered a second attack of acute rheumatic fever. During his first attack, the boy had been hospitalized for an extended period. The next time, however, Dr. Shute did not recommend hospitalization.

"The only treatment I used for the boy was 200 units of alpha-tocopherol daily," Dr. Shute reported. "In three days he was apparently well, and on the sixth day he walked into my office. He was able to return to normal farm activities. . . . This was the first case in all the world in which rheumatic fever had been treated with vitamin E."

Worldwide medical interest was aroused, of course, by this account. It was whetted even further in 1947 when the Canadian group reported on eighty-four patients of theirs treated with vitamin E. According to the group, all the patients had symptoms of angina pectoris—chest pain usually associated with coronary heart disease—and the majority had responded positively to vitamin E treatment.

Despite such growing accounts of vitamin E benefits, the vast majority of physicians today reject vitamin E as a treatment for heart disease (and for other ailments as well). The charge is repeatedly made that the medical profession turned thumbs down on vitamin E without even trying it out. This is simply false. Vitamin E was in fact tried out—and found wanting.

By 1950 thirteen studies had been published in medical journals, all reporting the worthlessness of vitamin E during clinical trials with patients who suffered from heart disease. These reports were written by thirty-two researchers, including eminent cardiologists and professors of internal medicine. They involved more than 450 patients—as compared with the eighty-four patients on whom Drs. Shute, Shute, and Vogelsang based their initial reports.

If any of those thirteen studies had verified the claims made in Canada, further trials of vitamin E would unquestionably have followed. News of a potential cure for heart disease compels medical attention, and no doctor or scientist could have ignored valid evidence in support of vitamin E. "We had indeed intended expanding our studies," a research group at Jewish Hospital in Philadelphia noted, "but the discouraging results presented in the preliminary report deterred us from carrying these investigations further."

Those sentiments were unmistakably representative of the medical community at large, as Dr. Herbert Eichert of Miami, Florida, confirmed during his studies of vitamin E and heart disease in 1948. In an attempt to determine the views of many heart specialists—including those who had not published any findings—Dr. Eichert sent questionnaires to department heads at medical schools throughout the United States. "Most of the clinicians," he reported, "abandoned their trials because of the utter lack of response during the preliminary phases of their investigations."

Then, in just one sentence, Dr. Eichert summed up all the medical evidence he had gathered on vitamin E's performance: "With the exception of the claims made by Shute and Vogelsang and their group, every published, written, or verbal report which this essayist has been able to obtain indicates that vitamin E has no value in the treatment of heart disease."

In the history of vitamin E research, only a handful of field trials have complied with the rigorous standards required in compiling scientific data—and most of those trials ended with negative conclusions. The claims made for vitamin E by Drs. Shute, Shute, and Vogelsang were not based on double-blind or even on simple blind trials. Indeed CU has seen no evidence that they were even based on trials comparing patients with controls. They are essentially the uncontrolled personal impressions of three physicians who have faith in their remedy and transmit that faith to their patients. Their claims, in short, have no scientific validity.

When vitamin E is tested by physicians who are *not* enthusiasts, however, the list of failures is long. Clinical trials have failed to show any vitamin E benefits for miscarriages, sterility, menopausal disturbances, muscular dystrophies, cystic fibrosis, blood disorders, leg ulcers, diabetes, and a variety of heart and vascular diseases. The June 1973 statement by the NRC was also negative about the supposed value of vitamin E supplements for the wide variety of ailments for which vitamin E is claimed to be of benefit.

A few studies suggest that vitamin E might be useful in the treatment of intermittent claudication—a vascular condition in which the blood flow to the lower limbs is reduced and pain, most often in the calves, is experienced during walking. However, the evidence for any such benefit from vitamin E is far from conclusive, in the judgment of CU's medical consultants who reviewed the studies. The *only* therapeutic use for vitamin E in humans established by a well-controlled clinical trial is one involving the treatment of an uncommon type of hemolytic anemia in certain premature babies. Beyond that, some doctors prescribe vitamin E simply as a precautionary measure in a few relatively rare diseases involving impairment of fat absorption. Vitamin E's value in a high-oxygen environment may possibly have validity but is still not established.

The efficacy of vitamin E in toilet soaps or cosmetics for skin care, despite advertised claims, has not been scientifically established. Its possible advantage in a deodorant was ruled out when the distribution of *Mennen E* was halted by its manufacturer as a result of a rash of skin complaints from unhappy users.

CU's medical consultants believe that research on vitamin E should continue, with the aim of better defining its role in human metabolism both in healthy people and in ill people. One double-blind pilot study from Canada on the use of vitamin E in treating angina pectoris was published in February 1974. The results showed no statistically significant benefits from the use of vitamin E; however, the researcher called for a larger study of vitamin E's potential in treating cardiovascular disease.

Meanwhile, CU's medical consultants discourage, as a waste of money, the use of vitamin E as a dietary supplement or as a medication for common ailments. More important, such self-medication could lead to postponing proper medical treatment. And the cost of that could be incalculable. For now, CU's medical consultants conclude, there is no convincing evidence that human beings need more vitamin E than they obtain in their ordinary diets, or that vitamin E is useful in the treatment of any but a few rare diseases.

19

THE ROAD TO SHANGRI–LA IS PAVED WITH VITAMINS

Reuben Bitensky, Ph.D.*

Much of the controversy that has raged over the medical worth of vitamins has neglected to consider why a scientific issue should stir up such vehemence. In the heat of battle the contestants have not paused to ask why they are involved in the fray. The passions that have been aroused seem more typical of religious and political conflicts than of the investigations of medical science. Not since the controversy over the flouridation of water, which has happily abated, has there been such polarization. In fact, "vitaminization" seems more apt to capture the minds and hearts of Americans than Vietnamization. Although I am not equipped to evaluate the therapeutic benefits of vitamins, nor do I wish to, it nevertheless seems to me that the whole subject could be approached more objectively if the psychological and ideological aspects of the vitamin crusade could be examined.

This was brought home to me when, in working with a number of patients in group therapy sessions, I suddenly found the vitamin cult to be an intruder in our midst. The rapid conversion of the group to this cult first struck me as a benign, if somewhat ironic, eccentricity. It was ironic because all the members of the group were attributing to vitamins some magical potency to ward off disease while they were being beset by various ailments. Indeed, as the group members became freer to disclose their be-

Reprinted from the *American Journal of Psychiatry*, November 1973, Vol. 130, pp. 1253–1256. Copyright 1973, the American Psychiatric Association.

* Dr. Bitensky is Associate Dean and Associate Professor, School of Social Work, Syracuse University, 926 South Crouse Ave., Syracuse, N.Y. 13210.

lief, they revealed their conviction that vitamins C and E would not only prevent disease but would restore youth. It seemed to me that in a sense such rallying under the banner of vitamins could be the cause célèbre of the older generation. If past generations could seek organ transplants from monkeys and if the young have their idiosyncracies, then why shouldn't today's older people see vitamins as the elixir of youth and the hope of the future?

However, I was soon to find out that treating the subject with tolerance and dispassion did not evoke a sympathetic chord. The group members interpreted my impartiality as a form of intellectual dilettantism. Moreover, they saw me as an agnostic who was undermining their faith in their tribal god. Thus, as time went on, I began to perceive that this was not merely a scientific dispute, but that it had distinct theological overtones. I began to be aware that a religion was at stake, with its high priests, its doctrines, and its rituals. To question the dogma was to contaminate the deep well of psychological gratification the cult offered its proselytes.

THE NATURE OF THE GROUP

To understand these psychological rewards, the nature of the group has to be considered. They were men and women of later middle age who, although they had achieved some successes in life, were frustrated in attaining the goals they had set for themselves in the sexual, social, and economic spheres, or in a combination of these. At the time they were still highly motivated for the future. What was common to them as a group was a high degree of emotional deprivation because of their failures and an intense investment in filling these lacunae. While these objectives seemed highly unrealistic given the passage of years, nevertheless they clung as a group to the illusion that in the near future—just around the corner—was the ideal love partner, the glittering pot of gold, or the stunning social coup. Unattainable as these goals were, it was maintaining the illusion that was paramount, and even the illusion was in danger of being dimmed by the approach of old age.

The character of this contradiction was brought home to the group members by their awareness that, while the attainment of their desires required ever greater expenditures of energy and will power, the onrush of time was depleting these precious resources. Psychologically, it became imperative to roll back or at least retard the aging process. For without their youth—or what was left of it—the ramparts of their dream worlds would be scaled by reality, and old age would have to be confronted. However, where there is a desire to be psychologically hoodwinked the answer is not long in coming. It was found in vitamins, particularly vitamin E.

Here was the panacea for disease, the talisman against the aging process, and the elixir to rejuvenate body and soul.

Although various reasons have been given for the resurgence of the vitamin cult, these explanations tend to be universal in scope and there has been little exploration of why particular groups resort to this psychological pattern. Given the nature of the group I worked with, why did they gravitate to vitamin E? Why not deep-breathing exercises, faith healing, or the transmigration of souls? To understand why a particular group seeks a specific resolution for a problem one must understand not only the problem but also the nature of the group. In this respect, awareness of the psychological needs of the group is a sine qua non; these needs have been identified and described in the psychological and sociological literature on the subject. What has received scant attention is the extent to which ideological imperatives and the value systems of the members of the group may influence the choice of a solution in attaining new psychological levels of adjustment.

This phenomenon was highly visible in the group that I worked with as therapist. All the members of the group were of a progressive inclination and in their youth had ascribed to liberal activism. However, the debilitating effects of the passing years were making it more and more difficult—physically and psychologically—to practice activism. It was becoming less and less inviting to attend meetings, participate in committees, and enter into the political fray. At the same time they were loath to give up their image of themselves as crusaders for progress, for this would lower their own self-esteem as well as imperil the adulation of children, relatives, and friends.

THE VITAMIN CULT AND THE ESTABLISHMENT

Vitamins offered a way out of this cul-de-sac. Adherence to the vitamin cult was a means of preserving their image of themselves as anti-establishment, particularly in regard to the medical sector of the establishment. Had not Linus Pauling postulated that vitamin C was being attacked as a cure for colds because the pharmaceutical companies had a vested interest in spurious cold remedies? Was not vitamin E being downgraded by the medical profession because of its investment in the perpetuation of disease? This charge against the medical establishment in the United States was given all the more credence because of the crisis in the delivery of health services and the resistance of the AMA to liberal solutions. Thus the vitamin evangelists could point to the medical profession's reservations about vitamins as one more example in a long history of opposition to progress in medical service for the populace. (It may be noted, however, that they seemingly took no cognizance of the fact that, with the growing popularity of vitamins, the same pharmaceutical companies were earning substantial profits from the boom in vitamins.)

In another respect the vitamin cult represented an attack upon the establishment through its link-up with the organic food zealots. This occurred because the therapeutic rationale for adding vitamins to the diet arose from the plausible charge that the food industry was processing the vitamins out of many foods. Therefore, the only effective method of getting sufficient vitamins was by the use of organic foods. The resulting alliance between the vitamin and organic food devotees (often they were the same people) brought the vitamin cult into confrontation not only with the medical empire but also with the food industry. Thus a Goliath had been created that would be a worthy adversary of any liberal David.

In such a conflict the image of the political crusader could be maintained and even strengthened with substantial rewards for one's self-concept. But it was crucial to this accomplishment that it involved only a minimal expenditure of energy. By ingesting vitamins one could fight the establishment with the kind of activism that required no more effort than swallowing. Moreover, the greater the dosage, the greater the witness to fervent liberalism and anti-establishment sentiments. The liberals in the group had discovered a holy rite comparable to the sacrament of the Eucharist. Through the substitution of vitamins they had created a political communion through which the dilemma of being a liberal activist without being active was resolved.

However, there was another way in which the vitamin cult answered the psychological needs of the group and this too arose from the anxieties, insecurities, and fears brought on by old age. As the years went by and as illness and thoughts of death loomed larger, the liberal ideology offered less and less consolation to the members of the group. Because of their beliefs it was difficult for them to seek the religious comfort of facing death in the promise of immortality. During their earlier years these liberals were either agnostics or atheists. This presented no problems during their youth and early middle age since illness and death were merely theoretical concepts and not concrete realities that required some psychological readjustment. But to resort to religious belief in later years would be a desertion of the liberal credo and a shattering of the crusading image that was at the core of their personalities. In this crisis it was once again the vitamin cult that unified the seemingly irreconcilable opposites of liberalism and religious orthodoxy.

The problem the group faced was that of staving off death without resorting to religious solutions. Since life in the hereafter could only be assured theologically, a dogma was necessary to provide immortality here on earth. Once again the vitamin cult came to the rescue by promising eternal youth, or at least postponement of the aging process. But why are vitamins more acceptable than other avenues to immortality? Here it becomes evident that the scientific emphasis inherent in the vitamin approach makes it compatible with the agnostic or atheistic value system of the group members. At the same time it also overcame the dilemma inherent in agnosticism and atheism, since it provided a rationale for dealing with death through the so-called youth-preserving properties of vitamins.

Here it is clear that the group members had to choose between two alternatives: they could retain their agnostic and/or atheistic beliefs or they could abandon their beliefs under the subterfuge that they were accepting a more scientific orientation in the vitamin cult. It is sufficient for our purposes to note that maintaining their agnosticism would have meant facing the limitations of old age and adapting to the realities of a new phase in their lives. On the other hand, the vitamin cult could preserve the illusion of youth and enable them to avoid—at least for some time—the necessity of regarding themselves as elderly. Interestingly enough, if character building is to be regarded as the outcome of confronting and dealing with the realities of living, it would have been adhering to their own beliefs rather than seeking the will-o'-the-wisp of eternal youth and the intimations of immortality promised by vitamins that would have contributed to their continued growth as individuals.

THE EFFECT ON THE GROUP

Given this new adjustment, how durable was it? Will this new homeostatic balance promote the cohesion of the group and will it foster the stability of the individual members? Already some stresses and strains are beginning to appear that augur ill for the psychological well-being of the group. There are signs that they are perplexed and uncomfortable with their status as a select group (one that has the quality of eccentricity rather than elitism) that is different from the remainder of society. It is a situation that conflicts with their cherished image of themselves as liberals since, although liberalism implies an advanced role in society, it is an integrated, not a deviant, position.

This insecurity in the group was mirrored in their doubts about the values of their colleagues. While each subscribed to the vitamin cult, they inwardly mistrusted their peers for adopting this stance and criticized them for abandoning the traditional tenets of liberalism. Differences between members of the group were thus exacerbated and they found it increasingly difficult to tolerate each other's company even though they held a common dogma. Only in dialogues about the curative powers of vitamins were they in harmony. However, when faced with the skepticism of friends and acquaintances outside the group, they tended to unite in categorizing the doubting Thomases as irredeemable, unenlightened pagans.

But why is the new psychological adjustment so tenuous? The ability to deal maturely with old age arises out of accepting its inevitability in order to philosophically and morally transcend its limitations. To live by the denial of old age, buoyed by fantasies of great expectations in the future, means to fail to live today. By giving up their value system and failing to face life's limitations the group first of all relinquished their tested liberal values and assumed the mantle of knowledge in an area in which they possessed no more expertise than the man in the street. They gave up being themselves and took on roles that were unbelievable to their friends. Far from being secure, they became threatened and defensive. Their behavior was guarded, with an increasing lack of variety, nuance, and spontaneity in their thoughts and actions. Previously, when the group sessions first began, their interaction demonstrated their interest in art, politics, and ideas. Now there was a perseverative discussion of their ailments, of vitamins, and of organic foods. Their intellectual horizons extended only far enough to include ecology as a topic of conversation since this was related to the future of organic farming.

In retrospect it is evident that, if the group had refrained from attributing magical therapeutic properties to vitamins and had accepted the inevitability of old age, they could have retained their self-respect and the esteem of their peers. They denied reality as fraught with antithesis and suffering. They chose instead the easy way—the dream of Shangri-La—and, in the frenetic pursuit of their youth, they are in danger of losing what remains of their old age.

20

BIOAVAILABILITY OF SYNTHETIC AND NATURAL ASCORBIC ACID

O. Pelletier, Ph.D., and M. O. Keith *

The ever-increasing number of synthetic fruit drinks on supermarket shelves indicates their successful competition with the natural juices. The synthetic drinks are usually fortified with synthetic L-ascorbic acid, but the efficacy of this form as a substitute for natural ascorbic acid in citrus juices has been questioned (1). Although natural and synthetic ascorbic acids are chemically identical, citrus fruits contain bioflavonoids (2) which could improve the bioavailability of ascorbic acid by protecting it from oxidation.

Bioflavonoids have been shown to improve the utilization and to increase the storage of ascorbic acid in guinea pigs (3–5).

This study investigated the relative bioavailability of ascorbic acid provided by orange juice or by synthetic L-ascorbic acid in man by measuring ascorbic acid in serum, leucocytes, and urine. The synthetic vitamin was provided with and without rutin, a commercially available bioflavonoid which has been shown to improve ascorbic acid utilization in guinea pigs (4).

EXPERIMENTAL PROCEDURE

Twelve healthy adult male volunteers, six smokers and six non-smokers, were randomly allotted to the different treatments specified in Table 1.

Reprinted from *Journal of the American Dietetic Association*, Vol. 64, No. 3, March 1974. © The American Dietetic Association. Printed in U. S. A.

* Food Research Laboratories, Health Protection Branch, Health and Welfare—Canada, Ottawa, Ontario, Canada. The authors acknowledge the technical assistance of R. Brassard and R. Madere.

Table 1: Treatments,* experimental format, and subject data

Subject	Age	Body weight	Smoking volume	1st * and 4th † weeks				2nd week ‡	3rd week #
				Day 1 (Mon.)	Day 2 (Tues.)	Day 3 (Wed.)	Day 4 (Thurs.)		
	yr.	kg.	Cigarettes/ Day						
Non-smokers									
No. 1	26	73	0	—	I ¶	III	II	I	—
No. 2	24	60	0	—	II	I	III	I	—
No. 3	29	70	0	—	III	II	I	I	—
No. 4	44	86	0	—	I	III	II	I	—
No. 5	23	79	0	—	II	I	III	I	—
No. 6	27	64	0	—	III	II	I	I	—
Smokers									
No. 7	24	65	8	—	I	III	II	I	—
No. 8	26	82	24	—	II	I	III	I	—
No. 9	24	75	11	—	III	II	I	I	—
No. 10	44	67	21	—	I	III	II	I	—
No. 11	24	95	16	—	II	I	III	I	—
No. 12	28	61	22	—	III	II	I	I	—

* Presaturation.

† Post-saturation.

‡ Saturation—1 gm. ascorbic acid daily.

No treatment.

¶ I = synthetic L-ascorbic acid; II = synthetic L-ascorbic acid + rutin; III = orange juice.

Diets.   During each week of dosing, the subjects' diets from Sunday noon until after the last urine sample on Friday morning (Table 1) included no foods containing ascorbic acid or only trace amounts (6).   Breakfast was light and consistent on the days of blood sampling.   Each subject recorded the complete intake of solids and liquids during the restricted dietary periods.

Dose preparation.   The juice of fresh oranges was prepared on Day 1 of the first and fourth weeks and refrigerated in a closed container during Days 2, 3, and 4.   The cold juice was weighed just before administration to provide 75 mg. ascorbic acid per dose.

Total ascorbic plus dehydroascorbic acid (TAA) concentrations measured on Day 1 of each week were assumed to be constant during the three following days because of the high stability of ascorbic acid in orange juice (7).   Actual TAA concentrations on Days 1, 2, 3, and 4 were: 51.6, 51.8, 50.2 and 49.0 mg. per 100 gm., respectively, in the first week and 51.7, 51.7, 50.4, and 48.8 mg. per 100 gm., respectively, in the fourth week.

A solution of L-ascorbic acid [1] (3.0 gm. in 1 liter water) was prepared daily before dosing, and subjects designated to receive the synthetic vita-

[1] Nutritional Biochemicals Corp., Cleveland.

min (Table 1) received 25 ml. (75 mg. ascorbic acid) with or without 400 mg. rutin.[2]

The total volume of each test dose, including water to rinse the containers, was 160 ml. for all treatments.

Collection and preparation of samples. On Days 2, 3, and 4, between 8:30 and 9:30 a. m., two 10-ml. blood samples were collected[3] from each subject. One tube contained disodium ethylene diamine tetra acetic acid (EDTA) and the other contained no anticoagulant. Immediately after blood sampling, each subject received 75 mg. ascorbic acid provided by orange juice or by synthetic L-ascorbic acid with or without rutin (Table 1). The increase in serum and leucocyte TAA concentrations produced by each ascorbic acid source was measured exactly 2 hr. later when the serum TAA concentration was near its peak (8). TAA was measured in the six collections of urine taken during the 24 hr. following each dose: (four of 2 hr. each, one of 5 hr., and one of 11 hr.) For control values, samples of blood and urine were collected on Day 1.

Blood serum was obtained using standard procedures. A 2-ml. volume of serum was added to a mixture of 3.5 ml. of 4.5 per cent metaphosphoric acid and 2.5 ml. of 95 per cent ethanol. Samples were frozen, then centrifuged and filtered before TAA assay.

Blood containing disodium EDTA remained at room temperature 10 to 20 min. before the leucocyte separation. Approximately 5 ml. were added to duplicate 20×150 mm. test tubes each containing 5 ml. of a solution of 6 per cent bovine fibrinogen[4] in 0.9 per cent sodium chloride (9). The tubes were mixed by inversion ten times and placed in a vertical position for 8 min. The top layers containing leucocytes and platelets were removed by aspiration, pooled in a 15-ml. conical graduated centrifuge tube with stopper, and thoroughly mixed. A 0.5-ml. aliquot was diluted in 1 ml. of 0.9 per cent sodium chloride and shaken momentarily, after which a leucocyte count was immediately done[5]. The volume of the remaining leucocyte solution was recorded after centrifuging at $1,200 \times G$ for 15 min.; the clear supernatant was discarded. About 1 ml. of 2 per cent metaphosphoric acid was added to the precipitate, which was transferred to the vessel of a tissue grinder[6] using a stainless steel spatula and a mixer[7]. Volume in the vessel totaled about 4 ml. after rinsing the centrifuge tube with three portions of about 1 ml. of 2 per cent metaphosphoric acid. The homogenized solution was returned to the centrifuge tube. The total vol-

[2] From buckwheat. Supplier: Nutritional Biochemicals Corp.

[3] Using Vacutainers ®, Becton, Dickinson and Co.

[4] Nutritional Biochemicals Corp.

[5] Model F_N, Coulter Electronics, Hialeah, Florida.

[6] Borosilicate glass vessel, 4 ml., size AA, with Teflon pestle, from A. H. Thomas Co., Philadelphia.

[7] Vortex Jr., Mixer, from Scientific Industries, Inc., Queen's Village, New York.

ume was about 8 ml. after rinsing the vessel with 2 per cent metaphosphoric acid. The exact volume was recorded after the sample was centrifuged as described above. The clear supernatant was frozen in polyethylene vials until assayed for TAA.

Urine was collected in polyethylene bottles containing enough metaphosphoric acid to make a 2 per cent concentration after the urine was diluted to about one-half concentration. Aliquots were frozen on the same day the urine was collected except for overnight collections.

The method of Pelletier (10) was used to measure TAA in urine. TAA in leucocyte and serum extracts and in orange juice was measured by the same method adapted to an automated Technicon system (11).

Statistical analysis. The experiment (Table 1) was designed statistically to evaluate the effects of treatments (source of ascorbic acid), smoking, subject variation, day of test, order of treatments, and the interactions of these factors. Covariate analysis was used because of the large variation in basal values between subjects; the concentration of TAA in serum and leucocytes immediately before the dose was administered was used as the respective covariate for serum and leucocyte TAA concentrations measured after the dose; the concentration of TAA in the urine for 11 hr. preceding each dose was used as the covariate for TAA concentration in the 24-hr. urine sample after each treatment.

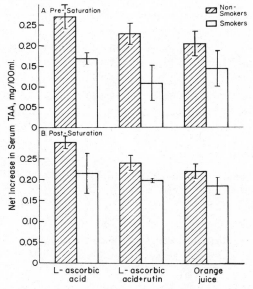

Figure 1: Effect of treatments and smoking on the net increase in TAA concentrations in serum obtained 2 hr. after ascorbic acid dose. Each bar represents the mean of six observations ± standard error of the mean.

When F-values were significant at or near the 0.05 level, further analysis using Student-Newman-Keul's (SNK) test was done to compare the adjusted means for each variable.

RESULTS

Ingestion of synthetic ascorbic acid without rutin caused a greater increase in serum TAA (Tables 2, 3) than ingestion of ascorbic acid with rutin or of orange juice in the presaturation period ($P<0.05$); a similar trend occurred in the post-saturation period ($P>0.05$). The test day affected serum TAA concentration ($P<0.05$) only in the presaturation period by causing higher levels after the first treatment (Table 3). The order of treatments and subject variation did not affect serum TAA concentration in either period. Smoking affected serum TAA concentration (Figure 1) by causing a smaller increase due to treatments, but the difference was significant ($P<0.05$) only in the presaturation period (Table 3).

Table 2: Effect of treatments on TAA concentrations in serum and leucocytes 2 hr. after the dose of ascorbic acid and in the urine collected during the first 24 hr. following each dose

Time of measurement	TAA *			F †
	Dose: ascorbic acid	Dose: ascorbic acid + rutin	Dose: orange juice	
	◄——— mg./100 ml. ———►			
Serum				
Presaturation				
before dose	0.67±0.06 ‡	0.70±0.05	0.69±0.06	—
after dose	0.88±0.08	0.86±0.08	0.87±0.08	6.08
Post-saturation				
before dose	0.88±0.04	0.90±0.04	0.93±0.05	—
after dose	1.13±0.05	1.11±0.04	1.14±0.05	3.19
	◄——— mcg./10^8 cells ———►			
Leucocytes				
Presaturation				
before dose	19.81±1.26	19.35±1.30	19.04±1.09	—
after dose	18.69±1.18	19.14±1.15	18.90±1.44	0.57
Post-saturation				
before dose	19.61±0.95	20.06±1.36	19.03±0.84	—
after dose	20.14±1.15	19.23±1.47	18.52±1.27	1.52
	◄——— mg./24 hr. ———►			
Urine				
Presaturation #	10.62±2.05	10.96±1.76	12.38±3.55	0.84
Post-saturation ¶	12.75±1.40	13.42±1.42	16.82±2.68	1.95

* Total ascorbic acid plus dehydro-ascorbic acid.

† F (2,21 df) = 3.47.

‡ Each value is mean of 12 observations ± standard error.

Basal excretion (Day 1) = 7.94±0.78.

¶ Basal excretion (Day 1) = 9.17±0.82.

Table 3: Application of Student-Newman-Keul's (SNK) test to the mean TAA concentrations * in serum obtained 2 hr. after an ascorbic acid dose

Effect	Mean TAA *								Number of observations per mean
	Ascorbic acid	Ascorbic acid + rutin	Orange juice	Smokers	Non-smokers	Day 2	Day 3	Day 4	
Presaturation period	← ——————————————————————— mg./100 ml. ——————————————————————— →								
Treatment	0.91[a]	0.85[b]	0.86[b]						12
Smoking				0.85[a]	0.90[b]				18
Days						0.82[a]	0.90[b]	0.89[b]	12
Post-saturation period									
Treatment	1.16[a]	1.12[a]	1.10[a]						

* Means with the same superscript within each variable are not significantly different (P>0.05). Each mean was adjusted by the respective covariate. See text.

Cumulative urinary excretion of TAA appeared to be slightly lower (P>0.05) in both periods after ingestion of L-ascorbic acid alone than after L-ascorbic acid plus rutin or after orange juice (Figure 2, Table 2). Urinary TAA was affected by subject variation in both periods (P<0.05) but not by smoking, order of treatments, or day of test.

In leucocytes, TAA concentration was not affected by treatments (Table 2), smoking, order of treatments, or day of test in either test period. Leucocyte TAA concentration was affected by subject variation in the post-saturation period.

Two subjects developed a cold during the third week (Table 1). Leucocyte TAA concentrations were not apparently affected in one. The other subject received antibiotic therapy; his leucocyte TAA concentration dropped slightly on Day 1 of the post-saturation period compared with presaturation levels, but returned to near presaturation levels on Days 2, 3, and 4.

There were no significant interaction effects (P>0.05) between sources of variation on TAA concentration in serum, leucocytes, or urine.

DISCUSSION

Higher serum concentrations in the presaturation (P<0.05) and post-saturation (P>0.05) periods 2 hr. after ingestion of synthetic ascorbic acid without rutin, compared with ascorbic acid plus rutin or orange juice, indicated a slightly greater bioavailability of synthetic ascorbic acid without rutin since more reached the systemic circulation. According to results of Todhunter *et al.* (8), peaks in serum ascorbic acid concentration would have occurred about 1.5 hr. after ingestion of either synthetic ascorbic acid or orange juice; consequently, the higher availability of syn-

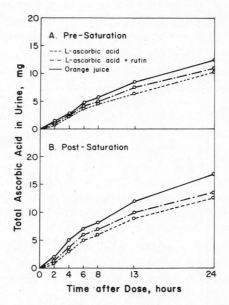

Figure 2: Effect of treatments on the cumulative excretion of TAA in urine at the end of each period. Points represent the mean of twelve observations.

thetic ascorbic acid apparently did not result from differences in absorption rates.

Although differences in the urinary excretion of TAA were not statistically significant, there was a tendency toward greater excretion of TAA after consumption of orange juice than after synthetic ascorbic acid without rutin (Figure 2). This was most evident in the post-saturation period when the differences in excretion showed within 2 hr. after dosing. A greater excretion of TAA after orange juice explains at least in part the lesser bioavailability evidenced by lower serum levels.

The higher serum levels and lower excretion of ascorbic acid that occurred with synthetic ascorbic acid alone compared with orange juice indicate slightly greater bioavailability of the synthetic vitamin. The synthetic L-ascorbic acid provided in freshly opened fruit drinks seems to be well utilized. However, based on this work, no claims can be made regarding the relative stability of ascorbic acid when the containers are opened and the contents allowed to stand for some time before consumption.

Ingestion of ascorbic acid with rutin apparently did not affect the urinary excretion of TAA, although it produced lower serum TAA levels. The rutin appeared to decrease the bioavailability of ascorbic acid, although the mechanism involved is not evident.

It is not surprising that bioflavonoids affect ascorbic acid utilization differently in man than in guinea pigs. In guinea pigs (12), ascorbic acid is rapidly broken down to carbon dioxide, producing a half-life of ascorbic acid of four days compared with eighteen days in man. The protection against oxidation afforded ascorbic acid by bioflavonoids should be more important for guinea pigs than man.

There were no treatment effects on leucocyte TAA concentrations. These levels are not likely to respond to short-term dietary influences, since leucocyte TAA concentrations indicate the amount of ascorbic acid stored in tissues (13), but they are expected to increase after saturation. However, seven subjects showed little or no increase in serum TAA concentration following saturation, indicating high initial ascorbic acid levels; leucocyte TAA concentrations in these subjects showed a similar pattern. In subjects whose serum TAA concentration increased after saturation, the magnitude of this increase was much greater than that in leucocyte TAA concentration. The latter indicated that there was little or no increase in body ascorbic acid status of individuals within each period of treatment, although the serum data reflected an increase (P<0.05) in TAA concentration between Days 2 and 3 in the presaturation period.

The net increase in serum TAA concentrations in the smokers was smaller (P<0.05) than in non-smokers in the presaturation period (Table 3, Figure 1). Smokers tend to store less ascorbic acid (14, 15), which could reflect a lower bioavailability.

SUMMARY

According to serum TAA concentrations, the bioavailability in human subjects of ascorbic acid provided by synthetic L-ascorbic acid is slightly superior to that of the natural vitamin provided by orange juice. A slightly higher urinary excretion of the vitamin after orange juice explains in part the lowering of the serum levels. A selected bioflavonoid, rutin, failed to promote better utilization of synthetic ascorbic acid.

REFERENCES

1. Hunter, B. T.: Consumer Beware! Your Food and What's Been Done to It. N.Y.: Simon & Schuster, 1971.

2. Harborne, J. B.: Comparative Biochemistry of the Flavonoids. N.Y.: Academic Press, Inc., 1967.

3. Cotereau, H., Gabe, M., Gero, E., and Parrot, J. L.: Influence of vitamin P (vitamin C_2) upon the amount of ascorbic acid in the organs of the guinea pig. Nature 161: 557, 1948.

4. Crampton, E. W., and Lloyd, L. E.: A quantitative estimation of the effect of rutin on the biological potency of vitamin C. J. Nutr. 41: 487, 1950.

5. Blanc, B., and Von der Muhll, M.: Interaction d'un facteur P (flavonoide) et de la vitamine C, son influence sur le poids du cobaye et le teneur en vitamine C de ses organes; effets de variations thermiques. Int. Z. Vitaminforsch 37: 156, 1967.

6. Heinz Nutritional Data, Fifth Edition. 2nd rev. prtg. Pittsburgh: H. J. Heinz Co., 1964.

7. Pelletier, O., and Morrison, A. B.: Content and stability of ascorbic acid in fruit drinks. J. Am. Dietet. A. 47: 401, 1965.

8. Todhunter, E. N., Robbins, R. C., and McIntosh, J. A.: The rate of increase of blood plasma ascorbic acid after ingestion of ascorbic acid (vitamin C). J. Nutr. 23: 309, 1942.

9. Skoog, W. A., and Beck, W. S.: Studies on the fibrinogen, dextran, and PHA methods of isolating leucocytes. Blood 11: 436, 1956.

10. Pelletier, O.: Differential determination of D-isoascorbic acid and L-ascorbic acid in guinea pig organs. Can. J. Biochem. 47: 449, 1969.

11. Pelletier, O., and Brassard, R.: A new automated serum vitamin C method. *In*: Advances in Automated Analysis. Technicon Intl. Congress, in press.

12. Burns, J. J., Dayton, P. G., and Schulenberg, S.: Further observations on the metabolism of L-ascorbic acid in guinea pigs. J. Biol. Chem. 218: 15, 1956.

13. Burch, H. B.: Methods for detecting and evaluating ascorbic acid deficiency in man and animals. Ann. N.Y. Acad. Sci. 92, Article I: 268, 1961.

14. Pelletier, O.: Smoking and vitamin C levels in humans. Am. J. Clin. Nutr. 21: 1259, 1968.

15. Pelletier, O.: Vitamin C status of cigarette smokers and non smokers. Am. J. Clin. Nutr. 23: 520, 1970.

21

DIETARY CALCIUM AND THE REVERSAL OF BONE DEMINERALIZATION

Leo Lutwak, M.D., Ph.D.*

The functions of dietary calcium and phosphorus have been considered repeatedly. We are now ready for a new look. Newer kinetic, endocrine, and nutrition knowledge may lead to a reevaluation of the role of dietary calcium in periodontitus and osteoporosis.

Almost 99 percent of the body's calcium is in the skeleton. The other 1 percent is found in extracellular fluid and participates in a number of life-support systems, i. e. blood clotting, hormone action, transport across cell membranes, and neuromuscular irritability. How does calcium move into and out of the body envelope?

Calcium can enter the body only through the diet. Several mechanisms exist, however, causing calcium to be continuously lost from the body. Renal excretion is relatively fixed for most individuals at between 100 and 200 milligrams daily under normal circumstances, relatively independent of dietary intake. Loss of calcium in the bile and pancreatic

Reprinted from *Nutrition News*, Vol. 37, No. 1, February 1974. Courtesy, National Dairy Council.

* Dr. Lutwak is Professor of Medicine at the University of California, Los Angeles, and Chief, Section of Endocrinology, Nutrition, and Metabolism in the Veterans Administration Hospital, Sepulveda, California. He has conducted extensive research in calcium, phosphorus, and magnesium metabolism; energy physiology; isotope kinetics; and clinical and space nutrition at Brookhaven National Laboratories, Yale University, Cornell University, and University of California. He is the author of many scientific articles and chapters in numerous scientific books. Dr. Lutwak has served as consultant to NASA and the National Institutes of Health.

juices, which are secreted into the gut and not reabsorbed, amounts to about 140 to 175 milligrams per day. Dermal losses of calcium average about 20 milligrams per day.

In the female, calcium may be lost in the development of the fetus during the last trimester of pregnancy and during lactation.

If the loss of calcium is less than the amount which is being absorbed from the diet, excess calcium will be present which can be deposited in the skeleton. If, however, the loss exceeds the intake, calcium then must be mobilized from the skeleton in order to maintain the homeostatic concentration in extracellular fluid necessary for life.

The mobilization of calcium is under the influence of various endocrine glands: pituitary, thyroid, adrenal, and parathyroid. Through the net effect of all of the hormone systems, calcium is deposited in or removed from the skeleton to help maintain the proper homeostatic concentration.

Are dietary calcium deficiencies sufficient to explain the development of periodontitis and osteoporosis?

Let's consider a hypothetical woman 50 years old and weighing about 135 pounds. Weighing almost the same at the age of 20, her skeleton would have contained about 1,500 grams of calcium. Now over the course of the past 30 years, having eaten a diet about average for middle-class American populations, daily dietary calcium would have dropped to 400 miligrams per day.

The National Research Council's Recommended Dietary Allowance for calcium is 800 milligrams. Many dietary surveys indicate that a vast majority of American adults, and particularly women homemakers, consume only about 400 milligrams daily. The range of absorption of a 400 milligram intake of calcium is between 10 and 50 percent.

If the losses are added (270) and the absorption (180) is subtracted, the difference is a 90 milligram negative balance per day. Over the course of 30 years, 90 *milligrams* per day totals 980 *grams* of calcium. With 1500 grams of calcium in the skeleton at age 20 and a negative balance of 980 grams of calcium by age 50, about one-third of the skeletal calcium remains.

Calcium absorption is greatly affected by the ratio of dietary calcium to phosphorus. In 1960 this ratio in the American diet was 1:2.8. U.S.D.A. figures at that time demonstrated that milk was the primary source of calcium. However, several major dietary sources of phosphorus exist. Milk provides some. Poultry, fish, and meat provide larger amounts. Significant changes in American diets have occurred since 1960. Milk consumption has decreased while meat consumption has increased. People who no longer drink milk substitute other liquids, which, in the last few years, have tended to be non-nutritious soft drinks some of which contain excess phosphorus in the form of phosphoric acid. Such dietary changes have caused an increase in phosphorus intake and a decrease in calcium intake so that the calcium/phosphorous ratio today approaches 1:4, a striking imbalance.

This imbalance in calcium/phosphorous ratio, decreased efficiency of the body to absorb calcium as age increases, coupled with an inadequate dietary calcium supply may lead to serious problems of skeletal health.

Coincidental appearance of severe periodontal disease with disruption of trabecular bone structure in the jaw as well as vertebral fractures and osteoporosis elsewhere in the body have been found. Review of hospital records indicates virtually a 1:1 ratio of patients having periodontal disease in association with osteoporosis. This has lead to the conclusion that some forms of periodontal disease with resorption of bone may very well be the long sought for preosteoporotic condition wherein the patient is still capable of regenerating bone.

A group of 90 patients with mild degrees of periodontal disease were selected as patients with possible preosteoporosis. Bone density was measured at the start of the study and at monthly intervals thereafter by photon densitometry. Patients were divided into groups that received either a one gram calcium supplement daily or a corresponding placebo for 12 months. There were only minor statistically significant differences measured in bone density of radius or ulna (arm bones) noted during this period of time.

Significant changes were seen in the jaw. The group receiving the placebo showed no significant change over the 12 months. The group receiving calcium supplements showed approximately 12½ percent statistically significant increase in bone density as a result of supplementation with dietary calcium.

What is the possible role of dietary calcium in bone metabolism? The usual individual eats three or four meals per day. Within half an hour to about two hours after the meal is eaten serum calcium rises, if calcium has been present in the food. This rise is slight, but detectable. Subsequently, serum calcium falls because of accretion processes and excretion. The resulting push-pull action continues through the day, with serum calcium rising and falling, and bone being formed and resorbed. If, however, the amount of dietary calcium is inadequate, if losses from the body exceed the amount that is being absorbed, there is no time during the day when bone resorption of calcium can take place. Thus, we may suggest a logical mechanism for the prevention and therapy of osteoporosis, is utilizing adequate amounts of dietary calcium to avoid bone resorption.

Periodontal disease, as defined by dentists, is any disease which affects any of the tissues surrounding the tooth, the periodontal tissues, the gingiva, the gum, the alveolar bone, the periodontal membrane, or the cementum that holds the tooth to the socket.

We have hypothesized that the primary disease causes a decrease in density of the alveolar bone in a significant number of patients with periodontal disease. Following a gradual continuous loss of calcium from this supporting bone, the teeth begin to move about in their sockets. Gradually, chewing beings to cause irritation and damage to the gingiva. The damaged tissue bleeds, shows inflammatory changes, and becomes readily infected with plaque. If our hypothesis is correct, some types of periodontal disease could be reversed by repleting dietary calcium. It should be mentioned, however, that certain types of periodontal disease affect only the gingiva and have no effect on the bone.

Based on our research findings there is a hierarchy of change when bones start to demineralize under osteoporotic conditions. First, decreases in bone density are detected in the jawbone, then in the vertebrae and other bones in the body. If periodontal disease is correctly diagnosed and correctly treated by increasing the dietary calcium at the time it's first found, then the vertebral disease (osteoporosis) doesn't progress to the point where fracture can occur.

People visit dentists on a regular basis but only go to physicians after trouble is well-established. An excellent example of preventive medicine in action can be illustrated by the dentist who detects early jawbone demineralization. If his diagnosis is substantiated, he can initiate proper therapeutic regimens to improve calcium intake before the disease has progressed to osteoporosis of the vertebrae.

This hypothesis is based on quite preliminary information from which we hope eventually to build a greater body of facts.

22

"NEWER" TRACE ELEMENTS IN HUMAN NUTRITION

F. H. Nielsen *

The ultimate goal of nutrition research is to assure the population of an optimal dietary intake of essential nutrients and to prevent overexposure to others. For some time, it was believed that this goal had been obtained and that a diet including a reasonable variety of foods would furnish an adequate intake of all the essential nutrients. However, the era of affluence we are experiencing today has resulted in the increased consumption of highly refined foods, food product analogs, and empty calories. Examples of the latter include some snack foods, alcoholic beverages, and soft drinks. Inappropriate excessive consumption of these nonnutritious food items may lead to nutritional deficiencies through their replacement of conventional foods.

It is also possible that deficiencies may occur when refined foods or food product analogs which are incomplete in nutrient content are used as the major constituents of the diet. The trace mineral content of such foods is of particular concern because, at the present time, knowledge of man's requirements for trace elements is incomplete. This is especially true for five elements—vanadium, nickel, silicon, fluorine, and tin—which have been found to be essential for laboratory animals since 1970. It seems probable that these elements are also essential for man. For the

Reprinted from *Food Technology*, January 1974, pp. 38–44.

Based on a paper presented at the 33rd Annual Meeting of the Institute of Food Technologists, Miami Beach, Fla., June 10–13, 1973.

* The author is with the Human Nutrition Laboratory, USDA/ARS, P.O. Box D, University Station, Grand Forks, N. Dak. 58201.

purpose of this report, silicon is considered as a trace element, even though it is apparently required in relatively high amounts.

VANADIUM ESSENTIAL FOR ANIMALS

Data supporting the view that vanadium is an essential element for animals was first reported by Hopkins and Mohr (1971a; b). The initial finding was a significantly reduced growth of wing and tail feathers in chicks fed a diet containing less than 10 ppb vanadium. Since then, several additional deficiency symptoms attributable to low levels of dietary vanadium have been reported in rats and chicks.

Strasia (1971) found that rats fed less than 100 ppb vanadium in the diet exhibited reduced body growth and a significantly increased blood packed cell volume when compared with controls receiving at least 0.5 ppm vanadium. He also noted an increase in blood and bone iron in deficient rats. About the same time, Schwarz and Milne (1971) found that rats fed a highly purified amino acid diet (containing an unknown amount of vanadium) demonstrated a growth response to 50–100 ppb vanadium. Chicks apparently require more than 30–35 ppb vanadium, as depressed growth occurs at that dietary level (Nielsen, 1973).

Vanadium appears to have a role in lipid metabolism, as shown in Table 1. Hopkins and Mohr (1971a; b) found that vanadium-deficient chicks had decreased plasma levels of cholesterol at 28 days of age, but that at 49 days their plasma cholesterol concentrations were greater than those of control chicks. Recently, increased plasma cholesterol levels have been found in vanadium-deficient chicks after only 28 days of deficiency (Nielsen and Ollerich, 1973a). Other recent data (Hopkins and Mohr, 1973) indicate that plasma triglyceride levels are also significantly increased in vanadium-deficient chicks.

In rats, reproductive performance is impaired by vanadium deprivation (Hopkins and Mohr, 1973). When five fourth-generation female rats were mated, there were significantly fewer live births and significantly more deaths of neonatal pups than with vanadium-sufficient controls.

Another recent finding has been the demonstration that vanadium deficiency retards bone development in chicks (Nielsen and Ollerich, 1973a). Histologically, the vanadium-deficient chick tibia shows severe disorganization of the cells in the epiphysis. The cells appear compressed and their nuclei seem flattened. These abnormalities apparently result in a shortened, thickened leg structure. The uptake and distribution of $^{35}SO_4=$ and hexosamine concentrations in the epiphysis are similar to those of the controls. It seems, therefore, that mucopolysaccharide metabolism is not affected by vanadium deficiency.

These data from 4 different laboratories, and on 2 different species, have established that vanadium is an essential nutrient for higher animals.

Table 1: Effect of vanadium deficiency on chick plasma lipids

Lipid	Vanadium-deficient diet	Vanadium-supplemented diet
Cholesterol, mg/100 ml		
(28 days) [a]	178	206
(49 days) [a]	249	224
(28 days) [b]	158(12) [c]	145(12)
(28 days) [d]	182(10)	163(10)
Triglycerides, mg/100 ml [e]	48.7(9)	25.4(9)

[a] Hopkins and Mohr (1971b).
[b] Nielsen and Ollerich (1973a).
[c] Number of chicks.
[d] Nielsen (1973).
[e] Hopkins and Mohr (1973).

VANADIUM INTAKE MAY BE INSUFFICIENT

Due to limited data, the level of vanadium required by rats and chicks to maintain health can only be estimated, but it appears that an intake of approximately 100 ppb is probably adequate. This is equivalent to about 34 µg/1,000 calories of experimental diet composed of 26% protein, 6% fat, and 57% carbohydrate (balance: minerals, vitamins, and non-nutritive fiber).

Information as to the amount of vanadium in natural feeds and foods is limited. This is in part due to the difficulty in accurately analyzing for low levels of vanadium. Soremark (1967) reported values obtained by activation analysis. These range from less than 0.1 ppb vanadium in peas, beets, carrots, and pears to 52 ppb in radishes. Milk generally contains less than 0.1 ppb (fresh basis), and liver, fish, and meat contain up to 10 ppb. Schroeder et al. (1963) found few foods rich in vanadium—these include bread, some grains and nuts, and a few root vegetables. These limited data indicate that many dietary items contain amounts of vanadium which are below 100 ppb. Table 2 gives representative levels of vanadium found in some foods.

Obviously, many additional data are needed before firm conclusions can be drawn; but enough data are available to suggest that the required intake of vanadium for animals will not necessarily be consumed in an ordinary diet. If man has a vanadium requirement which is similar to that of rats and chicks, adequate vanadium nutrition should not be taken for granted. A diet exclusively of milk, meat, and certain vegetables could contain less than 34 µg of vanadium per 1,000 calories.

Although the extrapolation of animal data to man can be misleading, the observation of altered lipid metabolism (i. e., increased plasma cholesterol and triglycerides) in vanadium-deficient animals makes one wonder if marginal vanadium deficiency indeed occurs in man and if it is in part responsible for the increased serum lipid concentrations which occur in some individuals. Obviously, this is highly speculative at present, as there are no data available which test the hypothesis.

Table 2: Levels of trace elements in selected fresh foods

Food	Vanadium (ppb)	Nickel [e] (ppb)	Silicon [f] (ppm)	Fluorine (ppm)	Tin [i] (ppm)
Milk	<0.1 [a]	0.0	1.4	0.1–0.2 [g]	0.19–0.68
Eggs	370–680 [b]	30	20–40	0.8–0.9 [h]	0.91
Red meat	<0.1 [a, b]	0–20	5–15	≃2.0 [h]	0.3 –3.0
Fish	0.0 [b]	20–50	≃5	5–10 [g, h]	0.49–3.0
Oysters	110 [b]	1,500	—	—	1.38
Corn oil	119 [c]	0.0	0.0	—	4.10
Rice	230–820 [b]	300–650	10,000 (dry)	1–3 [g]	0.28
Oats	1,630 [b]	1,710	5,700 (dry)	1–3 [g]	2.28
Wheat	0.0 [b]	0–160	200 (dry)	1–3 [g]	0.0
Bread	70 [b]	1,130	—	—	2.48
Peanuts	0.0 [b]	—	200 (meal)	—	—
Peas	<0.1 [a]	300	—	—	1.06
Lettuce	20 [a]	140	—	—	0.07
Apples	0.0 [b]	0–80	—	—	—
Sucrose	5 [d]	30	5–7	—	—

[a] Soremark (1967).
[b] Schroeder et al. (1963).
[c] Welch (1973).
[d] Nielsen (1973).
[e] Schroeder et al. (1962).
[f] Carlisle (1973b).
[g] Schwarz (1971).
[h] Underwood (1971).
[i] Schroeder et al. (1964).

NICKEL HAS PHYSIOLOGICAL ROLE

Until recently, only indirect evidence suggested that nickel has a physiological role in living organisms. Now, direct evidence has been provided which supports the hypothesis (Nielsen and Sauberlich, 1970; Nielsen, 1971; Nielsen and Higgs, 1971; Nielsen and Ollerich, 1973b). By using a diet containing 3–4 ppb nickel, and a trace element controlled environment, pathologic signs consistent with nickel deficiency have been produced in chicks and rats.

Day-old chicks fed the nickel-deficient diet for 3½ weeks showed few gross signs when compared with controls fed 3 ppm nickel. Their shank skin pigmentation was altered, and their livers were less friable than those of the controls. Other gross signs were inconsistent. In contrast, certain biochemical abnormalities were more consistently found. These included a decreased oxygen uptake by liver homogenates in the presence of α-glycerophosphate, an increase in liver total lipids, and a decrease in the liver phospholipid fraction (Table 3). The total lipids and the phospholipids of the heart were both increased (Table 3).

Table 3: Effect of nickel deficiency on liver oxidative ability and liver and heart lipids of chicks [a]

Group	No. of chicks	O$_2$ update [b] (μl/hr/mg protein)	Total lipid, liver [c] (%)	Lipid phosphorus, liver [c] (mg/g)	Total lipid, heart [c] (%)	Lipid phosphorus, heart [c] (mg/g)
Experiment 1						
Ni-def. (3 ppb)	12	4.7 [d]±0.2 [e]	6.21 [f]±0.10	—	—	—
+ 3 ppm Ni	12	5.5 ±0.2	5.78 ±0.11	—	—	—
Experiment 2						
Ni-def. (4 ppb)	11	5.4 [g]±0.2	6.27 [f]±0.18	1.327 [d]±0.016	4.09 [f]±0.06	0.942 [g]±0.007
+ 3 ppm Ni	11	6.0 ±0.2	5.87 ±0.05	1.379 ±0.016	3.85 ±0.11	0.898 ±0.010
Experiment 3						
Ni-def. (14 ppb)	12	5.5 [g]±0.1	5.71 ±0.09	1.318 ±0.016	—	—
+ 3 ppm	12	5.9 ±0.1	5.55 ±0.10	1.335 ±0.015	—	—

[a] Nielsen and Ollerich (1973b) and Nielsen (1973).
[b] Using liver homogenates and with α-glycerophosphate as the substrate.
[c] Fresh weight basis.
[d] Significantly different (P <0.025) from + 3 ppm Ni group.
[e] ± Standard error of the mean.
[f] Significantly different (P <0.05) from + 3 ppm Ni group.
[g] Significantly different (P <0.10) from + 3 ppm Ni group.

Ultrastructural abnormalities in the hepatocytes were also a consistent finding. These included dilation of the cisterns of the rough endoplasmic reticulum and swelling of the mitochondria. The swelling of the mitochondria was in the compartment of the matrix and was associated with fragmentation of the cristae. Other ultrastructural changes included a dilation of the perinuclear space and pyknotic nuclei. These findings extend earlier work in which Sunderman et al. (1972) found less severe ultistructural changes in the livers of chicks deprived of nickel.

NICKEL APPEARS TO BE ESSENTIAL

Results from rat studies are more preliminary (Nielsen and Ollerich, 1973b; Nielsen, 1973). Successive generations of rats have been raised. Thus, the animals have been exposed to deficiency throughout fetal, neonatal, and adult life. Reproduction apparently is affected, as seven first-generation nickel-deficient dams had a significant number of dead pups (15%), compared with no mortality in the young of six controls. Nine second-generation nickel-deficient dams had a 19% loss of pups. This finding was confounded by the fact that the eight controls had a 10% loss of pups; this was, however, roughly half the loss in the deficient group. The pups of the nickel-deficient dams also weighed less at 4 days and 24 days than those of the controls. In the third generation, the nickel-deficient pups showed a generally less thrifty appearance and were less active.

Nickel deficiency in rats, as in chicks, results in a decreased in-vitro liver oxidation of α-glycerophosphate. In addition, in the nickel-deficient rat liver, preliminary sucrose density gradients of liver postmitochondrial supernatants have been consistent with a decrease in polysomes and an increase in monosomes.

Thus, nickel also appears to be essential. The major effects of deficiency so far identified have occurred principally in the liver. Ultramicroscopic morphology, oxidative ability, and lipid levels have been affected.

NICKEL DEFICIENCY NOT A PROBLEM

As with vanadium, the level of nickel required by animals to maintain health can only be approximated. It has been suggested that an intake of 50–80 ppb of nickel, or approximately 16–25 μg/1,000 calories of experimental diet, is probably adequate for the rat and chick. The experimental diet contained 26% proteins, 11% fat, 47% carbohydrates, and 16% fiber, minerals, and vitamins.

Nickel is ubiquitous. Grains and vegetables are particularly rich in nickel (Table 2). Knowledge concerning the chemical form of nickel in foods of plant origin is limited (Tiffin, 1971). It has been shown that nickel translocates in plants as a stable anionic amino acid complex. Whether organic nickel complexes are the usual compounds of nickel in plant tissues, and whether they in any way influence the bioavailability of nickel, remain to be determined. It is important to note that grains, which are indeed rich in nickel, are also high in phytin. Nickel can form a stable complex with phytic acid. (Vohra et al., 1965). Thus, it appears possible that the phytate in grains and other vegetables may decrease the availability of dietary nickel for intestinal absorption. In contrast to foods of plant origin, those of animal origin contain relatively little nickel.

At present, it appears that nickel nutriture is not a practical problem for man. If animal data can be extrapolated to man, then the dietary requirement is probably in the range of 16–25 μg/1,000 calories. Most diets will provide this amount. On the other hand, nickel nutriture may conceivably be of concern in individuals with diseases which interfere with intestinal absorption, or who are under extreme physiological stress, or who have unusual dietary habits. It is known that the level of nickel in plasma is decreased in patients with cirrhosis of the liver or with chronic uremia (McNeely et al., 1971). Perhaps these findings are indicative of nickel depletion.

Another consideration is the relatively high concentrations of nickel in sweat (Horak and Sunderman, 1973). Conditions which result in large losses of sweat may conceivably increase the need for nickel. Finally, diets high in foods of animal origin and/or fats may be low in nickel. A human diet containing 1.3–4.3 µg of nickel per 1,000 calories has been prepared from meat, milk, eggs, refined white bread, butter, and corn oil (Schroeder et al., 1962); protein supplied 17.4% of the calories, carbohydrate 43.5% and fat 39.1%.

Studies are needed to define the level of nickel required by man, and to ascertain whether nickel deficiency occurs naturally.

SILICON ESSENTIAL FOR ANIMALS

Silicon is one of the newest elements to be shown essential for animals. It was first reported (Carlisle, 1970; 1971) that silicon is necessary for an early stage of bone calcification in rats and chicks. The first clear evidence that silicon is essential for animals was reported in 1972 (Carlisle, 1972a; b). Chicks fed a silicon-deficient diet had depressed growth. Pallor of the legs, combs, skin, and mucous membranes occurred. The subcutaneous tissue had a muddy to yellowish color in contrast to the white-pinkish subcutaneous tissue of the silicon-adequate control animals. The deficient chicks had no wattles, and their combs were severely attenuated. Feathering was retarded. Leg bones had a thinner cortex and were shorter and of small circumference than were those of controls. Femurs and tibiae fractured more easily, cranial bones were flatter, and beaks were more flexible. These latter gross signs supported the earlier suggestion that silicon is involved in some aspect of bone calcification.

It also was found (Schwarz and Milne, 1972a) that silicon deficiency in rats results in depressed growth and skull deformations. Recently, it has been shown (Carlisle, 1973a) that the skeletal alterations involve the cartilage matrix. In the silicon-deficient chick metatarsus and tibial epiphyses, epiphyseal plates, and spongiosae, there is a significant decrease in hexosamines.

A role for silicon in mucopolysaccharide metabolism is further supported by the finding that silicon is a constituent of certain glycosaminoglycans and polyuronides, where it is apparently bound to the polysaccharide matrix (Schwarz, 1973). Schwarz (1973) has reported 330–554 ppm of bound silicon in purified hyaluronic acid from umbilical cord, chondroitin 4-sulfate, dermatan sulfate, and heparan sulfate. These levels correspond to 1 atom of silicon per 50,000–85,000 molecular weight, or 130–280 repeating units. Lesser amounts (57–191 ppm) were found in chondroitin 6-sulfate, heparin, and keratan sulfate-2 from cartilage; hyaluronic acid from vitreous humor and keratan sulfate-1 from cornea were silicon-free. Schwarz has concluded from various biochemical studies that silicon is present as a silanolate, i. e., an ether (or ester-like) derivative of silicic acid, and has postulated that silicon has a structural role in the glycosamino-glycans and polyuronides. Silicon may link portions of the same polysaccharides to each other, or acid mucopolysaccharides to proteins. Thus, it has been suggested that silicon may function as a biological crosslinking agent, and may contribute to the structure and resilience of connective tissue.

SHOULD STUDY SILICON ROLE IN HUMANS

Carlisle (1973b) has estimated that the chick requirement for silicon as sodium silicate is in the range of 100–200 ppm, or approximately 26–52 mg/1,000 calories of experimental diet containing 26% amino acids, 5% fat, 62% carbohydrate, and 7% minerals and vitamins. It is probable that other forms of silicon are more available than the silicate. Thus, the absolute requirement probably is lower than suggested above. Foods high in silicon include unrefined grains such as unpolished rice (Carlisle, 1973b). For those who drink their calories, it should be reassuring that beer is a saturated solution of silicon, containing approximately 1,200 ppm. Dietary items of animal origin, except skin (i. e., chicken), are relatively low in silicon.

At present, a role for silicon in human nutrition can only be postulated. Its possible function in mucopolysaccharide metabolism suggests that certain connective tissue diseases should be studied with regard to their effects on silicon metabolism and the possibility that abnormal silicon metabolism may be a contributory factor in their occurrence. In addition, the effects of aging on silicon status should be assessed. Observations in the rat indicate that silicon levels of some tissues decrease with age (Charnot and Peres, 1971).

FLUORINE MUST BE CONSIDERED ESSENTIAL

A beneficial function of fluorine has been known since the late 1930s, when it was discovered that the fluoride ion can play a significant role in the prevention of human dental caries. In the 1960s, it was reported that treating patients suffering from osteoporosis and other demineralizing diseases with substantial amounts of sodium fluoride may result in beneficial effects upon back pains, bone density, and calcium balance. Epidemiological studies have shown that there is substantially less osteoporosis in high-fluoride areas than in low-fluoride areas.

Apparently, fluorine is not only beneficial for the maintenance of teeth, but also for the maintenance of a normal skeleton in the adult. These effects of fluorine have been reviewed by Underwood (1971). If an essential element is defined as one which is ordinarily required for health and well-being under the usual conditions in which individuals live, then in the light of the above evidence, fluorine must be considered as an essential element in human nutrition.

MORE FLUORINE RESEARCH NEEDED

Recently, interest in fluorine has been stimulated by unconfirmed reports that fluorine may be necessary for normal hematocrit levels, fertility, and growth. It was found that during the stress of pregnancy, feeding diets low in fluoride resulted in decreased hematocrits in mice (Messer et al., 1972b). Also, a marked decrease in fertility apparently occurred (Messer et al., 1972a). The number of litters produced by first- and second-generation females was reduced, but litter size was not affected. The condition was prevented by the addition of 50 ppm of fluorine in the drinking water.

It also was reported that fluorine could stimulate the growth of rats fed a highly purified amino acid diet and maintained in trace element controlled isolators (Schwarz and Milne, 1972b). This observation was received with reservation for the following reasons: • Experimental methods were inadequately described. • The control rats grew suboptimally, even though they were supplemented with fluorine. • Although significant, the differences in weight gain between the deficient and the control animals were small, approximately 6 g over 26 days, even though the diet contained all known essential elements including vanadium, silicon, and tin. • Others have not been able to confirm this finding even though they have fed diets containing less fluorine (Underwood, 1971). Clearly more research will be necessary before it can be stated that fluorine is essential for growth.

At present, a requirement for fluorine cannot be estimated. However, 1–2 ppm (0.23–0.46 mg/1,000 calories) in the diet (Schwarz, 1971; Schwarz and Milne, 1972b) or water (Underwood, 1971) appears beneficial. Foods high in fluorine include seafoods (5–10 ppm) and tea (100 ppm). Cereal and other grains contain 1–3 ppm. Cow's milk usually contains 1–2 ppm on a dry basis (Schwarz, 1971; Underwood, 1971).

An important source of fluorine is drinking water. On the basis of the above experimental studies in animals and studies in man with osteoporosis, it may well be that fluoridation of city water supplies is beneficial in ways other than the prevention of caries.

SUFFICIENT TIN IN CURRENT FOODS

Trace amounts of tin occur in many tissues and dietary items, but until recently, the element has been considered an "environmental contaminant" instead of an essential dietary factor. In 1970, it was reported that tin is essential for the growth of rats maintained on purified amino acid diets in a trace element controlled environment (Schwarz et al., 1970). Rats required 1 ppm tin as stannic sulfate, or approximately 0.23 mg of tin per 1,000 calories of experimental diet, for optimal growth.

Tin has a number of chemical properties which offer possibilities for biological function.   Tetravalent tin has a strong tendency to form co-ordination complexes with 4, 5, 6, and possibly 8 ligands.   Thus, it has been suggested by Schwarz et al. (1970) that tin may contribute to the tertiary structure of proteins or other components of biological impor-tance.   Schwarz et al. (1970) have also speculated that tin may partici-pate in oxidation-reduction reactions in biological systems because the $Sn+^2 \rightleftharpoons Sn+^4$ potential of 0.13 volt is within the physiological range. In fact, it is near the oxidation-reduction potential of flavine enzymes.

The levels of tin found to promote growth in rats are similar to the amounts found in many foods of plant and animal origin (Schwarz et al., 1970).   Therefore, tin nutriture is not of concern at present.   On the other hand, increased use of highly refined foods, or food product analogs con-taining little or no tin, may alter this judgment in the future.

SHOULD INCLUDE TRACE ELEMENTS IN FOODS

In summary, four new elements—vanadium, nickel, silicon, and tin—have been found essential and one—fluorine—possibly essential for ani-mals.   To date, these elements have not been shown essential for man. However, by extrapolation from animal data, it is possible to postulate their importance in human nutrition.   Moreover, the recognition of human deficiencies of other trace elements, such as zinc and copper, in certain populations and in patients with specific diseases, supports the concept that these less understood trace elements are probably also important for man.

Thus, human deficiency of one, or more, of the trace elements dis-cussed in this paper may be observed in the future.   If people are con-suming diets low in any of these elements, it is currently not clinically rec-ognized.   It is also unknown whether subclinical or marginal deficiencies occur.   In any case, prevention of marginal deficiencies may be prudent. Inclusion of reasonable amounts of these less well understood trace ele-ments in food product analogs and their replacement in refined foods may be desirable.

It is my opinion that the speculations and suppositions I have made today may be established as true in the not too distant future.   In addi-tion, thanks to improved experimental technology, trace element research is moving so rapidly that this discussion may be out of date by the time it is published and other trace elements will have been added to the list of "newer" trace elements which are probably essential for man.

REFERENCES

1. Carlisle, E. M.   1970.   Silicon: A possible factor in bone calcification. Science 167: 279.

2. Carlisle, E. M. 1971. A relationship between silicon, magnesium, and fluorine in bone formation in the chick (abstract). Fed. Proc. 30: 462.

3. Carlisle, E. M. 1972a. Silicon an essential element for the chick (abstract). Fed. Proc. 31: 700.

4. Carlisle, E. M. 1972b. Silicon: An essential element for the chick. Science 178: 619.

5. Carlisle, E. M. 1973a. A skeletal alteration associated with silicon deficiency (abstract). Fed. Proc. 32: 930.

6. Carlisle, E. M. 1973b. Personal communication. School of Public Health, Univ. of California, Los Angeles.

7. Charnot, Y. and Peres, G. 1971. Contribution to the study of the endocrine regulation of silicon metabolism (Fr.) Ann. Endocrinol., Paris, 32: 397.

8. Hopkins, L. L. Jr. and Mohr, H. E. 1971a. The biological essentiality of vanadium. In "Newer Trace Elements in Nutrition," p. 195, ed. Mertz, W. and Cornatzer, W. E. Marcel Dekker, Inc., New York.

9. Hopkins, L. L. Jr. and Mohr, H. E. 1971b. Effect of vanadium deficiency on plasma cholesterol of chicks (abstract). Fed. Proc. 30: 462.

10. Hopkins, L. L. Jr. and Mohr, H. E. 1973. Vanadium as an essential element. Submitted for publication in Fed. Proc.

11. Horak, E. and Sunderman, F. W. Jr. 1973. Scientific note: Fecal nickel excretion by healthy adults. Clin. Chem. 19: 429.

12. McNeeley, M. D., Sunderman, F. W. Jr., Nechay, M. W., and Levine, H. 1971. Abnormal concentrations of nickel in serum in cases of myocardial infarction, stroke, burns, hepatic cirrhosis, and uremia. Clin. Chem. 17: 1123.

13. Messer, H. H., Armstrong, W. D., and Singer, L. 1972a. Fertility impairment in mice on a low fluoride diet. Science 177: 893.

14. Messer, H. H., Wong, K., Wegner, M., Singer, L., and Armstrong, W. D. 1972b. Effect of reduced fluoride intake by mice on haematocrit values. Nature (New Biology) 240: 218.

15. Nielsen, F. H. 1971. Studies on the essentiality of nickel. In "Newer Trace Elements in Nutrition," p. 215, ed. Mertz, W. and Cornatzer, W. E. Marcel Dekker, Inc., New York.

16. Nielsen, F. H. 1973. Unpublished data. Human Nutrition Laboratory. USDA/ARS, Grand Forks, N. Dak.

17. Nielsen, F. H. and Higgs, D. J. 1971. Further studies involving a nickel deficiency in chicks. Proc. Trace Subs. Environ. Health 4: 241.

18. Nielsen, F. H. and Ollerich, D. A. 1973a. Studies on a vanadium deficiency in chicks (abstract). Fed. Proc. 32: 929.

19. Nielsen, F. H. and Ollerich, D. A. 1973b. Nickel: A new essential trace element. Submitted for publication in Fed. Proc.

20. Nielsen, F. H. and Sauberlich, H. E. 1970. Evidence of a possible requirement for nickel by the chick. Proc. Soc. Exp. Biol. Med. 134: 845.

21. Schroeder, H. A., Balassa, J. J., and Tipton, I. H. 1962. Abnormal trace metals in man—nickel. J. Chron. Dis. 15: 51.

22. Schroeder, H. A., Balassa, J. J., and Tipton, I. H. 1963. Abnormal trace metals in man—vanadium. J. Chron. Dis. 16: 1047.

23. Schroeder, H. A., Balassa, J. J., and Tipton, I. H. 1964. Abnormal trace metals in man—tin. J. Chron. Dis. 17: 483.

24. Schwarz, K. 1971. Trace elements newly identified as essential to animals (Fluorine as an essential element). Presented at the 138th meeting of the Am. Assn. for the Advancement of Science.

25. Schwarz, K. 1973. Recent dietary trace element research, exemplified by tin and fluorine. Submitted for publication in Fed. Proc.

26. Schwarz, K. and Milne, D. B. 1971. Growth effects of vanadium in the rat. Science 174: 426.

27. Schwarz, K. and Milne, D. B. 1972a. Growth promoting effects of silicon in rats. Nature 239: 333.

28. Schwarz, K. and Milne, D. B. 1972b. Fluorine requirement for growth in the rat. Bioinorg. Chem. 1: 331.

29. Schwarz, K., Milne, D. B., and Vinyand, E. 1970. Growth effects of tin compounds in rats maintained in a trace element controlled environment. Biochem. Biophys. Res. Comm. 40: 22.

30. Soremark, R. 1967. Vanadium in some biological specimens. J. Nutr. 92: 183.

31. Strasia, C. A. 1971. Vanadium: Essentiality and toxicity in the laboratory rat. Ph.D. thesis, University Microfilms, Ann Arbor, Mich.

32. Sunderman, F. W. Jr., Nomoto, S., Morang, R., Nechay, M. W., Burke, C. N., and Nielsen, S. W. 1972. Nickel deprivation in chicks. J. Nutr. 102: 259.

33. Tiffin, L. O. 1971. Translocation of nickel in xylem exudate of plants. Plant Physiol. 48: 273.

34. Underwood, E. J. 1971. "Trace Elements in Human and Animal Nutrition," p. 369. Academic Press, New York.

35. Vohra, P., Gray, G. A., and Kratzer, F. H. 1965. Phytic acid-metal complex. Proc. Soc. Exp. Biol. Med. 120: 447.

36. Welch, R. M. 1973. Personal communication. Soil & Nutrition Laboratory, USDA/ARS, Ithaca, N. Y.

D

The crisis surrounding certain foods
and unusual dietary practices

D The crisis surrounding certain foods

THIS CHAPTER reviews the value of certain foods in the diet. The first issue considered is athletes' diets. Athletes often stuff themselves with vitamins, protein pills and wheat germ oil in an attempt to ensure a victory. The author of the first article asked U. S. athletes from the 20th Olympic Games about their dietary practices. The answers, as might be expected, range from excessive intakes to a normal diet. The author concludes that genetics and physical training are more important determinants of athletic ability than diet. In the next article Dr. Mickelsen points out that the athletes do not need extra vitamins, and so forth. They get all they need from their higher caloric intake. The only problem they have is maintaining an adequate water intake.

Another subject of controversy is sugared cereal. Between 1970 and 1973, the U. S. Senate held many hearings on the value of sugared breakfast cereals. Robert Choate, a civil engineer turned nutrition advocate, damned cereals for their high sugar content and poor nutritional value. Many activist groups also wanted these cereals banned because they supposedly cause dental caries. The next articles examine this controversy.

E. B. Hayden traces the role of cereals as a provider of a balanced breakfast, especially for children. He also points out their importance in terms of low cost and addition to milk consumption.

Because of the growing concern over the value of the U. S. processed food supply, many young people have turned to special dietary regimens. Their choices often are based on religious, philosophical, sociological or political considerations rather than on nutritional soundness. One of these diets is the Zen Macrobiotic diet. The next article, a comment by the AMA Council on Foods and Nutrition on the Zen Macrobiotic diet, warns of the dangers involved. Following this is an excellent article on vegetarianism. The article reviews various types of vegetarian practices and gives diet recommendations on how to ensure good health.

One purveyor of special dietary supplements, health foods and organic foods was Adelle Davis, now deceased, who some called the grandmother of nutrition in the United States.   The final article in this chapter was prompted by her statement that eating perhaps one or two cups of yogurt daily for several weeks before vacationing in an area where food poisoning exists would prevent dysentary.   This study shows that the value of yogurt is comparable to that of skim milk and has no magical properties.

23

OLYMPIC ATHLETES VIEW VITAMINS AND VICTORIES

Elington Darden *

This past summer, I had the opportunity to question a number of American athletes who participated in the XXth Olympic Games in Munich, West Germany, about their practices and beliefs concerning nutrition and its relationship to maximum performance. Approximately 12,000 athletes and coaches from all over the world ate at least three meals a day in the Olympic Village cafeteria, which remained open continuously from 5:30 a. m. to 1 a. m. The menu changed daily and offered the athletes a choice of two soups, three entrees, five additional dishes, and ten desserts. Since the food was always marvelously prepared and everything was free, we may safely assume that no athlete went to bed hungry.

In talking with 27 of the American athletes, I asked this question, "Do you eat any special foods or take vitamin pills or other supplements in your training program?" These are the answers they gave me:

SPRINTERS

Rod Milburn—Olympic champion in the 110-meter high hurdles. "I eat no special foods. A lot of hard work is responsible for me winning the gold medal."

"Olympic Athletes View Vitamins and Victories," *JOURNAL OF HOME ECONOMICS*, Vol. 65, February 1973, pp. 8–11, copyright by the American Home Economics Association, Washington, D. C.

* Food and Nutrition Department, The Florida State University.

Eddie Hart and Robert Taylor—members of the gold medal winning 400-meter relay. "We don't eat any special foods. We just get out and run."

Kathy Hammond—bronze medal winner in the women's 400-meter run. "I take no vitamin or mineral pills other than iron. However, I avoid greasy foods in the meal preceding the race."

John Smith—world record holder for the 440-yard run. "I take a multivitamin/mineral supplement and a protein supplement each day. I figure it's better to have too much than not enough."

MIDDLE DISTANCE RUNNERS

Jim Ryun—holder of the world record in the 1,500-meter run and the mile run. "I eat no special foods and take no supplements."

Dave Wottle—world record holder and Olympic champion in the 800-meter run. "I don't take anything artificial except Rolaids."

Steve Prefontaine—American record holder in the 3,000- and 5,000-meter runs. "I take a multivitamin each day and a breakfast drink that includes wheat germ oil. I don't know if it helps me, but it sure doesn't hurt."

Leonard Hilton—national indoor champion in the three-mile run. "I'm a strong believer in additional vitamins C, E, and B-complex tablets each day."

LONG DISTANCE RUNNERS

Jeff Galloway—American record holder for the 10-mile run. "I'm a firm believer in three balanced meals a day. Even if there were magic pills which would make me run faster, I'd rather know that I did it on my own."

Jack Bacheler—1969 AAU cross-country champion. "I've gotten good results from eating a high carbohydrate diet several days prior to my competition. Also during my marathon running I will drink 64 ounces of uncarbonated Coke (eight eight-ounce plastic bottles) at intervals along the way. This seems to give me an additional kick."

Frank Shorter—Olympic champion in the marathon. "Three days prior to the marathon, I tried to load up on carbohydrates. I gained several pounds which I consider to be my advantage as I have more energy. However, generally speaking, training is more important than nutrition."

FIELD EVENTS COMPETITORS

Deanne Wilson—American champion in the women's high jump. "I take 12 different vitamin and mineral pills every other day. I think they help me."

Olga Connolly—former Olympic champion in the women's discus. "I just love whipping cream, but I can't seem to get it here at the Village." She takes no vitamin or mineral supplements.

Dwight Stones—bronze medal winner in the high jump. "I take a multivitamin, plus additional C and E tablets each day. I think these help me guard against colds and infections."

Ron Jourdan—1969 indoor national collegiate champion in the high jump. "I take a multivitamin and a B-complex tablet, plus a vitamin E pill each day. I've been taking them for the last year and a half. I really don't think they help unless you aren't eating three square meals a day. However, they are especially important to me because I try to lose four or five pounds before an important competition. Besides it's hard to really know what you're getting from most food you eat."

George Frenn—American record holder in the hammer throw. "I used to take vitamins by injection and eat many health foods, but not anymore. I think they are all a bunch of huey."

Al Feuerback—indoor record holder in the shotput. "Yes, I take most all the supplements including a time-released vitamin/mineral powder, wheat germ oil, and protein pills."

SWIMMERS

Mark Spitz—winner of seven gold medals. "No, I don't take any supplements. But I have been eating yoghurt to keep from getting diarrhea over here. Some of the swimmers are pill freaks, especially B_6 and B_{12}. I think it gives them just a mental lift or a type of placebo power."

Rick DeMont—holder of the world record in the 1,500-meter freestyle and disqualified winner of the 400-meter freestyle. "I take no food supplements in my training program."

Doug Northway—bronze medal winner in the 1,500-meter freestyle. "I take a multivitamin pill and several salt tablets daily during my training program."

Steve Genter—silver medal winner in the 200-meter and 400-meter freestyles. "I try to stay away from foods with little nutritional value. I take no food supplements as I try to eat a balanced diet each day."

OTHER SPORT COMPETITORS

Tom Burleson—U. S. basketball team member and tallest athlete at the Olympics at 7 feet 4 inches. "I eat lots of protein foods such as meat and milk. However, I take no pills or supplements."

Ray Seales—U. S. boxing team member and Olympic winner of the light welterweight class. "I don't eat any bread or starch. It makes me soft inside. I eat a lot of meat and green vegetables, and I also take a vitamin-mineral supplement."

Phil Grippaldi—U. S. weightlifting team member and several times American champion in the middle heavyweight class. "I take seven individual vitamin pills at each meal and also a liver protein supplement." When asked if he thought they did him any good, he said, "Well, I've been taking them for so long that I don't want to stop taking them now. I can definitely feel a lag in my endurance when I quit taking wheat germ oil."

Russ Knipp—U. S. weightlifting team member and former national champion in the middleweight class. "I adhere to a high protein/low carbohydrate diet during training. In addition I take a multivitamin/mineral pill and wheat germ oil."

Chris Taylor—U. S. wrestling team member and the current national collegiate wrestling champion and the heaviest athlete at the Olympics at 444 pounds. "I don't believe in supplements, just a lot of regular food."

WHO IS RIGHT? WHO IS WRONG?

Less than half of the athletes questioned felt that a diet of well-balanced meals alone, without supplements, would provide them with the energy and stamina needed for strenuous competition. Let's consider whether they were right or wrong in their beliefs.

Do athletes need quick-energy foods, and, if so, which foods? For swift surges of energy, the Olympic athletes tended to concentrate on oranges, dextrose, honey, chocolate bars, and Cokes. Research, however, indicates that high-carbohydrate foods benefit only those athletes who compete in long-endurance events. Most sports are of such short duration that pre-contest snacks offer no apparent physiological benefit (1, 2).

Furthermore, too much honey, dextrose, sugar, or other similar sweets may prove detrimental because they tend to draw fluid into the gastrointestinal tract from other parts of the body. Dehydration due to perspiration loss is a problem in endurance-type sports and may be aggravated further by the loss of fluid to the gastrointestinal tract. Actually the athlete who participates in short-term events probably does not need extra sweets but, in any case, should take no more than 50 grams of a sugar, i. e., three rounded tablespoons, in a liquid, during any one-hour period (3).

For athletes in long-term endurance contests, the preferred fuel, according to research, is glycogen (4). An athlete on a normal diet has enough glycogen stored to perform heavy exercise for two hours before exhaustion sets in. However, a carbohydrate-rich diet will allow him to work for another hour and 20 minutes. He will experience even greater results if he exercises for a prolonged period before eating the carbohydrate-rich diet. The effect will be still more pronounced if for three days prior to the high-carbohydrate diet, he abstains from carbohydrates and concentrates on fats and protein foods (5, 6).

Are large amounts of protein essential to athletes in training? Many athletes and coaches assume that vigorous physical activity results in protein loss because of "wear and tear" on the muscles. But if this assumption were true, the body, in breaking down the protein molecules, would excrete nitrogen in the form of urea. Numerous experiments on nitrogen balance indicate that the amount of nitrogen the body excretes after vigorous exercise is not significantly higher than the amounts excreted when the body has been resting. For example, research on cross-country skiers who raced 22 to 53 miles in one day showed no noticeable change in the nitrogen output from when the skiers had been sleeping or taking their ease, say, around the open fire (7).

Other investigators (8, 9, 10) who worked with rats found that the liver and kidney of rats showed stress-like reactions and hypertrophy as the protein intake increased. Whether or not the human body would react in a similar way has not been proved. We know, of course, that very active persons require more calories a day than do sedentary persons, but the calories may come from a variety of foods. The rule of thumb for maintenance appears to be one gram of protein a day for each kilogram of bodyweight.

Does wheat germ oil improve athletic performance and increase stamina? Although wheat germ oil is a potent source of vitamin E and polyunsaturated fats, we have little evidence that athletes benefit from wheat germ oil used as a supplement to a well-balanced diet. Some researchers have hypothesized that vitamin E facilitates the exchange of oxygen between cells and acts as a "cellular lubricant" to increase endurance, but these hypotheses have been difficult to validate (11). A medical team headed by I. M. Sharman found that young athletes receiving vitamin E did not differ from athletes receiving placebos in various performance measures (12). J. W. Siemann and R. Byrd reported similar findings in research using college men (13).

Do athletes in hard training need vitamin and mineral supplements? Nutritional scientists (14, 15, 16) have been unable to find evidence that strenuous exercise increases the body's requirements for vitamins or that excessive amounts of vitamins will supercharge the cells. The tissues do not store certain water-soluble vitamins and will therefore rapidly throw off any excess. A healthy athlete who eats sufficient amounts of a variety of foods probably receives all the vitamins he needs.

On the other hand, he may have to replenish sodium chloride that is lost in perspiration. Scientists (17, 18) generally agree that this is one mineral that warrants special attention. The daily requirement for salt may be increased by five to ten grams when vigorous activity produces profuse perspiration, particularly in hot and humid weather. Water alone merely accelerates the rate of perspiring that leads to fatigue. A salt water solution (0.1 to 0.2 percent concentration) taken frequently appears to be a more successful supplement than salt without water, which can cause nausea (19). There has been some promising work with slow-release, sodium chloride tablets that could be helpful in the future (20).

In conclusion, we have to remember that the human body requires 50 or more nutrients from which it synthesizes 10,000 different compounds necessary to health and performance. All the 50 or more nutrients work together; therefore, a lack of one nutrient could result in the underproduction of hundreds of the essential compounds. On the other hand, excessive amounts of any one or more of the nutrients could upset the balance.

Olympic and other athletes would do well to stay with balanced diets made up of a wide choice of foods and to realize that victory in the arena may depend more on genetic factors and hard training than on nutritional supplements.

REFERENCES

1. Karpovich, P. V. *Physiology of Muscular Exercise*. Philadelphia: W. B. Saunders Co., 1959.

2. Bergström, J., and Hultman, E. Nutrition for maximal sports performance. *JAMA*, Vol. 221 (Aug. 28, 1972), pp. 999–1006.

3. *Nutrition for Athletes: A Handbook for Coaches*. Washington, D. C.: American Association for Health, Physical Education, and Recreation, 1971.

4. Astrand, P. O. The physiology of maximal performance. *Modern Med.*, Vol. 40 (June 26, 1972), pp. 50–54.

5. Bergström, J., and Hultman, E. Muscle glycogen synthesis after exercise: An enhancing factor localized to the muscle cells in man. *Nature*, Vol. 210 (1966), pp. 309–310.

6. Bergström, J. Harris, R. C., Hultman, E., et al. Energy rich phosphagens in dynamic and static work. *Advances Exp. Med. Biol.*, Vol. 11 (1971), pp. 341–355.

7. Hedman, R. The available glycogen in man and the connection between rate of oxygen intake and carbohydrate usage. *Acta Physiol. Scand.*, Vol. 40 (1957), pp. 305–309.

8. Walter, F., and Addis, T. Organ work and organ weight. *J. Exp. Med.*, Vol. 69 (1939), pp. 467–483.

9. Samuels, L. T., Gilmore, R. C., and Reinecke, R. M. The effect of previous diet on the ability of animals to do work during subsequent fasting. *J. Nutr.*, Vol. 36 (1948), pp. 639–651.

10. Holt, Jr., L. E., Halac, Jr., E., and Kajch, C. N. The concept of protein stores and its implications in diet. *JAMA*, Vol. 181 (1962), pp. 699–705.

11. Cooper, D. L. Drugs and the athlete. *JAMA*, Vol. 221 (Aug. 28, 1972), pp. 1007–1011.

12. Sharman, I. M., Down, M. G., and Sen, R. N.   The effects of vitamin E and training on physiological function and athletic performance in adolescent swimmers. *Brit. J. Nutr.,* Vol. 26 (1971), pp. 265–276.

13. Siemann, J. W., and Byrd, R.   Vitamin E and human work efficiency. *Fla. J. Health, Physical Ed., Recreation,* Vol. 9 (August 1971), pp. 7–8.

14. Hillsendager, D., and Karpovich, P. V.   Ergogenic effect of glycine and niacin separately and in combination. *Res. Quart.,* Vol. 35 (1964), pp. 389–392.

15. Consolazio, C. F., et al.   Effects of aspartic acid salts (Mg and K) on physical performance. *J. Appl. Physiol.,* Vol. 19 (1964), pp. 257–261.

16. Osness, W.   The effects of the use of dietary supplements on high level performance.   Proceedings of the Scientific Congress of the XXth Olympiad, Munich, 1972.

17. Kuno, Y. *Human perspiration.* Springfield, Ill.: Thomas, 1956.

18. Kozlowski, S., and Saltin, B.   Effect of sweat loss on body fluids. *J. Appl. Physiol.,* Vol. 19 (1964), pp. 1119–1124.

19. Buskirk, E. R., and Bars, D. E.   Climate and exercise. *Science and Medicine of Exercise and Sports,* W. R. Johnson, ed. New York: Harper and Row, 1960, p. 311.

20. Clarkson, E. M., Curtis, J. R., Jewkes, R. J., et al.   Slow sodium: An oral slowly released sodium chloride preparation. *Brit. Med. J.,* Vol. 3 (1971), pp. 604–607.

24

NUTRITION AND ATHLETICS

Olaf Mickelsen, Ph.D.*

Despite the fact that athletics is seriously practiced by so many amateurs and professionals, there is relatively little information about the diets and food preferences of athletes. Most of the books on coaching and practically all journals devoted to sports do not even mention diet, pregame meals or water consumption. When these topics are alluded to, the only statement that appears is that a wholesome, varied diet should be consumed. This situation exists since the attitude of most coaches to nutritional advice is exemplified by the statement that "It is perfectly true that the nutritionist has a place where athlete's training is concerned. But one is forced to the conclusion that probably the body itself is as good a judge as any of what it requires in the broad manner; it is just in the finer points that the scientist can help." [1] From a pragmatic standpoint, it is easy to understand why coaches are reluctant to discuss the details of the dietary practices their players are required to follow. These frequently are regarded as trade secrets.

One of the outstanding characteristics of training tables is the large amount of protein served in the form of beef. This practice is based on a variety of psychological factors rather than physiological requirements. For many years, the evidence has been conclusive that athletes require no more dietary protein, even during strenuous training, than sedentary individuals. Although the training period is associated with the formation of additional muscle tissue, an ordinary good diet provides sufficient extra protein for that purpose.

Reprinted from *Food and Nutrition News*, Vol. 41, No. 7, April 1970.

* Department of Foods and Nutrition, Professor of Nutrition, Michigan State University, East Lansing, Michigan.

About 30 years ago, there were many reports suggesting that physical performance was improved by the ingestion of extra amounts of vitamins. This was especially true of the vitamin B complex. Theoretical support for these suggestions came from the involvement of these vitamins in the enzymatic reactions associated with the production of energy. Vitamin C also came in for its share of notoriety. There were reports that football players at a midwestern university lost large amounts of vitamin C in their sweat. Subsequent studies suggested that the probable explanation for the vitamin C loss in the sweat was the presence of compounds in the "sulphur bloom" on the rubber gloves used for collecting the sweat. These compounds behaved similar to vitamin C in the reaction with the dye used in estimating this nutrient. Again, it can be stated that athletics, even of the most strenuous type, does not increase the requirement for any of the vitamins above that needed by less active individuals.

Two nutrients may be required in increased amounts by individuals engaged in vigorous physical activity. The most important of these is water. The other is sodium chloride. For most individuals, the requirement for salt, even during periods of excessive perspiration, can be met by extra seasoning of the food.

The maintenance of water balance, especially during athletic performances, poses a problem since many coaches restrict the amount of water the players may consume during a meet. A number of reasons are given for this, but most of them revolve about the statement that too much water produces a "water-logged" condition. The latter interferes with a player's performance. To obviate this development, many coaches permit their players to rinse their mouths with water but this must not be swallowed.

Although the coaches have this attitude, there is considerable experimental and some practical evidence indicating that water consumed during an athletic event may be beneficial. Some of these are casual observations. Olympic cross country skiers are reported to drink as much as a liter of a glucose solution during a three-hour meet where they covered slightly more than 30 miles.[2] College football players receiving a 0.2 per cent sodium chloride solution *ad libitum* throughout a game played "in 80° heat"[3] impressed everyone including the sports writers with their performance. The latter commented on the fact that these players "showed the greater strength at the finish."

Strenuous physical activity has no adverse effect on absorption of water or solutes from the gastrointestinal tract. This is true whether the individual exercises on a treadmill,[4] on a track,[5] or in a swimming pool.[5] In these studies, the volumes of fluid used were extreme (e. g. 750ml). The rate of absorption of water and salt was normal, leading to the conclusion "that gastric emptying and intestinal absorption of saline solutions would be rapid enough to replace all of the losses of sweat incurred during heavy exercise, even in hot environments."[4]

The importance of maintaining water balance during an athletic competition stems from the fact that the primary accompaniment of dehydration is fatigue. That this is equally true of exercise in very cold weather is illustrated by the suggestion that Sir Edmund Hillary succeeded in conquering Mt. Everest because he and his men secured an adequate water intake during the final ascent.[6] Each member of the unsuccessful Swiss expedition, which preceded Hillary by one year, received less than a pint of water a day the last three days of the climb. The resulting dehydration may have contributed to the extreme fatigue of the Swiss. Sir Hillary profited from the Swiss experience and took sufficient fuel to melt enough snow to provide each man with a daily allowance of five to seven pints of water. He attributed the success of his expedition partly to the increased intake of water with its consequent reduction in fatigue.

Laboratory studies differ markedly from athletic contests. Just before and during the latter, the athletes are so high strung that many physiological reactions are likely to be affected. One of the more frequent disturbances that occur at mealtimes is vomiting. In an attempt to overcome this, Rose and coworkers[3] instituted a liquid pregame meal. A 16-ounce can of this fluid provided 925 kcal with 24 per cent of them from protein and most of the remainder from carbohydrates. On the day of the meet, the football players received a meal of toast, honey and sliced peaches at 9 o'clock. While they were briefed and taped, they were offered the liquid meal. No other food was served until after the game. When this program was followed, there were no problems with vomiting; the players commented that they felt much better both during and after the game. When offered the opportunity to return to the previous pregame meal of steak, eggs, cereal, etc., they chose to stay with the liquid meal.

The liquid meal left the stomach more rapidly than the steak meal served previously.[3] This plus the fact that the players were permitted to drink a 0.2 per cent sodium chloride solution throughout the game may have contributed to the improved performance attributed to the changed dietary program. It may also have eliminated the muscle cramps which had previously plagued the team.

Since water consumption during athletic contests is frequently forbidden, many athletes have looked for other anti-fatigue agents. There are a number of drugs used for this purpose. In addition, a number of nutrients have been suggested for the relief of fatigue. Wheat germ oil has received much notoriety in this respect. The daily consumption of 20 gelatin capsules each containing 175 mg. of wheat germ oil was reported to improve the running performance of physical education students.[7] However, no change was seen in members of the swimming team who followed the same regimen. Finally, controlled studies with animals indicated that wheat germ oil had no effect in improving either the time during which maximal physical activity could be maintained or the speed with which the animals ran.[8]

These reports indicate that a nutritious, normal diet should be adequate for extremely active athletes. The increased caloric intake of such individuals is likely to insure an adequate supply of all essential nutrients. The primary concern of athletes should be their water intake. This is especially important when strenuous exercise is undertaken or when the performance takes place on a hot day.

The principles discussed in this review can be documented by many additional studies. Whether they will convince a coach to change his dietary instructions is problematical. On this score, it should be recognized that coaching is an art with which only a few are sufficiently versed to be outstanding. For this reason, progress in the area of nutritional care of athletes may be slow and arduous.

REFERENCES

1. Leyton, R. N. A., *Brit. J. Nutr.* 2: 269 (1948).
2. Astrand, P. O., *et al, J. Appl. Physiol.* 18: 619 (1963).
3. Rose, K. D., *et al, J.A.M.A.* 178: 30 (1961).
4. Fortrand, J. S. and B. Saltin, *J. Appl. Physiol.* 23: 331 (1967).
5. Little, C. C., H. Strayhorn and A. T. Miller, Jr., *Res. Quart.* 20: 398 (1949).
6. Mickelsen, O., in *Yearbook of Agriculture* (1959), U.S. Dept. Agric. p. 168. U.S. Govt. Printing Office, Washington, D. C.
7. Cureton, T. K., *Res. Quart.* 26: 391 (1955).
8. Consolazio, F. C., *et al, J. Appl. Physiol.* 19: 265. (1964).

25

NEW MILEPOSTS IN NUTRITION

E. B. Hayden *

You are aware of today's widespread interest in nutrition, health, and the American food supply. There was a similar interest prior to 1940 when thousands of cases of pellagra and beriberi (vitamin-deficiency diseases) were present in the United States. This, together with the surprisingly poor physical development of many American young men reporting for World War II military service, called attention to serious deficiencies in the nation's nutrition.

Much more recently, findings of the Ten-State Nutrition Survey (1968–70) by the U. S. Dept. of Health, Education, and Welfare and other government studies provided new knowledge that current food consumption and dietary practices of many Americans still do not provide them with recommended amounts of important vitamins and minerals. U. S. Dept. of Agriculture studies showed that diets in 21% of American households were deficient in one or more nutrients. These newer findings and the White House Conference on Food, Nutrition, and Health, held three years ago, again focused strong attention on national nutrition needs.

These nutrient deficiencies occurred at all levels of income, in all age groups, in all sections of the country. The fact is that *America was a nation well-fed and malnourished.*

The White House Conference encouraged actions by the food industry and other groups to improve the nation's nutrition and health. The

Statement presented at a News Conference, New York Hilton Hotel, New York City, Feb. 6, 1973.

* President, Cereal Institute, Inc., Chicago.

cereal industry has been in the forefront of nutritional enhancement efforts since 1941, when the voluntary addition of several key nutrients to breakfast cereals was begun. There has been progressive enhancement of the nutrients in ready-to-eat cereals for more than 30 years since then.

Today we are reporting highly responsive industry actions to help meet nutritional needs pointed out at that Conference. *All major breakfast cereal manufacturers have substantially increased the amounts of key nutrients in ready-to-eat cereals and have added additional nutrients to their products.* This most-recent industry initiative is contributing importantly to national nutrition since more than 50,000,000 Americans make ready-to-eat cereals part of their breakfast each morning.

This accelerated enhancement of nutrition has involved both the introduction of new products and the vitamin fortification of large numbers of familiar brands—increasing the quantity of key nutrients from previous whole-grain levels to present levels that provide substantial quantities of the entire daily nutritional need. Included are such popular products as: General Mills' Cheerios, Wheaties, and Trix; Kellogg's Corn Flakes, Rice Krispies, and Sugar Frosted Flakes; Nabisco's 100% Bran Cereal; Post Grape Nuts, Super Sugar Crisp, and Raisin Bran; Quaker's Cap's Crunch; Ralston's Wheat Chex; as well as many others.

Today *more than 85% of all ready-to-eat breakfast cereals are fortified with the important B vitamins—thiamin (B_1) riboflavin (B_2) niacin, vitamins B_6 and B_{12}, and frequently vitamins A, C, and D. More than half of these products are also fortified with iron.*

**Percent of key nutrients in one ounce of a
typical vitamin-fortified cereal,
without milk**

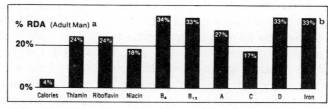

a RDA for vitamin D for the 18–22 year old male.
b About half of all vitamin-fortified cereals provide iron at 33 percent RDA or higher; the others are restored to provide iron at whole grain levels.
c Package labels state nutrient levels in percentage of established Minimum Daily Requirements (MDR) as required by Food and Drug Administration regulations now in effect. Recently FDA has proposed a change from MDR to "U.S. RDA", the latter having been derived from the RDA values developed by NAS–NRC.

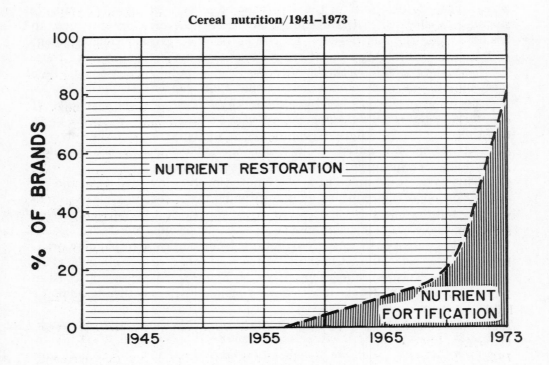

Cereal nutrition/1941–1973

Let's look at these vitamin-fortified cereals. A single serving without milk provides about 20% or more of the Recommended Dietary Allowances (RDA)[1] for five B vitamins and frequently vitamins A, C, and D. More than half of all vitamin-fortified cereals provide iron at 33% RDA or higher.

The vitamin-fortified cereals average just over 100 calories per serving, or only 4% of the day's recommended calories for an adult man. In a population where too many calories are frequently consumed for the amount of physical activity required by modern life, many people wish to reduce their caloric intake. Yet the quantity of nutrients they obtain from foods must be maintained. The much greater percentage of nutrients relative to calories in these cereals makes them highly desirable.

Today's *fortified* breakfast cereals have evolved from a long period of continuing nutritional emphasis.

Key nutrients (thiamin, niacin, and iron) were first added to breakfast cereals in 1941 in order to provide these nutrients at whole-grain

[1] Throughout this presentation the term "RDA" refers to daily nutrient intakes judged adequate for the maintenance of good nutrition in the U. S. population, developed by the Food and Nutrition Board of the National Academy of Sciences—National Research Council, 1968 (7th rev. ed.)

levels. This *restoration* program involved virtually all products and has been continued for more than 30 years.

The first successful fortified cereal was introduced in 1955 and other nutritionally fortified products followed. By 1969, at the time of the White House Conference, about 16% of all brands had already been nutritionally fortified.

Developing and perfecting good, taste-appealing fortified foods is complicated and takes a great deal of time and investment. Research must be conducted . . . new equipment designed and constructed . . . quality controls set up . . . products tested for long-time stability and consumer appeal. Yet in the three years since the White House Conference, the proportion of ready-to-eat cereals that are fortified has increased to more than 85% of all brands. These fortified cereals provide nutrients at higher levels than the products that had been nutritionally restored for many years.

These mileposts provide perspective on the continuing nutritional enhancement of ready-to-eat cereals for more than 30 years:

1941 Voluntary restoration of thiamin, niacin, and iron to whole-grain levels.

1955 Introduction of the first protein- and vitamin-fortified cereal. (Kellogg's Special K)

1961 The first cereal with 100% of the Minimum Daily Requirements for several vitamins. (General Mills' Total)

1969–72 Accelerated development of nutritionally fortified products.

1973 More than 85% of all ready-to-eat cereals vitamin-fortified.

Though we are reporting on the majority of products which are vitamin-fortified, some breakfast cereals offer extra protein and still others provide key nutrients at whole-grain levels. The nutritional facts about each are given on the package.

CEREAL AND MILK—AN EXCELLENT NUTRITIONAL COMBINATION

Since a bowl of cereal and milk is the entire breakfast for a substantial number of Americans, each of these foods carries a heavy nutritional responsibility. Let's look at the nutritional contribution of each component of this popular food combination.

These two foods are excellent companions, for each is a good source of *different* essential nutrients. Figure 1 illustrates how cereal and milk supplement each other to supply part of the daily need for key nutrients. For example, these cereals are important sources of the B vitamins, iron, carbohydrates, and vitamins A, C, and D, but they are low in several minerals.　Milk, however, is an excellent source of protein, calcium, and phosphorus, but is low in iron, niacin, and several important vitamins.　Both foods contain other nutrients, besides the 15 listed.

In addition to the quantitative way the nutrients in cereal and milk supplement each other, the key amino acids in milk make a most important contribution toward *improving the biological quality of the cereal proteins.* And that occurs routinely since breakfast cereals are consumed with milk about 95% of the time.

A number of popular cereals have been developed that offer extra protein—more than in the original grains.　These typically provide about 5.5 grams of protein per one-ounce serving, so with the 4.3 grams from the 4 ounces of milk, this serving provides approximately 10 grams of high-quality protein, or about 15% of the RDA.

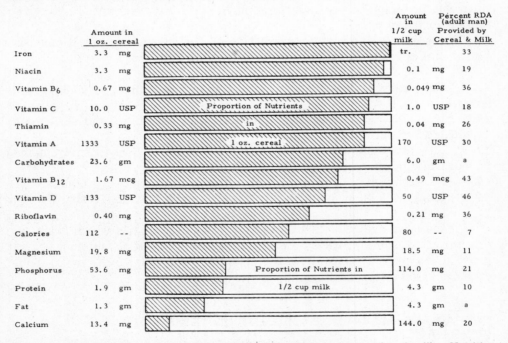

	Amount in 1 oz. cereal		Amount in 1/2 cup milk	Percent RDA (adult man) Provided by Cereal & Milk
Iron	3.3	mg	tr.	33
Niacin	3.3	mg	0.1 mg	19
Vitamin B$_6$	0.67	mg	0.049 mg	36
Vitamin C	10.0	USP	1.0 USP	18
Thiamin	0.33	mg	0.04 mg	26
Vitamin A	1333	USP	170 USP	30
Carbohydrates	23.6	gm	6.0 gm	a
Vitamin B$_{12}$	1.67	mcg	0.49 mcg	43
Vitamin D	133	USP	50 USP	46
Riboflavin	0.40	mg	0.21 mg	36
Calories	112	--	80 --	7
Magnesium	19.8	mg	18.5 mg	11
Phosphorus	53.6	mg	114.0 mg	21
Protein	1.9	gm	4.3 gm	10
Fat	1.3	gm	4.3 gm	a
Calcium	13.4	mg	144.0 mg	20

Figure 1: Several of the many nutrients provided by ready-to-eat cereal and milk.　Nutritive values for cereal are those of a typical group of vitamin-fortified RTE cereals.　Values for whole Milk [3.5% fat] are from *Food Values of Portions Commonly Used,* Bowes and Church, 11th edition and USDA Report No. 36.　Vitamin D fortified milk at 400 USP units per quart.　RDA for vitamin D for the 18–22 yr. adult male (ªstands for RDA not established).

GOOD NUTRITION AT LOW COST

The nutritional content and the cost of different foods vary greatly. This table shows the cost per serving and the amount of key nutrients in several popular foods.　A comparison of nutrient content and cost per

Cost and nutritional values of several popular foods

Food	Cost (in cents)	Percent recommended dietary allowances for an adult man													
		Thiamin	Riboflavin	Niacin	Vit. B$_6$	Vit. B$_{12}$	Vit. A	Vit. C	Vit. D	Iron	Calcium	Phosphorus	Magnesium	Protein	Calories
1 oz. rte cereal (vitamin-fortified)	4.5	23.6	23.5	18.3	33.5	33.4	26.7	16.7	33.3	33.0	1.8	6.7	5.7	2.9	4.0
1 egg (large)	4.6	4.3	9.4	0.6	3.0	22.0	12.8	0	6.8	12.0	3.6	13.8	1.7	10.8	3.1
4 oz. orange juice (frozen)	4.1	8.0	0.7	2.1	1.6	—	5.0	93.8	—	1.3	1.4	2.5	0	1.3	2.0
8 oz. milk (3.5% fat)	7.5	5.0	24.7	1.1	5.0	18.0	6.8	3.3	25.0	tr	36.0	28.4	10.6	13.1	5.7

Cereal costs based on A. C. Nielsen data, October 1972; other food costs, Estimated Retail Food Prices by Cities, U. S. Dept. of Labor, October 1972. Nutritive values for cereal are those of a typical group of vitamin-fortified RTE cereals. Values for other foods are from Food Values of Portions Commonly Used, Bowes and Church, 11th edition and USDA Report No. 36. Vitamin D fortified milk at 400 USP units per quart. RDA for vitamin D for the 18-22 year old male.

serving points out that vitamin-fortified breakfast cereals give a high nutritional return for the money spent.

The average per-ounce cost of a vitamin-fortified ready-to-eat cereal is only 4.5 cents. Yet the quantities of vitamins, minerals, and carbohydrates furnished are substantial relative to the other foods.

BREAKFAST—A SPECIAL NUTRITION NEED

Although good nutrition is vital to each of us, most Americans brush aside nutritional considerations in the hectic pace of modern life. Breakfast, the first meal of the day, is often not a real meal in a nutritional sense. Today about 50% of all women who have school-age children work outside the home. Breakfast is increasingly an individualized meal, prepared and eaten at different times by individual family members. It is only on weekends that breakfast may become the family social and communication occasion it once was.

Today's at-home breakfast may actually be quite different than you think. Here are the 11 most frequent choices of Americans at breakfast time: [2]

	% (Approx.)
No Breakfast	10
Coffee	4
Coffee, eggs, meat, toast	4
RTE cereal, milk	4
Coffee, toast	4
Juice, coffee, toast	2
Coffee, eggs, toast	2
RTE cereal, milk, coffee	2
RTE cereal, milk, juice	2
Juice, coffee, eggs, meat, toast	2
Milk, toast	2

About 10% of our population select no breakfast at all and another 4% choose coffee only—a total of 14% of our population. Each of the next three most-popular food combinations is served in about 4% of today's breakfasts; and each of the remaining is breakfast for 2% of modern America.

Ready-to-eat cereals are part of three of these nine most-frequently chosen food combinations. They are also consumed in combinations with many other foods and are included in about 25% of *all* breakfasts.

Ready-to-eat cereals have an important role in the nation's nutrition because they are a popular food that millions of people like to eat, and they combine convenience with nutrition at a cost of only a few cents per serving. They are present in more than 90% of all American homes.

TASTE APPEAL—VITAL TO NUTRITIONAL IMPACT

It is a fact of life that people choose foods with appealing tastes, flavors and textures. We eat what we like. Dr. Morris Fishbein, writing

[2] Third National Household Menu Census, Market Research Corporation of America.

recently in *Medical World News*, (November 24, 1972) emphasized the critical role that taste plays in getting foods consumed so their nutrients can be utilized. He said, "For most people, the primary factor in food selection is pleasure. For years we have been told that the way to avoid nutritional deficiency is to eat well-balanced meals, yet the average person selects what he eats without much regard for its nutrient value." Continuing emphasis has been given to taste appeal and consumer acceptance in the development of new products and in the nutritional fortification of old favorites.

Recognizing the frequency with which sugar is added to cereal by consumers, manufacturers have added it to some products during processing. These presweetened products make up slightly more than 30% of the total ready-to-eat cereal market. Thus consumers have a wide choice between presweetened cereals or those they sweeten themselves.

Manufacturers recognize the important nutritional role of presweetened cereals as a source of essential nutrients. *All* presweetened cereals are fortified with key vitamins to provide these nutrients in the same quantities as comparable non-presweetened products.

CEREALS—THE FOOD WITH THE MOST INFORMATIVE LABELS

Cereal packages have provided extensive nutritional information since 1941. Now other food manufacturers are beginning to move in this same direction. About two weeks ago the Food and Drug Administration published regulations for nutritional labeling to encourage many food manufacturers to provide nutrient information on food product packages. . . .

Ready-to-eat cereals show a complete list of ingredients; the quantity of all vitamins and minerals listed; the protein, fat, and carbohydrate content, and the number of calories in a typical one-ounce serving.

This informative labeling provides consumers with nutritional facts about each cereal.

DIMENSIONS OF THE BREAKFAST CEREAL INDUSTRY

Ready-to-eat and hot cereals have been part of the American breakfast scene for many years.

Hot oat and wheat cereals provide important levels of whole-grain nutrition. Newer quick-cooking and instant hot cereals have offered greater convenience with appealing flavor variations.

Ready-to-eat cereals have grown continuously in popularity. Their convenience has fit them well to the pace of modern America. Enhancement of their nutritional content has continued from restoration of several nutrients in 1941 to the more extensive nutritional fortification of recent years.

There has been interest recently in granola-type ready-to-eat cereals, primarily on the west coast of the United States. No one can predict at this time the extent to which they will become part of the ready-to-eat cereal market.

The following is a perspective on U. S. ready-to-eat cereals during 1972: [3]

Per capita consumption	Pound sales	Dollar sales
6.2 pounds	1,275,000,000	$850,000,000

Per capita consumption increased to 6.2 pounds during 1972, up from 5.9 pounds the previous year. Total pound sales increased 7%—the largest year-to-year increase since 1965. The average price paid by consumers for ready-to-eat cereals increased at a rate of less than one third the increase reported for all foods in the Consumer Price Index during 1972.

CONTINUING NUTRITION INFORMATION EFFORTS

The Cereal Institute has been committed to nutrition education since its founding 30 years ago. An Institute-funded film, released in 1944, reached millions of Americans through theater showings. A science-oriented television program provided special nutrition messages in the early 1950's. A continuing program of educational filmstrips for school use was started in 1956. More recently, the Institute has developed two filmstrip kits for Head Start and elementary grades that present concepts about nutrition and provide consumer information about today's foods. More than 100,000 prints of Institute filmstrips have been distributed without charge.

SPECIAL NUTRITION INFORMATION ON CEREAL PACKAGES

Breakfast cereal manufacturers have extended nutrition information to everyday life by providing special nutritional messages on product packages. More than 400,000,000 cereal packages have carried messages on the Four Food Groups. Recent messages emphasized the nutritional importance of breakfast, and others are stressing the nutritional role of cereals.

[3] A. C. Nielsen Company data.

CONCLUSION

This is a progress report of nutritional enhancement efforts that began in 1941, have continued for more than 30 years, and have been stepped up greatly since the White House Conference. The cereal industry has been in the forefront of efforts to meet nutritional needs emphasized at that Conference. The accelerated vitamin-fortification of ready-to-eat cereals helps meet documented nutritional needs, and each package gives the consumer the nutritional facts. This progress has been carried on within the framework of reality—the absolute autonomy of the consumer to accept or reject what he will eat, the intense competition within the industry, and the highest standards of product quality and safety.

26

DIET AND DENTAL CARIES

dental caries incidence and the consumption of ready-to-eat cereals

Robert L. Glass, D.M.D., Dr.Ph., and Sylvia Fleisch, M.S.*

The estimated amounts of regular and presweetened ready-to-eat cereals consumed by 949 children during two years were analyzed to determine the existence of an association between caries incidence and the consumption of these cereals. The average cereal consumption by type of cereal was estimated for each participant, and the children were classified as low, medium, or high consumers of cereals. Analysis of data on need for restorative treatment in permanent teeth and in permanent and deciduous teeth, by type and amount of cereal consumed, showed no association between caries incidence and cereal consumption. The cariogenicity of a food may be related to its consistency, the time of consumption, and the conditions under which it is eaten, as well as its sucrose content.

In view of attention focused recently in the United States on the sugar content of children's diets in relation to dental caries, it seemed worthwhile to analyze from this viewpoint, the records of a clinical trial designed to evaluate the cariostatic effect of 1% sodium dihydrogen phosphate added

Reprinted from the *Journal of the American Dental Association*, April 1974, Vol. 88, No. 4, pp. 807–813. Copyright by the American Dental Association. Reprinted by permission.

* Dr. Glass is an associate member of the staff of the Forsyth Dental Center, 140 Fenway, Boston, 02115. Miss Fleisch is assistant director, Boston University Computing Center, 111 Cummington St., Boston, 02115.

to ready-to-eat cereals, including presweetened cereals. The children participating in this study were provided with generous amounts of these cereals free of charge for two years. As no phosphate treatment effect on caries incidence was observed (unpublished data by Glass), a finding later corroborated by an independent study,[1] data for experimental groups could be combined for other types of analyses.

In the present study the amounts of cereals consumed, both regular and presweetened, were analyzed and their relationship to several measures of the caries incidence observed during the experimental period of two years was examined.

MATERIALS AND METHODS

A total of 1,199 children from 690 families participated in the clinical trial. At time of entry to the study, all children were between 7 and 11 years of age; they lived in eastern Massachusetts communities where the amounts of fluoride in the supplies of drinking water were not significant.

On entrance to the study, each participant was given an oral prophylaxis; comprehensive clinical and radiographic examinations of the teeth were made. Three examinations were carried out by the same dentist under standard conditions at annual intervals. Nutritional histories were made for the children through their mothers by trained nutritionists. Records were also made of the number and age of members of the immediate family. During the examination of a child the mother was instructed in the method of ordering supplies of ready-to-eat cereals that were provided free on request to all participants and their families. Fourteen types of cereal, eight regular and six presweetened, were made available to provide the variety considered necessary for continuing participation. All cereals were provided by the Kellogg Co. Mothers were asked to encourage their children to eat as much cereal as they liked, and at least one serving daily. All cereals were provided in the same style of packaging as that available on the open market.

Free dental care was offered to all participants at the Forsyth Dental Center to provide additional and continuing incentive to cooperate. The treatment philosophy was similar to that of a practicing pedodontist except orthodontics, prophylactic odontotomy, restoration of mobile deciduous teeth, and fluoride treatments were not provided.

The records of 979 children are included in the analyses for the present study. Although 1,011 of the original children were still participating when the study was terminated, the 979 participants included here met the additional conditions of having all their dental treatment provided under the supervision of the project director at the Forsyth Dental Center; also all the records of the families' cereal orders were available for the entire two-year span of participation. As no treatment effect due to the phosphate supplement was observed, data for children in the experimental and control groups were combined for the purpose of the present analyses.

A blank cereal order form and the types of cereal provided are shown in Figure 1. The amounts and types of cereal requested and shipped in

---

ORDER BLANK: You may order any assortment of cereals shown below. Write the number of packages of each product you wish to order opposite the product name. The TOTAL number of packages in your order should be a multiple of FOUR (4, 8, 12, etc.).

B0040   Date _____

_____01. CORN FLAKES   _____08. PEP (WHEAT FLAKES)
_____02. 40% BRAN FLAKES   _____09. COCOA KRISPIES
_____03. RAISIN BRAN   _____10. SHREDDED WHEAT
_____04. RICE KRISPIES   _____11. SPECIAL K
_____05. SUGAR POPS   _____12. OX_3 (OAT CEREAL)
_____06. SUGAR FROSTED FLAKES   _____13. FROOT LOOPS
_____07. SUGAR SMACKS   _____14. FROSTED STARS

                            _____ TOTAL NUMBER OF PACKAGES

Figure 1: Cereal order form showing types of cereal provided. All order forms were preprinted with participant's identification number, here B0040. Address for delivery station was printed on reverse side of form, with name and address of participant.

each order, participant identification number, and date of order were punched into machine records cards. All cereal order cards were sorted on date of order and family identification number and the information then coded on magnetic tape. Varieties of regular and presweetened cereals were identified and totaled to provide the number of boxes of regular cereal, boxes of presweetened cereal, and total boxes of cereal delivered to each family. Annual totals of each of the latter quantities were divided by the number of family members, excluding children under age 1, to estimate the average cereal consumption by type for each participant. These figures were verified on an individual basis through the dietary histories taken by nutritionists.

Findings of clinical and radiographic dental examinations were originally recorded on optically scanned, precoded examination records. These were processed by machine that encoded findings into punch cards to provide the data base for the calculation of caries increments. Caries increments are shown in terms of new decayed and/or filled (DF) surfaces. These are expressed as net new DF surfaces (observed minus changes in diagnosis), and net annual caries incidence rate per 100 surfaces at risk:[2] rate equals sd + sf + ud + uf − (ds + fs)/ss + us + sd + sf + ud + uf multiplied by 100, where the first letter in any pair indicates the surface status at an examination, the second letter indicates the status at a subsequent examination, and s equals sound, d equals decayed, f equals filled, and u equals unerupted. This caries incidence rate adjusts for any possible differences in tooth surface populations at risk. In addition, those tooth surfaces requiring resortation, according to each child's dental treatment plans made at the times of the dental examinations, were coded and punched into cards along with appropriate identification. These cards were processed by computer to obtain for each child, on an annual basis, the number of permanent tooth surfaces requiring restoration and the combined number of permanent and deciduous tooth surfaces requiring restoration. Summary cards containing this information were prepared for statistical analyses by computer.

Several methods were used to analyze the data. The mean age-specific counts of DMF teeth observed at each examination for each age group were plotted for inspection, along with the corresponding age-specific counts for all Massachusetts children. The DMF counts for the Massachusetts population used for comparisons were determined in an independent survey of 8,934 children of the same age distribution. The latter survey was carried out by the Dental Division of the Massachusetts Department of Public Health.[3]

The data on cereal consumption were used as continuous scale measurements in regression analyses of cereal consumption on age, caries increments, and needs for restorative treatment. In addition, this scale was collapsed to an ordinal scale to circumvent the difficulty involved in the exact measurement of cereal consumption. By means of this technique, children were classified as low, high, and medium consumers of cereal. Low consumers were defined as the lower 27% of users, high consumers as the upper 27%, and medium consumers as the middle 46%. This procedure utilizes a modification of a technique developed and validated by Kelley.[4] For these three groups, statistical analyses were carried out by analysis of variance for these variables: age; annual counts of new decayed and/or filled surfaces; annual caries incidence rate; annual counts of permanent tooth surfaces requiring restoration; and annual counts of permanent and deciduous tooth surfaces requiring restoration.

RESULTS

The distribution of the 979 children is shown by age and sex in Table 1. Their caries prevalence as characterized by mean age and sex-specific counts of DMF teeth is shown in Table 2. The mean age-specific DMF counts are plotted by age and examination in Figure 2, along with corresponding mean age-specific values for 8,934 children (one examination only) from representative communities in Massachusetts.

Table 1: Distribution of children by age and sex at the time of the first examination

Age	Boys	Girls	Total
7	66	78	144
8	129	126	255
9	121	115	236
10	110	97	207
11	79	58	137
Total	505	474	979

Table 2: Mean counts of DMF teeth by age and sex of 979 children at times of three examinations, each one year apart

	Age	Boys Mean	SD	Girls Mean	SD	Total Mean	SD
First examination							
	7	2.20	1.77	2.23	1.79	2.22	1.78
	8	2.73	1.91	2.66	1.66	2.69	1.79
	9	3.13	1.87	3.70	1.69	3.41	1.80
	10	4.14	2.07	4.69	2.66	4.40	2.38
	11	5.34	2.82	5.03	3.14	5.21	2.95
Second examination							
	8	2.89	1.68	3.27	1.62	3.10	1.65
	9	3.60	1.98	3.51	1.72	3.56	1.85
	10	3.84	1.85	4.74	2.62	4.28	2.30
	11	5.18	2.74	5.96	3.53	5.55	3.15
	12	7.58	4.00	7.24	4.66	7.44	4.28
Third examination							
	9	4.02	1.56	4.40	1.81	4.22	1.71
	10	4.94	2.80	4.73	2.38	4.84	2.60
	11	5.62	3.48	7.26	4.12	6.42	3.88
	12	7.57	3.94	9.11	5.50	8.30	4.78
	13	11.04	4.75	9.55	4.95	10.41	4.87

The caries prevalence of those in the study approximates that of the Massachusetts population. The growth curves resulting from the mean age-specific DMF counts from the three examinations of study participants increase at a rate similar to that of the Massachusetts population.

Analyses of cereal consumption in terms of boxes per child per year are shown in Table 3. On the average, consumption of regular varieties was slightly less than that of the presweetened cereals. However, a considerable range in estimated amounts consumed is evident for both regular and presweetened types. Cereal consumption generally was reduced somewhat during the second year. Each box of cereal on the average contained 10 oz. of cereal, so numbers of boxes should be multiplied by 10

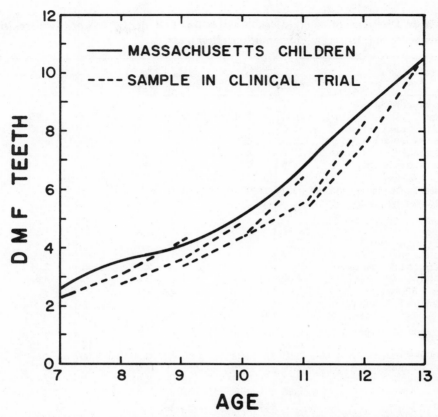

Figure 2: Mean counts of DMF teeth in Massachusetts children, 7 to 13 years of age, and sample participating in clinical trial. Solid line connects mean age-specific counts of DMF teeth for 8,934 Massachusetts children.[3] By age group, dashed lines connect mean age-specific counts of DMF teeth observed at three examinations carried out a year apart for 979 children in present study. For example, 7-year-old children were aged 8 at second examination and aged 9 at third examination.

Table 3: Number of boxes of cereal consumed per child per year, for 979 children

	Regular	Presweetened	Total
First year			
Mean	16	18	34
SD	10	11	18
Minimum	1	0	6
Median	14	16	31
Maximum	115	90	206
Second year			
Mean	14	15	29
SD	10	11	18
Minimum	0	0	2
Median	12	13	26
Maximum	72	68	138

Table 4: Analyses of age, caries increments, and dental restorative treatment needs according to cereal consumption: first year

	Low consumers		Medium consumers		High consumers		
	Mean	SD	Mean	SD	Mean	SD	F
Regular cereals							
Age	9.94	1.30	9.93	1.27	9.94	1.25	0.02
Net increment *	1.96	3.27	2.23	3.18	2.25	2.90	0.79
Caries incidence rate †	2.35	4.09	2.74	3.79	2.80	3.64	1.16
Permanent treatment	1.88	2.75	2.34	3.28	2.19	2.74	2.04
Total treatment	2.75	3.46	3.55	4.28	3.25	3.64	3.53
No. children	264		451		264		...
Range of consumption in boxes per year	1–9.2		9.3–19.1		19.2–115		...
Presweetened cereals							
Age	10.01	1.26	9.90	1.28	9.93	1.28	0.67
Net increment	2.01	3.89	2.15	2.80	2.34	2.82	0.73
Caries incidence rate	2.34	4.31	2.70	3.73	2.88	3.50	1.36
Permanent treatment	2.13	3.47	2.13	2.77	2.31	2.91	0.33
Total treatment	3.05	4.29	3.32	3.84	3.33	3.64	0.48
No. children	261		453		265		...
Range of consumption in boxes per year	0–9.8		9.9–21.7		21.8–90.0		...
All types of cereal							
Age	9.99	1.30	9.91	1.27	9.93	1.25	0.40
Net increment	2.02	3.83	2.05	2.80	2.50	2.87	2.12
Caries incidence rate	2.36	4.26	2.55	3.67	3.11	3.62	2.83
Permanent treatment	2.02	3.33	2.18	2.92	2.32	2.80	0.65
Total treatment	2.92	4.04	3.39	3.94	3.36	3.73	1.33
No. children	264		446		269		...
Range of consumption in boxes per year	6–20.7		20.8–39.8		39.9–206		...

* New decayed and filled surfaces.

† New decayed and filled surfaces per 100 surfaces at risk.

to determine intake in terms of ounces of cereal. More than 33,000 boxes were consumed by participating children during the first year and more than 28,000 boxes during the second year. The cumulative percentage distributions of children were plotted against amounts of cereal consumed (not shown); the shapes of the curves are similar for regular and presweetened cereals for each year.

Tables 4 and 5 show analyses of age, incremental caries, and needs for restorative treatment in permanent teeth and in permanent and deciduous teeth according to type and amount of cereal consumed. Low, medium, and high consumers are defined as previously specified.

During each of the two years of the study, the mean age of consumers in each category was nearly identical, differing only by no more than 0.1 of a year. Statistical analyses by analysis of variance resulted in

Table 5: Analyses of age, caries increments, and dental restorative treatment needs according to cereal consumption: second year

	Low consumers		Medium consumers		High consumers		
	Mean	SD	Mean	SD	Mean	SD	F
Regular cereals							
Age	10.91	1.31	10.92	1.26	10.99	1.25	0.32
Net increment *	4.24	4.87	3.84	4.16	3.53	3.93	1.79
Caries incidence rate †	4.30	4.54	3.88	3.86	3.55	3.92	2.26
Permanent treatment	4.38	5.42	3.81	4.72	3.52	4.07	2.23
Total treatment	5.06	5.67	4.36	4.88	4.12	4.30	2.65
No. children	263		451		265		. . .
Range of consumption in boxes per year	0–7.4		7.5–17.1		17.2–72.0		. . .
Presweetened cereals							
Age	11.01	1.28	10.91	1.30	10.91	1.21	0.64
Net increment	4.04	5.02	3.68	4.01	4.01	4.04	0.80
Caries incidence rate	3.91	4.56	3.81	3.90	4.07	3.86	0.34
Permanent treatment	4.48	5.95	3.73	4.38	3.57	3.98	2.90
Total treatment	4.98	5.99	4.35	4.64	4.21	4.33	1.89
No. children	263		452		264		. . .
Range of consumption in boxes per year	0–7.6		7.7–19.2		19.3–68.0		. . .
All types of cereals							
Age	10.94	1.30	10.95	1.28	10.90	1.24	0.14
Net increment	4.22	5.09	3.82	4.11	3.59	3.76	1.46
Caries incidence rate	4.14	4.61	3.92	3.94	3.65	3.73	0.98
Permanent treatment	4.33	5.81	3.89	4.52	3.45	3.94	2.27
Total treatment	4.90	5.92	4.46	4.74	4.12	4.27	1.68
No. children	263		446		270		. . .
Range of consumption in boxes per year	2.0–16.2		16.3–35.7		35.8–138.0		. . .

* New decayed and filled surfaces.
† New decayed and filled surfaces per 100 surfaces at risk.

F ratios less than the critical values, demonstrating that observed differences in age by group were nonsignificant.

Statistical analyses by analysis of variance of the two measures of incremental caries demonstrate no statistically significant differences among levels of incremental caries during the first or second year of the study. Examination of the rank order of the measures of caries increments during the two years encompassed by the study shows no consistent trend of caries incidence that suggests an association with cereal consumption.

Statistical analyses of the need for dental restorative treatment of permanent tooth surfaces demonstrate no statistically significant differences among groups with different levels of consumption. During the first year of the study, the difference among groups of regular cereal consumers in the need for restorative treatment of combined permanent and deciduous tooth surfaces is significant ($P=0.05$). (According to statistical theory, 1 F ratio in 20 is expected to be significant because of chance alone.) However, no significant differences are observed among mean treatment needs of permanent and deciduous teeth according to grouping based on consumption levels of presweetened and all cereals. Examination of the rank orders of the mean levels of need for dental treatment in all catgories of consumption during both years of the study reveals no consistent trend that suggests any association between caries incidence and cereal consumption.

Regression analyses of cereal consumption with the several measures of caries increments also showed no association between cereal consumption and caries incidence. The observed correlation coefficients were near zero, ranging from $+\ 0.08$ to $-\ 0.07$ and equally divided between positive and negative values. The correlations between age and cereal consumption were also near zero.

DISCUSSION

As seen in Figure 2, the caries prevalence of the sample of participants is quite similar to that of the Massachusetts population. This similarity is remarkable in that the two sets of data are derived from two completely independent studies with two sets of examiners operating under their own diagnostic criteria. The data in Table 2 plus the plots in Figure 2 demonstrate that the participating children were suspectible to dental caries and that their caries prevalence was typical of that of children in a nonfluoride area.

As mentioned in the previous section, the cereal consumption of individual children was estimated from family size and orders of cereal. It is impossible to determine with accuracy the exact amount of food ingested except in metabolic ward studies where food intake is weighed. Although the procedure for estimating cereal intake in the present study may not provide exact measures of individual consumption, it does facilitate a rank ordering of participants according to level of consumption. This provides a means of categorizing children as low, medium, and high consumers. Interviews carried out by nutritionists verified this correlation between volume of cereal ordered and amounts consumed by the individuals.

Although some of the participating children consumed large amounts of cereals containing up to 45% sucrose, the results of the several analyses carried out demonstrate no association between dental caries and cereal consumption. During the two years, no significant differences nor any consistent pattern of differences in incremental caries were observed between children eating small amounts and those eating large amounts of cereal. This lack of differences is apparent in two measures of incremental caries, as well as in the needs for dental restorative treatment in permanent and deciduous teeth. No differences are observed in mean ages according to level of consumption; therefore, age is not a confounding factor.

These findings are not inconsistent with existing knowledge concerning caries etiology and findings of human dietary studies. Almost all of the studies on diet and caries have been carried out with experimental animals. The extrapolation of the findings to humans may or may not be appropriate because of significant differences in eating habits. Few long-term prospective studies have been reported in relation to diet and dental caries. The most comprehensive of these is the Vipeholm dental caries study,[5] carried out during five years in a Swedish mental institution. The authors of this classic study concluded that, although increased sugar consumption may increase caries activity, the risk is greater if the sugar is contained in a vehicle that tends to stick to the teeth and if the sugar is consumed between meals. They found that increased sugar consumption in solution at meals resulted in no increase in dental caries activity.

Finn and Jamison [6] concluded that a sugar-coated cereal does not produce a significant change in dental caries incidence when compared to noncoated cereals or fruits. The same conclusion of lack of demonstrable cariogenicity of cereals is drawn from the results of the present study. However, this conclusion must not be construed to dilute in any way the evidence associating dental caries with sucrose in general. Although some ready-to-eat cereals contain up to 45% sucrose, these cereals are eaten with milk 94% of the time.[7] The presence of milk may reduce the retentive characteristics of the cereals so that remaining food particles may be more rapidly cleared from the mouth. For the most part, cereals are eaten at mealtime. As shown in the Vipeholm study, sucrose taken at mealtimes and in other than a sticky vehicle failed to produce increased caries activity.

Many observational studies on diet and dental caries have been reported; these include findings of significant increases in caries experience in populations exposed to dietary changes involving increased consumption of highly refined carbohydrates.[8-10] However, the eating habits and the specific foodstuffs involved were not considered.

The results of the present study and those of other prospective dietary studies suggest that the cariogenicity of foods depends on factors other than sucrose content alone. The consistency of a food, the time of eating (at meals or between meals), plus accompanying foods (for example, milk) may somehow affect the cariogenicity expected as a result of sucrose content.

Certain dietary restrictions of highly refined carbohydrate intake may be extremely important in the control of rampant dental caries. However, it is impractical to eliminate all such foods from the diet, especially the diets of children. More extensive research in humans will be required to identify and to establish the rank order of the cariogenicity of different foods and eating habits. Such research is difficult, time-consuming, and expensive. This type of research is further complicated by the problems of obtaining approval from committees on studies involving human subjects, as there is a tendency to pass judgment on the cariogenicity of all highly refined carbohydrates before evidence from controlled experiments is available.

CONCLUSIONS

Under the conditions of the present study, no association was observed between dental caries incidence and the consumption of ready-to-eat cereals. In spite of the children's free access to unusually large quantities of regular and presweetened cereals, no increase in caries incidence was observed. The observed lack of cariogenicity of cereals may be due to their ingestion with milk and at mealtimes.

The cariogenicity of a foodstuff may not be highly correlated with the sucrose content alone. The time of eating, the consistency of the food, and the conditions under which a particular food is eaten may be as significant as its sucrose content in the determination of its relative cariogenicity.

REFERENCES

1. Peterson, J. K.   North Dakota field test of cariostatic effect of 1% sodium dihydrogen phosphate and disodium hydrogen phosphate added to presweetened breakfast cereals.   J Dent Res 48:1308 Nov-Dec 1969.

2. Glass, R. L.; Alman, J. E.; and Fleisch, S.   The measurement of caries increments by counts and rates.   Abstracted.   IADR Program & Abstracts of Papers No. 633 March 1971.

3. Wellock, W. D.   Dental Div. Massachusetts Dept of Public Health.   House Doc No. 3902, 1967.

4. Kelley, T. L.   The selection of upper and lower groups for the validation of test items.   J Educ Psych 30:17 Jan 1939.

5. Gustafsson, B. E., and others.   The Vipeholm dental caries study.   The effect of different levels of carbohydrate intake on caries activity in 436 individuals observed for five years.   Acta Odontol Scand 11:232 Sept 1954.

6. Finn, S. B., and Jamison, H.   The relative effect on dental caries of three food supplements to the diet.   Abstracted, IADR Program & Abstracts of Papers No. 667 March 1969.

7. National Family Opinion.   Cereal consumption study.   Toledo, Ohio, National Family Opinion, 1972.

8. Toverud, G. The influence of war and post-war conditions on the teeth of Norwegian school children. II. Caries in the permanent teeth of children aged 7–8 and 12–13 years. Milbank Mem Fund Q 35:127 April 1957.

9. Holloway, P. J.; James, P.M.C.; and Slack. G. L. Dental disease in Tristan da Cunha. Br Dent J 115:19 July 2, 1963.

10. Harris, R. Biology of the children of Hopewood House, Bowral, Australia. 4. Observations on dental-caries experience extending over five years (1957–61). J Dent Res 42:1387 Nov–Dec 1963.

27

ZEN MACROBIOTIC DIETS

Council on Foods and Nutrition

The American Medical Association's Council on Foods and Nutrition is deeply concerned over the increasing popularity, particularly among adolescents of "Zen Macrobiotics" and its nutritional implications. The Zen Macrobiotic diet was originated by a Japanese, Georges Ohsawa. The philosophy of Zen Macrobiotics is outlined in two of Ohsawa's books, *Zen Macrobiotics* and the *Philosophy of Oriental Medicine*.

The Macrobiotic diet represents an extreme example of a general trend toward natural and organic foods. One of the reasons given for the popularity of these unusual diets is that they are considered to be a means of creating a spiritual awakening or rebirth. Some persons have undertaken these diets as a form of protest against the establishment which, in their minds, is represented by the food industry, or even as a means of protest against war or man's inhumanity to man. Regardless of the underlying reasons or motives, however noble and sincere, the concepts proposed in Zen Macrobiotics constitute a major public health problem and are dangerous to its adherents. Unusual diets have existed in all societies since ancient times and appear to be a universal phenomenon. The Zen Macrobiotic diet, however, is one of the most dangerous dietary regimens, posing not only serious hazards to the health of the individual but even to life itself. According to Ohsawa, there is no disease that cannot be cured by "proper" therapy which consists of natural food, no medicine, no surgery, and no inactivity. Thus the diet (or "cult") may interfere with the application of established medical principles.

Reprinted from the *Journal of the American Medical Association*, October 18, 1971, Vol. 218, No. 3. (c) 1971 American Medical Association. Reprinted by permission.

Ohsawa states that there are ten ways of eating and drinking through which an individual can establish a healthy and happy life. This can only be attained through a proper balance of Yin and Yang. Certain foods are categorized as Yin, whereas others fall into the Yang category. A diet composed of natural foods is advocated. The prescribed diets are predominantly vegetarian with a great emphasis being placed on the inclusion of whole-grain cereals. In addition, fluids are to be avoided as much as possible.

The dietary regimen proposed basically comprises ten diets, ranging from the lowest level (diet–3) which includes 10% cereals, 30% vegetables, 10% soup, 30% animal products, 15% salads and fruits, and 5% desserts, to the highest level (diet 7), which is made up of 100% cereals.

Ohsawa recommends that followers of Zen Macrobiotics who cannot achieve the desired state of well-being at any one stage of the diets proposed, should progress from one level of dieting to another until they reach the highest level, diet 7. This all-cereal diet is supposedly the easiest, simplest, and wisest diet in achieving that state of well-being, one which will serve as a panacea for all diseases known to man. For example, the management of cancer is handled as follows:

> No illness is more simple to cure than cancer [this also applies to mental disease and heart trouble] through a return to the most elementary and natural eating and drinking: Diet No 7.

For those who have no faith in the teaching of Jesus (prayer and fasting), suggestions are given for macrobiotic external treatment of symptoms; namely, apply 801 and 802 to painful area (ginger compress and albi plaster [albi=yucca+ginger]).

The following statement is made regarding appendicitis: "No Macrobiotic person can be a victim of this illness. Diet No. 7 is best. External: Ginger compress (801) followed by albi plaster (802)." Herein lies the greatest danger for followers of the Zen Macrobiotics philosophy—medical consultation is not advocated; every individual must be his own doctor. The tragedy associated with application of this philosophy is well documented.

Individuals who persist in following the more rigid diets of Zen Macrobiotics stand in great danger of incurring serious nutritional deficiencies, particularly as they progress to the highest level of dieting. Cases of scurvy, anemia, hypoproteinemia, hypocalcemia, emaciation due to starvation, and other forms of malnutrition, in addition to loss of kidney function due to restricted fluid intake, have been reported, some of which have resulted in death.[1, 2]

To merely brand as food faddists those individuals whose dietary beliefs are not in accord with what is ordinarily considered sound nutritional practice serves no useful purpose. There is no doubt that some of these philosophies provide satisfying emotional, spiritual, and physical experiences for their followers.

A great deal of research still needs to be done to evaluate, on a scientific basis, the effect of nutrition on many disease states. It would be premature, at this time, to categorize all "unusual" dietary philosophies as hazardous without evaluating their nutritional contributions. But, when a diet has been shown to cause irreversible damage to health and ultimately lead to death, it should be roundly condemned as a threat to human health. The Council on Foods and Nutrition believes that such is the case with the rigid dietary restrictions placed on followers of the Zen Macrobiotic philosophy.

REFERENCES

1. Zen Macrobiotic diet hazardous: Presentment of Passaic grand jury. *Public Health News* (New Jersey State Department of Health), June, 1966, pp. 132–135.
2. Sherlock P. Rothschild EO: Scurvy produced by a Zen Macrobiotic diet. *JAMA* 199:794–798, 1967.

28

THE VEGETARIAN DIET

**U. D. Register, Ph.D., R.D., and
L. M. Sonnenberg, R.D.***

Large populations of the world have lived for centuries on diets considered near-vegetarian because of economic necessity and availability of little or no animal products. Today, however, in an affluent society where food supplies are abundant, an interesting trend has been developing in that more and more Americans, particularly young adults, are becoming vegetarians.

There are a number of reasons which vary as to the type of diet adopted, adherence to it, and other characteristics of life style. A common objective appears to be that of promoting health and a sense of well-being, although many individuals turn to vegetarian diets for their own personal reasons without adequate information of food values and nutritional principles. The use of Zen macrobiotic diets is a well known example of problems that potentially may develop when the diet is improperly selected.

The Zen macrobiotic regimen basically consists of ten diets, ranging from the lowest level (Diet—3) which includes fruits, vegetables, and some animal products in addition to cereals, to the highest level (Diet 7) made up entirely of cereals. Individuals who persist in following the more rigid diets are in great danger of developing serious nutritional deficiencies. Cases of scurvy, anemia, hypoproteinemia, hypocalcemia, emaciation due to starvation, and other forms of malnutrition, in addition to loss

Reprinted from *Journal of The American Dietetic Association*, Vol. 62, No. 3, March 1973. © The American Dietetic Association. Printed in U. S. A.

Presented at the 55th Annual Meeting of The American Dietetic Association in New Orleans, on October 11, 1972.

* Department of Nutrition, School of Health, Loma Linda, University, Loma Linda, California.

of kidney function due to restricted fluid intake, have been reported, some of which have resulted in death (1).

There is a vast difference between people who are vegetarians by choice and those who have no other alternative because of economics and available food supplies. Both groups can benefit from the assurance that their diets can be adequate and healthful. To understand and to be prepared to provide professional counsel and assistance are challenges to all involved in nutritional care.

PROTEIN IN THE VEGETARIAN DIET

Quantitative aspects. German physiologists recommended high protein intakes based on their opinion that protein need was proportionate to muscular activity (2). Voit based his recommendation for an intake of 120 gm. protein on his survey among German workers who were eating a high-protein diet (3). However, controlled experiments using the nitrogen balance method showed that normal subjects can maintain nitrogen equilibrium on protein intakes of from 30 to 35 gm. per day (4).

In 1946, Hegsted *et al.* studied adults on an all-plant diet in which cereals provided 62 per cent of the protein. They concluded (5) that on this type of diet, 30 to 40 gm. protein per day would meet minimal requirements of a man weighing 70 kg.

A comprehensive nutritional study by Hardinge and Stare (6) in 1954 compared nutritive intake and nutritional, physical, and laboratory findings of 200 subjects on three types of diets: twenty-six pure vegetarians, who used *no* animal products; eighty-six lacto-ovo-vegetarians, who used milk and eggs; and eighty-eight non-vegetarians. No evidence of deficiency was found, and each group met or surpassed the Recommended Dietary Allowances. These results showed that the average protein intake of the adult men on the pure vegetarian diet was 83 gm.; on the lacto-ovo-vegetarian diet, 98 gm.; and on the non-vegetarian, 125 gm. Results for women were 61, 82, and 94 gm., respectively. Dietitians accustomed to computing meatless menus find it difficult not to exceed the protein allowances when caloric needs are met.

Hegsted and the Harvard group have commented (7) that for adults "it is difficult to obtain a mixed vegetable diet which will produce an appreciable loss of body protein without resorting to high levels of sugar, jams, and jellies, and other essentially protein-free foods." Similar experiences have been found in our laboratories.

Total serum protein, albumin, and globulin values and the hematologic findings for the vegetarian and non-vegetarian groups in Hardinge and Stare's study were not statistically different. The pure vegetarians averaged 20 lb. less in weight than the others who average 12 to 15 lb. above their ideal weight.

Although protein has been singled out for attention in populations where malnutrition is prevalent, the problem is often compounded by a total caloric deficit. Even when an adequate amount of protein is provided, symptoms of protein deficiency may still appear if the diet does not also provide sufficient calories since, under these circumstances, some of the protein is utilized for energy.

In a review of cereal diets in which 10 per cent or less of the protein calories were derived from animal sourves, Ohlson reported (8) that the adult protein requirements, as analyzed by FAO, probably could be met if sufficient calories were available. She found that 2,500 kcal from such a food mixture would, on the average, supply 67 gm. protein—almost 50 per cent more protein than estimated to be adequate for 98 per cent of the adult population.

In India, the average caloric intake is about 2,050 kcal per day, supplying a total of 57 gm. protein, of which 51 gm. come from plant sources (9). By contrast, in the United States, the average intake is approximately 3,200 kcal with a total of 97 gm. protein, of which 31 gm. is from plant sources. By increasing the Indian diet 1,000 kcal (comparable to the caloric level in American diets), there would be an increase of 25 gm. plant protein. With this caloric increase, the total protein level in the Indian diet would be 82 gm. considerably exceeding recommendations.

In a review of current concepts of protein, nutrition, Scrimshaw of Massachusetts Institute of Technology asks (10) : "How do we allow adequately for individual variation without recommending a wasteful margin of safety?" To answer this question, at least for young adults, he studied 100 young men, all university students, who were given a diet adequate in calories but lacking in protein. His studies indicated that generally an amount less than 30 gm. protein daily is adequate for normal activities. Nitrogen balance at these low levels of intake was possible only because a protein of excellent quality, that of freeze-dried whole egg, was used. A correction for the lesser protein quality of ordinary mixed diets must be made. Scrimshaw makes the point that absolute requirements for protein in healthy adults are much lower than commonly suggested, provided the quality is good.

Scientific studies continue to confirm Sherman's findings (11) that 1 gm. protein per kilogram body weight provides a liberal margin of safety for adult maintenance. This is reflected in the 1968 revision of the Recommended Dietary Allowances, which are practical and desirable levels. The importance of planning adequate diets to meet these allowances has been amply substantiated, not only by research but by clinical studies and human experience. Table 1 shows how easily protein needs can be met on a lacto-ovo-vegetarian diet. It will be noted that the protein total for two meals is about 60 gm., approximately twice the minimum requirement for adult man.

Qualitative aspects. The extensive fund of knowledge supplying information in regard to the amino acid composition of foods has been achieved through a number of methods of experimentation. Among these are animal growth studies, biologic value methods, nitrogen balance studies, and dietary surveys, as well as chemical and chromatographic determinations.

A number of the very early studies used the rat growth method for evaluating the quality of single proteins. By this method, the quality of plant proteins was generally undervalued. However, the concept of mutual supplementation evolved. As pointed out in *The Lancet* (12): "For-

Table 1: Two menus to meet protein needs from typical lacto-ovo-vegetarian meal patterns *

Food	Protein
Menu I	gm.
Oatmeal and raisins	4
Milk, 1 glass	8.5
Bread, 2 slices whole wheat toast	5
Fruit, 1 serving	1
Egg or meat analog (1–2 oz.) or nuts (½ oz.), or peanut butter (1 Tbsp.)	5–6
Total	24
Menu II	
Lettuce and tomato salad	2
(with cottage cheese)	(15)
Entrée	12
Peas	5
Potato	3
Bread, whole wheat	2.5
Milk, 1 glass	8.5
Dessert	3
Total	36

* Total for two meals = approximately 60 gm. protein; values for the third meal are not included.

merly vegetable proteins were classified as second-class and regarded as inferior to first-class proteins of animal origin; but this distinction has now been generally discarded. Certainly some vegetable proteins, if fed as the *sole* source of protein, are of relatively low value for promoting growth; but many field trials have shown that the proteins provided by suitable mixtures of vegetable origin enable children to grow as well as children provided with milk and other animal proteins."

Bressani and Behar have stated (13): "From a nutritional point of view, animal or vegetable proteins should not be differentiated. It is known today that the relative concentration of the amino acids, particularly of the essential ones, is the most important factor determining the biological value of a protein. . . . By combining different proteins in appropriate ways, vegetable proteins cannot be distinguished nutritionally from those of animal origin. The amino acids and not the proteins should be considered as the nutritional units."

Since wheat is so widely used, early studies (14) of the supplementary value of wheat protein with other proteins were carried out in this laboratory. Because wheat is low in lysine, foods that are relatively high in this amino acid were tested. We found that when 70 per cent of the protein in the diet was from wheat protein and the remaining 30 per cent from milk, yeast, nuts, soybeans, and other legumes, excellent supplementary action occurred as judged by rat growth.

In a study by Sanchez, Porter, and Register (15), a week's hospital vegetarian diet containing milk and eggs was fed to a group of animals, and their growth was compared with that of a group of animals receiving the same diet in which meat replaced the plant protein entrées. The results showed no significant difference. The average growth of the animals on the meat and meatless diets was 39 and 37 gm. per week, respectively.

Sanchez *et al.* designed a study (16) to evaluate by the biologic value method the protein content of complete meals. All basal meal patterns consisted of portions from plant foods and were tested together with supplements of lysine, soybean milk, cow's milk, or a combination of these supplements. When diets were formulated to contain grain-legume mixtures as eaten in most countries, biologic values were above 70 and compared favorably with diets containing meat, milk, and lysine. These results suggest the possible supplementary value of proteins in diets of peoples of many countries which include large quantities of cereals, some legumes and possibly some other vegetables, fruits and nuts, and little or no animal foods.

Using the nitrogen balance method, Register *et al.* evaluated (17) in human subjects the protein quality of diets containing vegetable protein mixtures prepared to simulate meat products. The results were compared with similar diets containing milk and beef. Six university students served as subjects in each of four tests. At an approximately 60-gm. protein level, selected diets containing prepared vegetable protein mixtures with soybean milk or cow's milk maintained nitrogen balance. Such diets also compared favorably with the non-vegetarian diet in maintaining nitrogen balance.

The metabolic response of eighteen-year-old adolescent girls to a lacto-ovo-vegetarian diet was studied by Marsh and co-workers (18). The calculated essential amino acid intake was far in excess of the minimal requirement for women for every amino acid.

Edwards *et al.* did nitrogen balance studies on twelve men at the beginning and end of four, fifteen-day intervals following the ingestion of wheat diets containing 46 gm. protein per day. They found (19) that nitrogen balance was maintained over a period of sixty days.

In studying vegetarians, Hardinge, Crooks, and Stare analyzed (20) the essential amino acids of the dietary proteins of the subjects. Their figures showed that the intake of all groups ranged from more than twice to many times the minimum essential amino acid requirements (Table 2).

Table 2: Essential amino acids in diets of adult male vegetarians and non-vegetarians*

Amino acid	Non-vegetarian	Lacto-ovo-vegetarian	Pure vegetarian	Recommen-dation †
Isoleucine (gm.)	6.6	5.4	4.0	1.4
Leucine (gm.)	10.1	8.2	6.0	2.2
Lysine (gm.)	8.3	5.4	3.7	1.6
Phenylalanine + tyrosine (gm.)	10.4	8.8	7.0	2.2
Methionine + cystine (gm.)	4.3	3.2	2.7	2.2
Threonine (gm.)	5.0	3.8	2.9	1.0
Tryptophan (gm.)	1.5	1.2	1.1	0.5
Valine (gm.)	7.1	5.6	4.3	1.6
protein intake (gm.)	121.3	97.2	81.5	65.0

* Taken from Hardinge, Crooks, and Stare (20).
† Recommendation is twice the minimum requirements.

Evaluating protein quality by various methods has resulted in a large body of information that provides scientific basis for planning vegetarian diets that are quantitatively and qualitatively adequate. Understanding of protein nutrition has progressed to the point where an all-vegetable combination, such as Incaparina, is completely adequate in feeding very young children even those suffering from malnutrition.

In the developing countries, this concept of mutual amino acid supplementation has sparked investigations into many single plant sources to determine combinations of available supplies which supplement each other. Rao and Swaminathan summarized (21) a number of these studies: peanut proteins supplement wheat, oat, corn, rice, and coconut proteins to a significant extent; being rich in lysine and valine, soybean proteins supplement those of wheat, corn, and rye; a mixture of soy and sesame proteins has a high nutritive value comparable to milk proteins; and the proteins of legumes and leafy vegetables remarkably supplement those of cereals.

In a paper on current concepts of protein nutrition, Scrimshaw declares (10): "Vegetable mixtures supplying the amino acids in appropriate proportions are as efficient in meeting protein needs at minimum levels of intake as proteins of animal origin." Recent advances in our understanding of protein requirements, he says, free us "from dependence on the concept of the need for animal protein or amino acids from conventional food alone and allows us to concentrate on ways of most efficiently and economically meeting man's need." He further states that the "bulk of present and future needs will be met by conventional plant proteins."

Information from studies on the supplementary relationship of plant proteins has resulted in the development and marketing of a number of formulated plant protein foods referred to as "meat analogs." A number of these products combine various proportions of legumes, nuts, and cereals. One advantage of all of these foods is that, since they are made of plant sources, they do not contain cholesterol or saturated animal fats.

SOY PRODUCTS

Vegetable proteins that are finding special consumer interest are the spun soy and textured soy protein products. They offer great potential and versatility because they can be formulated to any protein, fat, or carbohydrate level desired, and proteins may be blended to accomplish a very favorable amino acid composition.

Since spun soy isolates are the purified protein fraction of soybeans, it is important that they be fortified or used in combination with foods which contain the essential nutrients, such as iron and a number of the B vitamins which meat proteins provide in the diet. The U. S. Department of Agriculture's Agricultural Research Service has set up compositional requirements for textured vegetable protein products for use in the school lunch program (22).

Based on casein as a standard with a protein efficiency ratio (PER) of 2.50, ham analog has a PER of 3.10; smoked turkey analog, 2.81; plant protein wieners, 2.50; textured protein sausage, 2.40; and chicken analog, 2.34. Meat analogs also usually contain less fat than their meat counterparts. Ham analog has only 12 per cent fat compared with about 30 to 35 per cent for ham; plant protein wieners, 12 per cent compared with up to 30 per cent for meat wieners; and beef analog, 12 per cent compared with 18 to 23 per cent for beef (23).

In a study by Koury and Hodges (24), prison volunteers were hospitalized and placed on a diet for twenty-four weeks with soy protein foods as the only source of protein. The diet was well accepted, weight was maintained, and all subjects remained in good health. Laboratory results showed normal findings for hemoglobin, hematocrit, and urea nitrogen, indicating that the protein was well utilized. Serum cholesterol and triglyceride values were markedly influenced by the diets. The average decrease in serum cholesterol was approximately 100 mg. per milliliter.

Bressani *et al.* compared the protein quality of textured soy protein with meat and milk in experimental animals and children (25). Growth was the same for dogs fed soy protein as for those fed meat. Even when large amounts of soy protein were given, no adverse physiologic effects were observed. Nitrogen absorption and retention were essentially the same for both the milk and soy protein diets of children. It was concluded that the protein quality of soy protein is high, about 80 per cent of the protein quality of milk, with adequate digestibility.

As the world protein supply dwindles in relation to the population growth, textured protein products will be used to supplement and extend existing protein sources. A recent Cornell University study (26) forecasts that meat analogs and extenders may reach 10 per cent of all domestic meat consumption by 1985, certainly by year 2000. This would represent an increase from the present level of 145 million lb. per year to approximately 2.45 billion lb. in fifteen years.

ADEQUATE AND INADEQUATE VEGETARIAN DIETS

World-wide studies of properly selected vegetarian diets support the adequacy of such a dietary pattern. True, many reports have been published of nutritional diseases prevalent in underprivileged areas of the world. These generally show that the diseases are due, not to a vegetarian diet as such, but to a gross shortage of food, or to a diet consisting largely of such foods as refined cornmeal, cassava root, tapioca, or white rice, with practically no milk, eggs, leafy vegetables, legumes, or fruits. Lack of suitable post-weaning foods affects young children, particularly. Parasitic infestations frequently accentuate the symptoms of nutritional diseases in these areas.

Hardinge and Crooks reviewed the scientific literature on vegetarian and near-vegetarian diets (27). Tables 3 and 4 summarize their findings. They conclude that "widely differing dietary practices appear among vegetarians and near-vegetarians. A reasonably chosen plant diet, supplemented with a fair amount of dairy products, with or without eggs, is apparently adequate for every nutritional requirement of all age groups.

"Pure vegetarian diets, the use of which produced no detectable deficiency signs, contained adequate calories obtained mainly from unrefined grains; legumes; nuts and nut-like seeds; a variety of vegetables, including the leafy kinds; and usually an abundance of fruits.

"Vegetarian and near-vegetarian diets that have proved inadequate include: (a) vegan diets which have been reported to produce vitamin B_{12} deficiency in some individuals; (b) grossly unbalanced near-vegetarian diets in which as much as 95 per cent of the calories were provided by starchy foods extremely low in protein, such as cassava root; (c) diets dependent too largely on refined cereals, such as cornmeal or white rice, even though small amounts of animal foods were included: and (d) intake of total calories insufficient for maintenance requirements."

PLANT DIETARIES AND SERUM LIPIDS

Experimental studies and epidemiologic findings on the lipid-lowering effect of plant dietaries may have great significance for current prob-

Table 3: Examples of adequate and inadequate near non-flesh and non-flesh diets of population groups reported in the literature *

Investigator	Population group	Characteristics of the diet
Adequate-diets		
McCarrison	Hunza	Wheat, barley, millet, maize, legumes, vegetables, apricots, milk, meat occasionally
Richards	Bemba	Finger millet, maize, sweet potatoes, legumes, plantains, vegetables, little animal food
Steiner	Okinawans	Rice, sweet potatoes, soybeans, vegetables, some milk, meat infrequently
Adolph	North Chinese	Wheat, millet, barley, corn, soybeans, other legumes, vegetables
Anderson *et al.*	Otomi Indians, Mexico	Corn (mainly as tortillas, up to 80% of total calories) legumes, vegetables, fruit, animal protein low
Toor *et al.*	Yemenite Jews	Large quantities of "pita" (flat bread) and vegetables, sunflower seeds, legumes, nuts, little meat
Walker	South African Bantu	50–90% whole-ground or lightly milled cereals, corn, sorghum and wheat, legumes, vegetables and greens; a little milk, eggs, and meat
FAO/WHO Report	Lebanese	56% of calories from cereals—wheat, barley, millet, rice; milk, cheese, legumes, fruits, vegetables, olive oil, and ghee; meat intake very low
Inadequate diets		
McCarrison	India, poor southern	Mostly white rice, some legumes, vegetables, fruits, little or no milk or meat
Gillman	poor Bantu	Diet largely maize meal (mealie pap) and sour milk when available
Oomen *et al.*	Papua, Highland	Sago, sweet potato, or taro, often providing 90% of total calories
Bailey	Java (cassava area)	Poor man's diet; cassava root providing 95% of calories, vegetables 4%, and beans 1%; total calories, 1,600; total protein, 9 gm.
Collis *et al.*	Nigeria (Yoruba)	Starchy roots and starchy portion of grains, fruit rarely eaten, low intake of pulses and animal products
Orr and Gilks	Africa (Kikuyu)	White millet, maize, some legumes and vegetables, a little milk, but taboo for women from puberty to menopause
de Wijn	Central Celebes	Rice providing 82% of calories, coconut 11%, vegetables 1%, a little fish and coconut oil

* From Hardinge and Stare (27).

lems in nutrition and public health. The pure vegetarians in a study by Hardinge and Stare (28) had significantly lower serum cholesterol than either the lacto-ovo-vegetarians or non-vegetarians.

Serum cholesterol and the dietary habits of a voluntary group of 466 Seventh-Day Adventists (SDA) were studied to determine the influence of diet on serum cholesterol in an adult population whose main environmental differences related to their adherence to a vegetarian diet. West and Hayes matched vegetarians with non-vegetarians from the same base population and examined the effects of various levels of meat, fish, and fowl consumption (degrees of non-vegetarianism) on serum cholesterol levels (29). The difference between serum cholesterol of the vegetarians and non-vegetarians was statistically significant. Several degrees of non-vegetarianism were noted, and the evidence was clear that as the degree of non-vegetarianism increased, the serum cholesterol increased.

Lemon and Walden, in their study of California Adventists, showed (30) that male SDAs suffered their first heart attack a full decade later than most Americans and the incidence of heart disease was only 60 per cent of the average California male population. Hodges *et al.* fed a diet to men in which the source of protein was meat analogs; they reported (31) a significant decrease in serum cholesterol.

Although the type and amount of fat, as well as the cholesterol content of the diet, have usually been singled out in relation to elevated serum lipid levels, within recent years a number of studies have suggested that people with diets rich in fiber have lower blood cholesterol levels.

Leguminous seeds, twice as rich as cereals in fiber content, have been considered in animal experiments (32) and in human subjects (33). In India, male volunteers ate 247 gm. Bengal gram (chick peas), consuming 16.0 gm. fiber daily. Even while eating a high-fat diet (156 gm. butter fat per day), they had a decrease in mean serum cholesterol from 206 mg. to 160 mg. per 100 ml. (34). It was necessary to eat the diet for twenty weeks to produce the maximal hypocholesteremic effect. Excretion of all bile salts was significantly increased on the high-fiber diet.

In 1963, a Japanese dietary survey reported (35) an average daily per capita consumption of 5.7 gm. ordinary beans—similar to the United States figure of 7.5 gm.—but a total of 69.4 gm. leguminous seeds, used largely as *miso, tofu,* and other processed forms. Since leguminous seeds appear to have a cholesterol-depressing effect, this feature of the Japanese diet may contribute to the maintenance of the low serum cholesterol level characteristic of that population.

PRACTICAL CONSIDERATIONS FOR DIETARY CHANGE

It is fortunate that the planning of a vegetarian diet is not difficult. In essence, it is the application of the basic concepts of good nutrition with a relatively few but important modifications. If one were to state the fundamental consideration, it would be to choose a wide variety of foods with a minimum number of refined products. (This basic principle is appropriate to the planning of any type of diet.)

The lacto-ovo-vegetarian diet. The Basic 4 food pattern provides a reliable guide for planning vegetarian diets with the major change in the meat or protein-rich group. In applying the Basic 4 pattern to a lacto-ovo-vegetarian diet, the following recommendations are important:

(a) Since in a vegetarian diet fewer concentrated sources of protein, such as meat, are used frequently, it is necessary to decrease significantly the "empty" calories. It has been estimated (36) that approximately 35 per cent of calories in the typical American diet are from sugars and visible fats. Unrefined foods, on a caloric basis, with few exceptions, supply their quota of protein to the diet. In evaluating the diet of anyone changing from a non-vegetarian to a vegetarian diet, the dilution of nutrients by empty calories should be checked and corrected.

(b) Meat in the protein group will be replaced by a generous intake of a variety of legumes, nuts, meat analogs made from wheat and/or soy proteins, and other formulated plant proteins. Although commercially prepared plant proteins are not essential to a well balanced vegetarian diet, these products do facilitate menu planning and preparation. Their use in the meal replaces the meat entrée with little further change in the menu needed. A number of canned, dehydrated, and frozen meat analogs are available in an expanding number of markets. Many combinations, consisting of legumes, cereals, and nuts, with or without milk and eggs, can be made in the home. Vegetarian recipe books are available, and a homemaker can make many tasty vegetarian entrées.

(c) In the milk group, greater use of nonfat or low-fat milk products, such as cottage cheese, contribute to protein intake and provide vitamin B_{12}. The recommendation of the milk group will supply vitamin B_{12} sufficient to meet the average adult need.

(d) Since the cereal and bread group also supplies some protein, as well as iron and B vitamins, intake of this group, preferably in the whole grain form, should be somewhat increased. However, care must be observed that this increase does not take place at the expense of the other food groups.

(e) The fruit and vegetable group is usually well represented in the vegetarian diet. Perhaps because of this, a vegetarian diet is often associated in the minds of the general public as consisting largely of vegetables. This class of foods is an important part of the diet, but other food groups are an integral part of a balanced vegetarian diet.

Actually, the lacto-ovo-vegetarian diet does not differ markedly from the average Western diet. The main difference is that it replaces meat with a variety of legumes, meat analogs, cereals, and nuts and more generous intake of milk and milk products and some eggs. In practice, the nutritional composition of this type of diet is strengthened by the variety of foods which replace meat. Ohlson has pointed out (8) that "many

Americans, particularly adult men, eat diets which are poorly balanced because of the large intakes of muscle meat, sweets, and fats and almost complete omission of cereals, except as refined flour entering into the preparation of sweet rolls or desserts. The vegetables and fruits used are limited in both amount and variety."

The pure vegetarian diet. Several difficulties may be encountered when diets completely devoid of animal foods are eaten. In the first place, many plant foods are low in calories; consequently, the sheer bulk of food to meet caloric needs can become a problem if the selection is not well planned. Second, although a lacto-ovo-vegetarian diet provides adequate amounts of vitamin B_{12}, no presently known practical source of vitamin B_{12} is present in plant foods. Some individuals appear to maintain good health for many years on a pure vegetarian diet without developing symptoms of deficiency, while others develop symptoms in a shorter time (27). The reason for this variation is not clear. Until more information is available, a pure vegetarian should include a source of vitamin B_{12} in his diet.

The following recommendations are important in changing from a lacto-ovo-vegetarian diet to a pure vegetarian diet:

The same consideration for the protein and cereal-bread groups which has already been made applies to a pure vegetarian diet. There will be, of course, increased use of the foods of these two groups, as well as from the fruit-vegetable group, to meet caloric needs. An adequate intake of calories is important. When caloric intake is inadequate, the body will preferentially use protein to meet its energy needs.

The milk group requires special attention. In the lacto-ovo-vegetarian diet, the milk group supplies 75 per cent of the calcium, 43 per cent of the riboflavin, 22 per cent of the protein, and practically 100 per cent of vitamin B_{12}. One way to obtain an adequate intake of these nutrients is to use sufficient quantities of fortified soybean milk. For an adult, this would be a minimum of two glasses a day. The label must be checked to make certain that the soybean milk is *fortified.*

Green leafy vegetables, on a weight basis supply as much calcium and riboflavin as milk (Table 4). A large serving (about 1 cup, 200 gm.) of such greens as collards, kale, turnip, and mustard, provides as much calcium as 1 cup milk. It is interesting that the Chinese Medical Association (37) recommended an intake of 500 gm. green leafy vegetables per day. In addition to greater consumption of dark green leafy vegetables, the use of cabbage, broccoli, and cauliflower will contribute lesser amounts of calcium but more than most other vegetables. Other plant sources which are fair to good sources of calcium include: legumes, particularly soybeans; some nuts, particularly almonds; and dried fruits. An evaluation of a pure vegetarian diet must be made to determine how often and in what quantity these plant sources are used. Occasional use cannot be counted on to replace the calcium and riboflavin of milk.

Table 4: Greens compared with milk as sources of nutrients

Food *	Protein	Calcium	Riboflavin	Iron	Vitamin B$_{12}$
	gm.	mg.	mg.	mg.	meg.
Milk	7.0	234	340	0.2	1.2
Soymilk †	6.0	60	120	1.5	0.6
Broccoli	7.2	206	460	2.2	
Turnip greens	6.0	490	480	3.6	
Greens, average ‡	6.7	305	390	3.0	
Soybeans, green	19.6	120	260	5.0	

* 1 cup or 200 gm.

† Commercial.

‡ Greens included: broccoli, Brussels sprouts, collards, dandelion greens, kale, mustard greens, spinach, and turnip greens.

Hardinge and Stare found (6) that diets of the pure vegetarians they studied usually consisted of cooked cereals and bread, legumes, nuts, large quantities of fruits and vegetables, especially large salads, vegetable oils, and olives. Minimal quantities of refined and commercially prepared foods were used. Few desserts were eaten. Table 5 shows the caloric distribution of selected foods from their study.

Table 5: Caloric distribution of selected foods of adult men on various diets *

Food	Per cent calories		
	Non-vegetarian	Lacto-ovo-vegetarian	Pure vegetarian
Milk	10.6	16.6	2.1 †
Meat	12.9	—	—
Cereal			
Dark	5.5	16.0	13.8
White	8.8	4.5	1.4
Legumes	1.2	4.0	5.7
Nuts	3.4	4.5	15.0
Fruits	9.3	19.0	30.8
Fat, visible	10.8	8.2	11.3
Desserts (sweets), including honey, sirup, molasses, soft drinks	25.0	11.9	7.0

* From Hardinge and Stare (6). Similar values were found for women.

† Soymilk.

Properly selected lacto-ovo-vegetarian diets are tasty and attractive and require no supplementation. A pure vegetarian diet can be planned that is adequate in quantity and quality of protein, as well as all other known nutrients, if supplemented with vitamin B_{12}. The approximate values of certain essential nutrients and amino acids for a one-day vegetarian diet are given in Tables 6 and 7.

Table 6: Approximate nutrient composition of one-day vegetarian diet

Nutrient	Lacto-ovo-vegetarian	Pure vegetarian	Recommended allowance *
Kilocalories	2,030	2,040	2,000
Protein (gm.)	78	75	55
Fat (gm.)	76	77	—
Carbohydrate (gm.)	260	265	—
Calcium (mg.)	1,110	740	800
Iron (mg.)	18	24.8	18
Vitamin A (I.U.)	12,600	14,600	5,000
Thiamin (mg.)	2.5	2.9	1.0
Riboflavin (mg.)	2.2	2.3	1.5
Niacin (mg.)	18.6	22.9	13.0
Ascorbic acid (mg.)	185	185	55

* For woman, 22 to 35 years of age.

Table 7: Amino acid content of one-day lacto-ovo-vegetarian and pure vegetarian diets

Amino acid	Lacto-ovo-vegetarian	Pure vegetarian	Minimum	Recommendation *
Isoleucine (gm.)	3.74	3.40	0.7	1.4
Leucine (gm.)	6.59	5.66	1.1	2.2
Lysine (gm.)	3.39	4.09	0.8	1.6
Methionine (gm.)	1.36	1.08	—	—
Cystine (gm.)	1.15	1.27	—	—
Total sulphur (gm.)	2.51	2.34	1.1	2.2
Phenylalanine (gm.)	4.13	3.76	—	—
Tyrosine (gm.)	3.10	2.56	—	—
Total aromatic (gm.)	7.23	6.32	1.1	2.2
Threonine (gm.)	2.93	2.75	0.5	1.0
Tryptophan (gm.)	0.92	0.89	0.25	0.5
Valine (gm.)	4.34	3.74	0.8	1.6

* For average man.

The dimensions of change in food patterns and products, in attitudes and habits during the 1960's have been extensive. The seventies and eighties will continue to present challenges to the dietetic practitioner to become concerned and involved in meeting the nutritional needs of the changing life style of our contemporary world.

One-day vegetarian menu

Breakfast	Noon meal	Evening meal
Orange juice—4 oz.	Soy patties with tomato	Vegetable soup—1 c. (200 gm.)
Cooked oatmeal—1 c.	sauce—2	Sandwich
Milk (LV)*—4 oz.	Baked potato—1	whole wheat bread—2 slices
Soymilk (PV)†—4 oz.	Margarine—1 pat	garbanzo-egg filling (LV)
Whole wheat toast—1 slice	Cooked fresh or frozen	Savory garbanzos (PV)
Peanut butter—Tbsp.	peas—⅔ c.	Sliced peaches—½ c.
Clear hot cereal beverage,	Shredded carrot salad—	Walnut-stuffed dates—4
if desired	½ c., scant	Milk (LV)—8 oz.
	Dressing—½ Tbsp.	Soymilk (PV)—8 oz.
	Wheat roll	
	Margarine—1 pat	
	Strawberries, fresh or	
	frozen without sugar—	
	¾ c.	
	Milk (LV)—8 oz.	
	Soymilk (PV)—8 oz.	

* LV = lacto-ovo-vegetarian.
† PV = pure vegetarian.

REFERENCES

1. Council on Foods and Nutr.: Zen macrobiotic diets. J.A.M.A. 218: 397, 1971.

2. Lusk, G.: The Elements of the Science of Nutrition. Philadelphia: W. B. Saunders Co., 1906.

3. Womack, M., and Kade, C. F.: Amino acids and proteins in nutrition. *In* Sahyun, M., ed.: Outline of the Amino Acids and Proteins. N.Y.: Reinhold Publishing Corp., 1944, p. 221.

4. Boeher, L. E.: Economic aspects of food protein. *In* Sahyun, M., ed.: Protein and Amino Acids in Nutrition. N.Y.: Reinhold Publishing Corp. 1948, p. 158.

5. Hegsted, D. M., Tsongas, A. G., Abbott, D. B., and Stare, F. J.: Protein requirements of adults. J. Lab. Clin. Med. 31: 261, 1946.

6. Hardinge, M. G., and Stare, F. J.: Nutritional studies of vegetarians. 1. Nutritional, physical, and laboratory findings. Am. J. Clin. Nutr. 2: 73, 1954.

7. Hegsted, D. M., Trulson, M. F., White, H. S., White, P. L., Vinas, E., Alvistur, E., Diaz, C., Vasquez, J., Loo, A., Roca, A., Collazos, C., Ch., and Ruiz, A.: Lysine and methionine supplementation of all-vegetable diets for human adults. J. Nutr. 56: 555, 1955.

8. Ohlson, M. A.: Dietary patterns and effect on nutrient intake. World Rev. Nutr. Dietet. 10: 13, 1969.

9. Jansen, G. R., and Howe, E. E.: World problems in protein nutrition. Am.J. Clin. Nutr. 15: 262, 1964.

10. Scrimshaw, N. S.: Nature of protein requirements. J. Am. Dietet. A. 54: 94, 1969.

11. Sherman, H. C.: Protein requirement of maintenance in man and the nutritive efficiency of bread protein. J. Biol. Chem. 41: 97, 1920.

12. New sources of protein. Lancet 2: 956, 1959.

13. Bressani, R., and Behar, M.: The use of plant protein foods in preventing malnutrition. *In* Livingston, E. S., ed.: Proc. 6th Intl. Congress of Nutrition, 1964, p. 182.

14. Porter, G. G.: Some supplementary studies with wheat proteins. Master's thesis, Loma Linda Univ., 1957.

15. Sanchez, A., Porter, G. G., and Register, U. D.: Effect of entrée on fat and protein quality of diets. J. Am. Dietet. A. 49: 492, 1966.

16. Sanchez, A., Scharffenberg, J. A., and Register, U. D.: Nutritive value of selected proteins and protein combinations. 1. Biological value of proteins singly and in meal patterns with varying fat composition. Am. J. Clin. Nutr. 13: 243, 1963.

17. Register, U. D., Inano, M., Thurston, C. E., Vyhmeister, I. B., Dysinger, P. W., Blankenship, J. W., and Horning, M. C.: Nitrogen-balance studies in human subjects on various diets. Am. J. Clin. Nutr. 20: 753, 1967.

18. Marsh, A. G., Ford, D. L., and Christensen, D. K.: Metabolic response of adolescent girls to a lacto-ovo-vegetarian diet. J. Am. Dietet. A. 51: 441, 1967.

19. Edwards, C. H., Booker, L. K., Rumph, C. H., Wright, W. G., and Ganapathy, S. N.: Utilization of wheat by adult man: nitrogen metabolism, plasma amino acids and lipids. Am. J. Clin. Nutr. 24: 181, 1971.

20. Hardinge, M. G., Crooks, H., and Stare, F. J.: Nutritional studies of vegetarians. 5. Proteins and essential amino acids. J. Am. Dietet. A. 48: 25, 1966.

21. Rao, M. N., and Swaminathan, M.: Plant proteins in the amelioration of protein deficiency states. World Rev. Nutr. Diet. 11: 116, 1969.

22. Food & Nutr. Serv., USDA: FNS Notice 219, Feb. 22, 1971.

23. Robinson, R. F.: What is the future of textured products? Food Tech. 26: 59, 1972.

24. Koury, S., and Hodges, R. E.: Soybean protein for human diets? Wholesomeness and acceptability. J. Am. Dietet. A. 52: 480, 1968.

25. Bressani, R., Viteri, F., Elias, L. G., de Zaghi, S., Alvarado, J., and Odell, A. D.: Protein quality of a soybean textured food in animals and children. J. Nutr. 93: 349, 1967.

26. Hammonds, T. M., and Call, D. L.: Utilization of protein ingredients in the U.S. food industry. Dept. of Agric. Economics Res. 320 and 321. Ithaca, N.Y.: Cornell Univ., 1970.

27. Hardinge, M. G., and Crooks, H.: Non-flesh dietaries. 3. Adequate and inadequate. J. Am. Dietet. A. 45: 537, 1964.

28. Hardinge, M. G., and Stare, F. J.: Nutritional studies of vegetarians. 2. Dietary and serum levels of cholesterol. Am. J. Clin. Nutr. 2: 83, 1954.

29. West, R. O., and Hayes, O. B.: Diet and serum cholesterol levels. A comparison between vegetarians and non-vegetarians in a Seventh-Day Adventist group. Am. J. Clin. Nutr. 21: 853, 1968.

30. Lemon, F. R., and Walden, R. T.: Death from respiratory system disease among Seventh-Day Adventist men. J.A.M.A. 198: 117, 1966.

31. Hodges, R. E., Krehl, W. A., Stone, D. B., and Lopez, A.: Dietary carbohydrates and low cholesterol diets: effects on serum lipids of man. Am. J. Clin. Nutr. 20: 198, 1967.

32. Devi, K. S., and Kurup, P. A.: Effects of certain Indian pulses on the serum lipids, liver and aortic lipids in rats fed a hypercholesterolemic diet. Atherosclerosis 11: 479, 1970.

33. Grande, F., Anderson, J. T., and Keys, A.: The effect of carbohydrates of leguminous seeds, wheat and potatoes on serum cholesterol concentration in man. J. Nutr. 86: 313, 1965.

34. Mathur, K. S., Khan, M. A., and Sharma, R. D.: Hypocholesterolaemic effect of Bengal gram: a long-term study in man. Br. Med. J. 1: 30, 1968.

35. Keys, A.: Diets of middle-aged farmers in Japan. Am. J. Clin. Nutr. 23: 212, 1970.

36. Economic Res. Serv., USDA: National Food Situation, NFS 134, Nov. 1970.

37. Comm. of Nutrition, Council on Public Health, Chinese Med. Assoc.: Minimum nutritional requirement for China. Chinese Med. J. 55: 301, 1939.

29

YOGURT

is it truly Adelle's B vitamin factory?

K. M. Acott and T. P. Labuza *

The most interesting claim made for yogurt since Metchnikoff's 1907
"prolongation of life" theory is that made by Adelle Davis in the book,
Let's Eat Right to Keep Fit (*1*). She claims that, "yogurt offers a factory
of hard working bacteria willing to produce B vitamins for future needs,"
so one should eat plenty of it everyday. She cites research by Seneca et
al. (*21*), who found that, "when yogurt is eaten over a long period of
time no other bacteria except those from yogurt are found in the stools."
An example of how this is applied appeared in the *Minneapolis Tribune* of
Sunday, June 25, 1972. Here Adelle Davis states that eating yogurt
daily for several weeks before going to Europe will prevent any attacks of
dysentery or food poisoning while there.

Others have claimed magical properties for yogurt, including its use
as a daily enema in a cancer cure (New Hope for Cancer Victims, Dr. W.
D. Kelly, D. D. S., Kelly Research Foundation, 1969, Grapevine, Tex.) to
provide useful nutrition for the liver.

Statements such as these appear believable in this modern-day atmosphere of strong consumer concern for good nutrition. But what they
really show is the need for well qualified, specific evidence to support
health claims.

Reprinted from *Food Product Development.* © November 1972.

* Department of Food Science and Nutrition, University of Minnesota, St. Paul.

Concerning the claims made for yogurt by Davis, three questions must be answered:

1.   Do the bacteria present in yogurt produce and excrete B vitamins into this food during their growth?
2.   Do these organisms produce B vitamins in a sufficient quantity in terms of the human vitamin requirements?
3.   Do the viable bacteria become established at the site of the gastrointestinal tract where B vitamins could be absorbed?

Yogurt is a cultured product made from milk.   The starting point is either evaporated milk or milk to which nonfat dry milk solids have been added to concentrate the solids (*2, 3*).   It is first pasteurized and then a mixed culture of two bacteria is added for controlled fermentation. Symbiosis occurs between two organisms, *Steptococcus thermophilus* and *Lactobacillus bulgaricus*, during the incubation in the pasteurized, concentrated milk.   *S. thermophilus* has a short lag phase and outgrows *L. bulgaricus* until the ratio of *S. thermophilus* to *L. bulgaricus* is about 3:1. At this point, lactic acid has accumulated and inhibits further growth of *S. thermophilus*.   *L. bulgaricus* begins growing and, being more tolerant to a low pH, proliferates through the lag phase.   As the population increases, more lactic acid is produced.   When the acidity finally inhibits further growth of *L. bulgaricus* the ratio of *S. thermophilus* to *L. bulgaricus* is about 1:1 (*3*).   After incubation the bacteria have produced a protein-coagulated, bacteriologically stable, sour milk product.   Flavorings, sugar, and fruit may be added along with potassium sorbate, which increases the product's resistance to degradation by mold (*3*).

As a nutritional food, yogurt is similar to milk, having a higher protein and calcium content resulting from its higher concentration of milk solids.   Table I compares the standard analysis of two popular brands of yogurt to milk.   Table II compares the vitamin content of whole fluid milk to yogurt.   Vitamin A, a fat-soluble vitamin, is 56 per cent lower in yogurt because of yogurt's lower fat content.   Vitamin C content is 71 per cent lower in yogurt because of the heating of the milk during pasteurization and the higher milk solids level it contains.   Addition of fruit, however, often will increase the level of vitamin C present in the yogurt. The level of choline in yogurt is less than that of milk by about 95 per cent. Choline is required by *L. bulgaricus* (*2*), probably for the synthesis of phospholipids for membranes, thus, it is consumed during fermentation (*6, 8*).   If one depended on yogurt for his choline source, this loss would be important.

Yogurt is inferior to milk with respect to nearly all other vitamins. A most interesting comparison is that yogurt contains 72 per cent less vitamin B_{12} than that of whole fluid milk.   Rasic and Panic (*9a, 9b*) found a loss of 55 to 77 per cent of vitamin B_{12} to be due to the heating of the milk before addition of the starter culture. In addition, *L. bulgaricus* and *S. thermophilus* are large consumers of B_{12} from the milk during fermentation and growth (*2, 3, 7*). Thus, since yogurt bacteria require vitamin B_{12} for growth, they do not increase the B_{12} content in the yogurt as has been claimed.

Table I: Standard analysis of two commercial brands of yogurt and whole milk

	Glamour (4) yogurt		Dr. Gaymont's (5) yogurt		Whole (6) milk
	Plain	Fruit	Plain	French	
Protein, %	5.5	4.8	4.2	4.7	3.0 to 4.0
Carbohydrate, %	7.8	19.0	5.78	9.0	4.5 to 5.0
Fat, %	2.0	1.5	2.0	2.0	3.5 to 5.0
Calories/oz	22.0	30.0	15.0	22 to 25	20

Table II: Vitamin composition comparison

	Whole fluid milk	Plain yogurt	Difference from milk, %
Vitamin A (IU/100 g)	156.	69.	—56
Thiamine (mg/1)	.44	0.37	—16
Riboflavin (mg/1)	1.75	1.40	—20
Nicotinic Acid (mg/1)	0.94	1.3	+12
Biotin (mg/1)	0.031	0.012	—61
Vitamin B_{12} (mg/1)	0.0043	0.0012	—72
Choline (mg/1)	121.	6.	—95
Vitamin C (mg/1)	21.1	6.2	—71

Source: Ref. (7).

With respect to question one, the production of vitamins if any is not a supported claim for yogurt.

As to question two, in all cases the vitamin content is reduced significantly from that of milk. Usually one does not consume quantities of yogurt as large as one does of milk because yogurt seems to have a filling effect. Thus, if one depended solely on yogurt for vitamins, the loss of nutrition would be significant. If it is used merely as a partial meal substitute, however, yogurt is a useful food.

In any case it is still necessary to answer question three for those instances where yogurt is eaten in large quantities either as stated earlier, for nutritional purposes, or to prevent food poisoning. It is possible that eating could transport the viable bacteria supplied to a place in the gastrointestinal (GI) tract where they could become implanted or occupy a suitable ecological niche. Attempts to implant the lactic acid bacteria, *Lacotbacillus acidophilles*, contained in acidophilus milk were reported by Kapeloff (*10*) and Rettger (*11*). They could show no implantation of *L. bulgaricus,* and "implantation" after ingesting *L. acidophilus* was short term, and the diet required supplementation with large amounts of lactose and dextrin (*10, 11*). Since then some workers have concluded that *L. acidophilus* will implant temporarily (by taking acidophilus milk with 4 x 10^8 organism/ml), because it is a normal inhabitant of the lower intestinal tract, and when conditions are right, this species can increase. These lactic acid bacteria would be of therapeutic use if put into the econiche of the lower GI tract especially after antibiotic therapy until normal balance for the tract is reached. At this time most of the *L. acidophilus* (*12*) are replaced by other microorganisms normally present.

Demonstration of implantation of *L. bulgaricus* or *S. thermophilus* has not been possible (*11*). In fact, a remarkable property of the GI tract is its ability to maintain a balance of normal flora in spite of variation in diet (*13, 14*). Haenal did experiments involving feeding a certain group or type of food for an extended period of time (*13*). Diets of meat and egg, or milk and vegetables, or only vegetables, or 40 g lactose and 1 kg of true Bulgarian yogurt/day resulted in no significant variation in fecal bacteria. This assumes GI tract flora would be represented in the feces (*14*). Bulgarian yogurt is made with *L. bulgaricus;* therefore, apparently the number of *L. bulgaricus* ingested did not multiply and were merely diluted in the vast balance of flora of the GI tract. Had *L. acidophilus* been used possibly an increase of that species would have been observed.

Even grossly changing the diet does not give evidence of any proliferation of *L. bulgaricus*. It is not likely that *S. thermophilus* would implant because it is not as tolerant to acidic conditions as *L. bulgaricus* (*3*). Implantation requires that viable bacteria endure the stomach pH of 1.0 to 2.0 (*8*) for the residence time of the yogurt in the stomach (30 min. to 1 hr.) (*15*). The following experiment attempts to determine the effect of acidic stomach-like conditions on the viable lactic acid bacteria in a cup of commercial yogurt.

MATERIALS AND METHODS

Two commercial brands of plain yogurt were used to determine the normal bacterial population. One brand was contaminated with mold spores (7 x 10^3 spores/ml) of a species forming white colonies on lactic agar. The large size of the mold colonies which resulted interfered with counting bacterial colonies, so this brand of yogurt was eliminated as a test medium.

All platings were made by pour plate technique with lactic agar (Table III) carrying out serial dilutions in 0.85 per cent NaCl saline. The HCl solution used was 0.12 N, pH 1.3. A milk coagulation test for the organisms was made using sterile nonfat milk (NFM) of 11 per cent solids content.

Table III: Lactic agar composition

Tryptone	20.0 g
Yeast Extract	5.0 g
NaCl	4.0 g
NaOOCCH₃	1.5 g
Gelatin	2.5 g
Lactose	5.0 g
Sucrose	5.0 g
Dextrose	5.0 g
Agar	15.0 g
Water	1 liter
pH adjusted to 7.0	

Plain yogurt, 38.7 g (pH 3.9), was diluted with 60 ml of the acid solution to give a final pH of 2.0 at 37°C (all components were tempered to 37°C prior to pH adjustment). An initial plating was made to determine original population before acid was added. This plating was made on yogurt diluted with saline by the same factor as when diluted by 0.12 N HCl, (i. e. 38.7 g yogurst plus 60 ml saline). Yogurt at pH 2.0 was held at 37°C, sampled at regular intervals for 3.5 hours and plated in duplicate on lactic agar.

RESULTS

Three types of colonies appeared on lactic agar. These were transferred to sterile milk (11%) and streaked onto lactic agar. Gram stains were made for isolated colonies taken from lactic agar plates. The observations are shown in Table IV. Without further biochemical tests iden-

Table IV: Colony observations

Colony type	1	2	3
Gram stain	g+	g+	g+
Morphology	cocci	rod	rod
Coagulates milk	yes	yes	no
Appearance of the colony on lactic agar	tiny, white	tiny, white	white, watery, spreader

tification of the bacteria cannot be certain, but Types 1 and 2 colonies were presumed to be *S. thermophilus* (cocci) and *L. bulgaricus* (rod) on the basis of their presence in yogurt and the coagulation of milk that occurred. The Type 3 organism was not identified but was probably a contaminant in the yogurt. Differentiation between Types 1 and 2 colonies was impossible on lactic agar so a total count is reported in Figure 1.

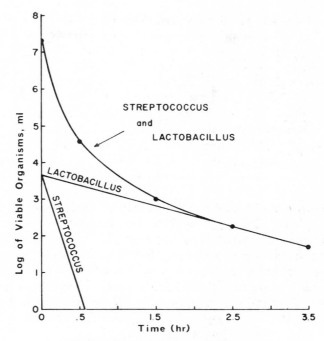

Figure 1: Log of viable organisms per ml

As seen from Figure 1, the number of survivors dropped suddenly in the first 30 min.   This was probably due to death of all the *S. thermophilus* organisms since they represent half the initial population and are more sensitive to low pH than is *L. bulgaricus* (*3*).   The viable population of *L. bulgaricus* decreased, until after 3.5 hours the yogurt had only 50 organisms/ml of diluted yogurt.   Presumably, the curve represents two superimposed exponential death processes.   Extrapolation of the lower part of the curve back to the origin shows that about 50 per cent of the population is *L. bulgaricus* as would be expected and as observed in plating the culture.

DISCUSSION

If the residence time of yogurt in the stomach is between 30 min. to 1 hr.   (*14*), the survivors may number from 10^4 to 10^3 organisms/ml of diluted yogurt assuming that pH alone is the critical factor.   Other components of gastric juice such as enzymes and mucous also may have some effect.

The next most influential factors are the environment and normal flora of the GI tract beyond the stomach.   Dixon (*16*) and others (*17*) have reported on the relative lack of bacteria in the stomach and in the small intestine. Peristalsis and possibly other inherent antimicrobial factors (such as immunoglobulins) prevent the growth of microbes in the place where most digestion and absorption occur (*18*). Thus, they are restricted to growth, primarily, in the large intestine (*19*).

Bornside et al. (*17*) aspirated the contents of stomach and small intestine of patients during abdominal surgery and found predominantly aerobes. Streptococci averaged 10^3 organisms/ml of aspirate and occurred in nearly all individuals sampled. Occasionally, lactobacillus was found in the jejunum (upper small intestine) where the pH is higher than that of the stomach but lower than the pH found in the ileum (lower part of the small intestine). The lactobacillus occurred in very few people, and when it did the population was very low. Thus, in answer to question three, it is possible that some lactobacillus organisms reach the small intestine and could grow. However, it seems incredible that they could have any effect on the presence of *Salmonella* food poisoning organisms which might be ingested and certainly would not prevent food poisoning from bacterial toxins present such as those produced from staphlococci organisms. Yet, it is possible that lactobacillus organisms may be transported to the large intestine and become the dominant microflora. As previously discussed, however, this seems unlikely.

The role of intestinal flora in nutrition of the host has been demonstrated in cows, horses, and rabbits (*6, 19*), and a major fraction of man's biotin and vitamin K requirement is thought to be supplied by the intestinal flora of the large intestine (*6*). The actual effect of bacterial metabolic activities on man is not clearly known and can only be suggested on the basis that metabolites are produced and absorbed.

The large intestine bacterial flora are predominantly anaerobic, as has been determined from feces. Lactobacillus is represented in anaerobic flora as well as the aerobic (*18, 19, 20*). Gall discussed vitamin production and use by the anaerobes in terms of the synergism that results. Vitamin production is significant only because it plays a role in the symbiosis between the organisms, thus, maintains a normal balance of the GI flora. Vitamins might be directly beneficial to the host if their production took place in a part of the gut where absorption could result. However, it is generally accepted that water is the only product of digestion absorbed by the large intestine (*8*). If B vitamins were produced by organisms and absorbed in the large intestine, there would never be an incidence of B vitamin deficiencies in individuals having normal GI microflora. This is Adelle Davis' hypothesis in her claim for yogurt.

In the paper "Bacterial Properties of Yogurt" by Seneca referred to earlier, research by Fykow and Meyer is mentioned. These latter workers fed *L. bulgaricus* sour milk to infants for 12 years by which time *L. bulgaricus* was the only organism in the stool and diarrhea was not present. When yogurt feeding stopped, the *L. bulgaricus* was replaced by a normal GI microflora. Seneca et al. (*21*) studied "in vitro" the bacteriocidal and bacteriostatic action of yogurt on a variety of pathogenic and nonpathogenic bacteria. He observed that bacteriocidal properties were very strongly correlated to the final pH of the yogurt. When yogurt was neutralized with sodium hydroxide to pH 7, the bacteriocidal property was lost. The pH effects of yogurt do not apply to "in vivo" situations where the gastric juice and pancreas control the pH of the GI contents. Seneca's discussion of this, however, was not reflected in Adelle's conclusion of the magical properties of yogurt.

Adelle Davis' comments about yogurt and accompanying bacteria reveal her lack of understanding of scientific literature on this subject. The reference she uses to validate her point is meaningless in terms of "in vivo" situations. The real problem is her widespread purveyance of this misinformation.

Vitamin assays of yogurt show the actual food is not as rich in B vitamins as is milk. Actually, yogurt bacteria are users not producers of B vitamins. An experiment to determine survival of the bacteria in yogurt suggests that if pH were the only controlling factor low populations of viable bacteria, most likely *L. bulgaricus*, could enter the small intestine. Implanting these bacteria offers no benefits in terms of B vitamins. It may even be possible that *L. bulgaricus* would compete with the host for B vitamins. There are microbes present in the normal flora of the intestines which have demonstrated the ability to produce B vitamins, but this effect is probably only part of the symbiotic relationship occurring among the normal microflora. Certainly, the bacteria common to yogurt do not prevent food poisoning.

One should not write off yogurt as a useless food, however. It has an interesting flavor and mouthfeel and can make a useful contribution to the diet in terms of calcium and protein nutrition, especially for those on reducing diets.

REFERENCES

1. Davis, A. 1970. Let's Eat Right to Keep Fit. The New American Library, Inc. New York. pp. 64, 93.

2. Pelczar, M. J. Jr. and R. D. Reid. 1958. Microbiology, McGraw-Hill Book Co., Inc., New York, pp. 82, 544.

3. Humphreys, C. L. and M. Plunkett. 1969. Yogurt: A review of its manufacture. *Dairy Sci. Abstr. 31*, pp. 607–22.

4. Glamour Yogurt. Bulletin from Mid America Dairymen, Inc., St. Paul, Minn.

5. Dr. Gaymont's Yogurt, Bulletin from Old Homes Food, Inc., University Avenue, St. Paul, Minn.

6. White, A., P. Handler, and E. L. Smith. 1959. Principles of Biochemistry. McGraw-Hill Book Co. Inc., New York. pp. 718, 929, 972.

7. Hartman, A. M. and L. P. Dryden. 1965. *Milk and Milk Products: A Review.* American Dairy Sci. Assoc. U.S.D.A. Beltsville, Maryland. pp. 15, 21, 38, 46, 61, 70.

8. Conn, E. E. and P. K. Stumpf. 1964. Outlines of Biochemistry. John Wiley and Sons, Inc. New York. pp. 55, 311–312.

9a. Rasic, J. and B. Panic. 1961. *Ach. Poljopr. Nauk. 14,* pp. 94. [DSA 23 (3326)].

9b. Rasic, J. and B. Panic. 1963. *Dairy Indus. 28,* p. 35.

10. Kapeloff, N. 1926. Lactobacillus Acidophilus. The Williams & Wilkens Co., Baltimore, Maryland.

11. Rettger, L. F. 1935. Lactobacillus Acidophilus and Its Therapeutic Application. Yale Univ. Press, New Haven, Conn. pp. 5, 6, 178–185.

12. Storrs, A. B. and R. M. Stern. 1967. *Lactobacillus acidophilus* concentrates. In Microbial Technology. H. J. Peppler, Ed. Reinhold Publ. Corp., New York. pp. 76–81.

13. Haenal, H. 1970. Human normal and abnormal gastro-intestinal flora. *Amer. J. Clin. Nutr. 23,* pp. 1433–1439.

14. Conn, H. O. and M. H. Floch. 1970. Effects of lactose and *Lactobacillus acidophilus* on the fecal flora. *Amer. J. Clin. Nutr. 23,* 1588–1594.

15. Sharp, H. University of Minnesota Hospital. Personal communication.

16. Dixon, J. M. 1960. The fate of bacteria in the small intestine. *J. Pathol. Bacterial. 79,* p. 131.

17. Bornside, G. H., J. S. Welsh and I. Cohn, Jr. 1966. Bacterial flora of the human small intestine. *J.A.M.A. 196,* pp. 125–127.

18. Hersh, T., M. H. Floch, H. J. Binder, H. D. Conn, R. Prizont, and H. M. Spiro. 1970. Disturbances of the jejunal and colonic bacterial flora in immunoglobulin deficiencies. *Amer. J. Clin. Nutr. 23,* pp. 1595–1601.

19. Gall, L. S. 1970. Normal fecal flora of man. *Amer. J. Clin. Nutr. 23,* pp. 1457–1465.

20. McBee, R. H. 1970. Metabolic contributions of the cecal flora. *Amer. J. Clin. Nutr. 23,* pp. 1514–1518.

21. Seneca, H., E. Henderson and A. Collins. 1950. Bactericidal properties of yogurt. *Amer. Pract. and Digest of Treatment. 1,* pp. 1252–1259.

E

The overweight

crisis

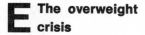

E The overweight crisis

THE OVERWEIGHT PROBLEM is one that involves almost 60 million people in the United States. In the first article, Dr. C. Gastineau of the Mayo Clinic attempts to define obesity, that is how much overweight constitutes obesity, and then examines its various causes. His list of causes includes genetics, impaired metabolism, loss of appetite control, fat cell size and environment. As he points out, no one factor is completely to blame.

Regardless of the cause of obesity, a majority of our population goes on a weight reducing diet at some time. The next two articles discuss the relative merits and dangers of weight-reducing diets. Dr. Fineberg's article provides an excellent overview, and the AMA's critique of Dr. Atkins' low carbohydrate diet indicates specific dangers.

30

OBESITY

risks, causes, and treatments

C. F. Gastineau, M.D.*

The risks imposed on health and life by obesity are not readily measured. Although mortality data from life insurance studies demonstrate clearly increased death rates among the obese from cardiovascular-renal disease, diabetes mellitus, and some diseases of the digestive system,[19] when factors such as hypertension or hyperlipidemia are removed, the risks are not as readily demonstrable.[12, 14] Even so, the possibility that obesity may contribute to coronary artery disease, for example, is of concern to physicians because of the number of deaths resulting from coronary artery disease and perhaps the intuitive belief that a large amount of adipose tissue should be reflected by a corresponding accumulation of fat lining the arteries. Postmortem studies suggest an increased incidence of coronary atherosclerosis among the obese, but again, the relationship is not as striking as one might think.[25]

Nevertheless, in obese persons diabetes, hypertension, and increased levels of blood lipids often do develop—all factors which contribute to coronary artery disease. The commonly observed lessening of both hypercholesterolemia and hypertriglyceridemia with weight reduction supports the view that obesity can contribute to vascular disease and, moreover, that correction of obesity can improve prospects for a longer life. Mortality rates (derived from insurance data) among men who successfully lost weight after having been obese are about the same as for men who were never obese.[19] Perhaps, therefore, in considering the risks of obesity it is appropriate to approach the subject of the hazards and the mortality

Reprinted from *Medical Clinics of North America*—Vol. 56, No. 4, July 1972, by permission of W. B. Saunders Company.

* Mayo Clinic, Rochester, Minnesota.

among the obese by taking an overview rather than by attempting to differentiate the separate roles of the various contributory factors.

THE RISKS OF OBESITY

A major problem in assessing the role of obesity in disease is the determination of who is obese and by how much the normal weight is exceeded. Height-weight tables are only approximate guides. Although skin-fold measurements are better, measurements of body composition with total body radioactive potassium or deuterium oxide dilution techniques are the best means of estimating obesity. Using such measurements as a reference, we have gained the impression that physicians tend to underestimate ideal weights for young adult obese subjects and to overestimate ideal weights for those later in life. Thus, a grossly obese man 25 to 30 years old may have a surprisingly large lean body mass; and his physician, guided by height-weight tables and perhaps by his own height-weight proportions, might estimate for him an ideal total body weight which is less than the actual lean body mass. In order to achieve the goal thus calculated, the subject would then have to lose not only all of his adipose tissue but also part of his muscle mass. In contrast, an older woman may be regarded by ordinary standards as only moderately overweight, when in reality 50 per cent or more of her body may consist of adipose tissue.[20] To reach a "normal" proportion of fat (15 to 25 per cent of the body weight), many older persons would need to reduce to a weight appreciably less than that recorded by them in their third decade of life.[12]

In our culture we commonly accept as normal a gradual weight gain year by year; but because with aging there is a decrease in muscle and other lean body-mass components, in order to keep the same proportion between fat and body structures, we should lose weight slowly once we have passed the age of 30. Many middle-aged and elderly obese patients have difficulty comprehending that it is not "right" for them to be 20 to 30 pounds heavier than they were when they were in the army or on their wedding day, two common reference points for remembering weights in young adult life. Men are in relatively good physical condition during their military service, and most women like to consider themselves as having been neither unattractively underweight nor overweight at their marriage.

Accordingly, the majority of older persons are in fact obese, rather than of ideal weight. Thus when we compare morbidity and mortality rates for older persons of different weights we usually are dealing with differences between greater and lesser degrees of obesity rather than differences between the obese and the non-obese.

Perhaps for some diseases moderate obesity may have almost as adverse an effect as severe obesity, whereas the distinctly lean person may

not be threatened.   Expressed in another way, the relation between obesity and a given disease, if it exists, may not be linear; and because of
practical difficulties in measuring degrees of obesity and excluding other
risk factors, the hazards of being obese may not be readily proved.

Some of these hazards are clear.   Thus, extreme obesity can cause
severe impairment of ventilation.   Alveolar hypoventilation, hypercapnea,
hypoxemia, and secondary polycythemia result; and clinically, somno-
lence, cyanosis, and congestive heart failure characterize the cardiorespiratory syndrome of obesity.[17]

The risks of surgery in the obese seem to be greater than normal.
However, a precise estimate of this risk cannot be made because obesity
in a patient influences the surgeon's decision whether or not to operate.
The difficulties of caring for the obese person postoperatively also seem
obvious.   Yet, objective measurements do not readily confirm these.

The mechanical effects of obesity in accelerating degenerative joint
disease of the knees and hips have also contributed to much disability
among the elderly.   It is not surprising that patients needing total surgical
replacement of the hip are among the best motivated and most successful groups of persons who lose weight by dieting, for they are told that
their obesity must be substantially corrected before surgery can be considered.   Another consideration is the insulin resistance imposed by obesity and the worsening effect of obesity on diabetes.   These are well documented.   Obesity may also cause diabetes to appear at an earlier age.[3]

Many other handicaps imposed by obesity cannot be measured by
mortality statistics.   The list of handicaps is virtually endless.   But consider just the following: the obese person is likely to find himself less
sought-after for employment and for marriage; many forms of physical
exercise and sport are not feasible for the overweight person; and attractive clothes are difficult to find.   To the patient, such handicaps are as
meaningful as the hazards to life.

ETIOLOGY

Metabolic factors

As possible explanations for obesity, differences in the metabolic
pathways of the obese person, insulin resistance, and elevated levels of
insulin and changes in adipose cell number and size have been examined.[3-5, 22]   The trend toward obesity in some families and in some strains
of animals has suggested a genetically determined difference in metabolism.[11]   The obesity of Cushing's disease is commonly cited as an example
of a metabolic cause of obesity; yet this is not so much an absolute increase in fat as a wasting away of structures composed of protein and
an accumulation of fat on the face and supraclavicular areas.   As the rest
of the body may be covered with little adipose tissue, the total picture

sometimes is that of a plump-faced but lean-limbed person with a protuberant abdomen.

The incidence of obesity in persons in whom diabetes is discovered during middle age or later years is sometimes explained by postulating that hyperinsulinism causes excessive fat accumulation and is an integral part of early diabetes. Yet it is more likely that the increased values of serum insulin often found in obese diabetics are an effect of obesity [16] rather than a cause. Further, it is likely that the increased levels of insulin still are lower than would be anticipated for similar levels of plasma glucose in the nondiabetic person of similar adiposity, and that diabetes is characteristically a disorder of defective insulin release.[16]

It seems almost unnecessary to argue that the obese person has eaten more than he requires; the obvious storage of fat provides prima facie evidence of this. The person who is 100 pounds overweight has approximately one third of a million calories of fuel stored in his excess adipose tissue. Many obese patients and not a few physicians keep looking for some anomaly in the assimilation and metabolism of food as an explanation for the excessive accumulation of adipose tissue and poor response to dietary efforts. An important observation which was made a half-century ago, when basal metabolic rate (BMR) standards were being developed,[22] and was verified recently in our laboratories, is that even grossly obese persons have normal basal metabolic rates. The mean and standard deviation of the BMR for a group of very obese persons are nearly identical with those of the normal population. Since the BMR is related to surface area, the values for oxygen and fuel consumption and carbon dioxide production in the obese person will be perhaps 20 to 30 per cent greater than for the counterpart of the same sex, height, and age, but of normal weight, the increase being proportional to the greater surface area. Thus, the obese person can be thought of as hypermetabolic. Even with a BMR of −15 or −20, the obese person will usually exhibit a "calorie-burning rate" which is greater than the mean for the person of the same sex, height, and age but of normal weight. No special economy or alteration of efficiency in use of food by the obese during exercise or during the digestive phase has been demonstrated.[11, 22] It therefore appears that the obese person actually requires, for the same activity, more food (often several hundred calories per day) to maintain himself than does his lean counterpart.

Appetite-regulating factors

If we reject metabolic factors as an unlikely explanation of obesity, we must postulate some disorder of the appetite-regulating mechanism. Here we find fertile ground, for any number of explanations have a reasonable ring, and they cannot readily be disproved.

Simple conditioning of eating habits in infancy and childhood would explain the familial occurrence of obesity. Attitudes of what constitutes an appropriate weight and appearance are also culturally determined, and these are powerful influences. Environmental factors show their influence as well in the form of greater variations in weight among siblings reared in different circumstances than among members of a family growing up and maturing in the same home and community.[18]

That genetic factors may influence weight is supported by observations that identical twins tend to be of similar weight even when they are reared in different homes.[18] Genetic forces may operate through appetite-controlling mechanisms situated in the hypothalamus. Injury to the hypothalamus also modifies eating patterns. In experimental animals, satiety centers in the ventromedial nuclei seem to inhibit and control a pair of appetite-stimulating centers situated in the lateral portions of the hypothalamus. These appetite-controlling centers in turn appear capable of modifying or producing gastric hunger contractions.

As to how these centers might sense the need for food and then signal that a meal providing sufficient energy had been ingested, an early proposal was that the temperature of the hypothalamus rose as a result of the specific dynamic action of food. Mayer subsequently proposed the glucostatic theory, according to which fluctuations in blood sugar provide the stimulus by which the hypothalamus perceives the need for fuel and measures the ingestion of food.

Striking similarities between obese persons and rats which became obese after lesions had been induced in the ventromedial nuclei were noted by Schachter. He observed that obese humans and rats had in common the following differences from their normal counterparts: they were less active and more "emotional," they ate less often but more rapidly and in larger amounts, and they were not inclined to work for their food unless it was visible or otherwise evident, though quite ready to perform tasks for food when it was apparent. Also, they were likely to eat less than normal if their food did not taste good. Schachter concluded that eating by obese persons is unrelated to any internal visceral state such as gastric distention or recent eating, and that it depends rather on external stimuli such as the sight, smell, and taste of food. It appears that if food is removed from his surroundings, the obese person can fast with less distress than the person of normal weight, whereas in the presence of food he seems to have more difficulty in fasting.

Some obese persons maintain a remarkably constant weight. Even after brief periods of weight loss, their weight tends to return to the original figure within a few months. Similarly, rats with hypothalamic lesions, once they have become obese, seem to maintain constancy of weight.

Adipose tissue cell size

Adipose tissue cells in obesity are often increased in number as well as in size,[4, 5] particularly if the obesity began in childhood or is of extreme degree. It has been suggested that a greater number of adipose tissue cells means an increased adipose cell mass, even when individual cells are normal in lipid content. If an obese person mobilized lipid from these normal-sized but more numerous adipose tissue cells, he would still have a relatively large mass of adipose tissue cells containing relatively little lipid. This would constitute a barrier to weight reduction.[5] A possible mechanism for the maintenance of constant weight is sensing by the hypothalamus of the average size of the adipose cells. The young obese person, for example, might have a larger number of adipose cells of relatively normal size; the hypothalamus would then govern appetite to maintain a normal adipose tissue cell size and thus there would be difficulty in restricting the intake of food. The manner in which signals as to cell size would reach the hypothalamus, however, is unclear.

Personality factors

As intriguing as these physiologic mechanisms are, we must remember that the consumption of food is ultimately under conscious control. Each bite of food is another decision, often an agonizing one, for the dieter. Emotional and personality factors are often interwoven with obesity, and these are remarkable for their complexity and diversity. Thus, the problem of the causes of obesity remains both simple, in that it is a matter of the obese person consuming more calories than are needed, and complex, as to why he is driven to consume that increased amount of food.

THERAPY

Many forms of treatment for obesity have been used, some of them potentially harmful, and most of them only partially successful. The ease with which a person can be weighed affects our concept of the problem and the way in which we are likely to evaluate the results of treatment. Without really thinking, we and our patients generally assume that loss of weight means loss of a corresponding amount of adipose tissue, but not all weight lost is fat. For instance, if desiccated thyroid, thyroxine, or triiodothyronine is given in greater than physiologic amounts, some degradation of muscle and other components of the lean body mass may occur. A similar loss of lean body mass can occur with fasting, and the magnitude of such lean tissue loss may be appreciable.[2] Weight loss resulting from degradation of lean body mass or from dehydration does nothing to correct the excess of adipose tissue. Yet the scales give an illusion of accomplishment.

Thyroid preparations

Since the obese person is already hypermetabolic, the risks of inducing a state of exogenous hyperthyroidism by the treatment for obesity are
not negligible.   Physiologic or smaller doses of thyroid extract or a synthetic thyroid preparation might be expected to have no metabolic effect
on the euthyroid person, since endogenous thyroid function would be
decreased in proportion to the dose.   Amounts greater than physiologic
would cause exogenous hyperthyroidism in proportion to the dose.

Pronounced loss of body weight can occur with initiation of a fast and
to a lesser extent with the beginning of a low-calorie diet.   This is probably a result of rapid losses of labile protein of hepatic glycogen and perhaps changes in hydration of body tissues.[6]   A correspondingly rapid repair of this tissue can occur when a fast is discontinued and a normal or
low-calorie diet is instituted.   This explains the paradoxical gain in weight
which sometimes occurs during the first several days of a nutritionally
complete low-calorie diet.   The risks of fasting are surprisingly small and
yet not to be ignored.   A physician choosing to use this mode of treatment
should familiarize himself with more detailed reports.[15]

Intestinal by-pass operations

Intestinal by-pass procedures are currently being employed rather
widely.   Surgical techniques have been improved and are becoming better
standardized.[21]   But the metabolic derangements resulting from these
procedures are likely to be complex, and are not entirely predictable.   The
threat of serious liver damage, perhaps a result of formation of an abnormal bile acid, is one problem not resolved.[7, 9, 13]

Amphetamines

Amphetamines are becoming less popular, because first, we are now
more aware of their potential for abuse, and second, the results of their
use have been generally discouraging.[8]

Chorionic gonadotropin

A. T. W. Simeons of Rome has devised a scheme for treatment of obesity which includes a 500-Kcal diet of prescribed foods in two meals with
a minimum intake of 2 quarts of fluids daily, as well as daily deep intra-
muscular injections of 125 units of chorionic gonadotropin.   It is claimed
that the use of chorionic gonadotropin in exactly this fashion makes the
low-calorie diet more tolerable and causes abnormal fat deposits to be lost
while normal fat is retained.[11A]

Proof is lacking, however, that this scheme of treatment is effective in any way other than through caloric restriction and facilitation of adherence to diet by means of the elaborate ritual.[1A]

The physician's responsibilities

Perhaps our greatest responsibilities are to explain to the patient the nature of the problem, to correct misconceptions, and to supply the nutritional information relating to a proper dietary program. A nutritionally complete, low-calorie diet is nearly without risk, and if adhered to will inevitably cause less of adipose tissue. We should point out the hazards of amphetamines, diuretics, and digitalis preparations. The risks and problems of total fasting, and of the ileojejunal shunt procedures should be discussed. For all of this, the physician should prepare himself by keeping abreast of the pertinent literature.

Frank psychiatric problems should be treated. In many cases, the obesity is just one aspect of a personality disorder, but psychiatric therapy is often disappointing if judged only by pounds lost. Group therapy is often useful—not instead of the efforts of physician and dietitian, but as a complement. Such groups can be formed in a variety of ways, but the benefits seem to be gained in basically the same fashion as that of Alcoholics Anonymous or Synanon. Perhaps the best results would be obtained when the patient lives within a special community which exists for handling his variety of problem. This arrangement has perhaps been the most effective situation for control and care of patients suffering from drug addiction.[10] Groups operating on a more social and informal level meeting at intervals are also remarkably effective in some instances.[24]

Massage, weighted belts, and inflated garments have all been commercially successful through promises of loss of adipose tissue in desired anatomic locations, but objective proof that any device or procedure will cause loss of fat from any particular portion of the body is lacking.

Although the long-term treatment of obesity, as judged by pounds of weight lost, is often disappointing, the physician can count himself as having been at least partially successful if he can help the patient avoid potentially injurious or futile and expensive modes of treatment.

REFERENCES

1. Albrink MJ: Cultural and endocrine origins of obesity. Am J Clin Nutr 21:1398–1403, 1968

1A. Albrink MJ: Chorionic gonadotropin and obesity? (Editorial.) Am J Clin Nutr 22:681–685, 1969

2. Ball MF, Canary JJ, Kyle LH: Comparative effects of caloric restriction and total starvation on body composition in obesity. Ann Intern Med 67:60–67, 1967

3. Bierman EL, Bagdade JD, Porte D Jr: Obesity and diabetes: the odd couple. Am J Clin Nutr 21:1434–1437, 1968

4. Björntorp P, Sjöström L: Number and size of adipose tissue fat cells in relation to metabolism in human obesity. Metabolism 20:703–713, 1971

5. Bray GA: The myth of diet in the management of obesity. Am J Clin Nutr 23:1141–1148, 1970

6. Dole VP, Schwartz IL, Thorn NA, et al: The caloric value of labile body tissue in obese subjects. J Clin Invest 34:590–594, 1955

7. Drenick EJ, Simmons F, Murphy JF: Effect on hepatic morphology of treatment of obesity by fasting, reducing diets and small-bowel bypass. N Engl J Med 282:829–834, 1970

8. Edison GR: Amphetamines: a dangerous illusion. Ann Intern Med 74:605–610, 1971

9. Editorial: Drastic cures for obesity. Lancet 1:1094, 1970

10. Etzioni A, Remp R: Technological "shortcuts" to social change: can major segments of contemporary social problems be handled efficiently by technology? Science 175:31–38, 1972

11. Gordon ES: Metabolic aspects of obesity. Adv Metab Disord 4:229–296, 1970

11A. Gusman HA: Chorionic gonadotropin in obesity: further clinical observations. Am J Clin Nutr 22:686–695, 1969

12. Heyden S, Hames CG, Bartel A, et al: Weight and weight history in relation to cerebrovascular and ischemic heart disease. Arch Intern Med 128:956–960, 1971

13. Juhl E, Christoffersen P, Baden H, et al: Liver morphology and biochemistry in eight obese patients treated with jejunoileal anastomosis. N Engl J Med 285:543–547, 1971

14. Keys A: Relative obesity and its health significance. Diabetes 4:447–455, 1955

15. Lawlor T, Wells DG: Metabolic hazards of fasting. Am J Clin Nutr 22:1142–1149, 1969

16. Lerner RL, Porte D: Insulin secretion in diabetes and other pathological states. *In* Diabetes Mellitus: Diagnosis and Treatment. Vol 3. New York, American Diabetes Association, 1971, pp. 31–37

17. Lillington GA, Anderson MW, Brandenburg RO: The cardiorespiratory syndrome of obesity. Dis Chest 32:1–20, 1957

18. Mayer J: Overweight: Causes, Cost, and Control. New York, Prentice-Hall, Inc., 1968

19. Metropolitan Life Insurance Company: Major findings and implications of the "Build and Blood Pressure Study, 1959." Stat Bull, Metropol Life Ins Co, 41:4–7 (Jan); 6–10 (Feb); 1–4 (Mar); 1–3 (Apr); 3–6 (May), 1960

19A. Nelson RA, Anderson L, Gastineau CF, et al: Physiology and natural history of obesity (abstract). Fed Proc 31:673, 1972

20. Novak L: Unpublished data

21. Payne JH, DeWind LT: Surgical treatment of obesity. Am J Surg 118:141–147, 1969

22. Rynearson EH, Gastineau CF: Obesity . . . Springfield, Illinois, Charles C Thomas, Publisher, 1949

23. Schachter S: Some extraordinary facts about obese humans and rats. Am Psychol 26:129–144, 1971

24. Stunkard A, Levine H, Fox S: A study of a self-help group for obesity. *In* Excerpta Medica, Proceedings of the Eighth International Congress of Nutrition. Prague, Number 213, 1969, pp 223–225

25. Viel B, Donoso S, Salcedo D: Coronary atherosclerosis in persons dying violently. Arch Intern Med 122:97–103, 1968

31

THE REALITIES OF OBESITY AND FAD DIETS

S. K. Fineberg, M.D.*

The foundation of the treatment of obesity must be the physician's unremitting effort to teach his patients the necessity of adhering religiously to a diet that is restricted in calories but balanced in terms of nutrient content.

"Calories" and "balance"—these are the key words. There is no other way to treat—or, more accurately put, to control—obesity. The patient must be made to understand that if he is to reduce his weight, keep it down, and not harm himself in the process, he must practice the self-discipline that is needed to adhere to a balanced diet of reduced caloric content. This requires strong motivation on his part. He must not waver in his determination to change his style of life and eating habits. Once he has made the change, he must abide by the new regimen no matter how great the temptation to stray from this straight, narrow path.

These are the harsh, plain realities. And perhaps because they are so stark and simple, obesity is for the physician one of the thorniest problems he has to tackle in his daily practice.

Although there are many fine points involved in the effective application of the simple rules of caloric restriction and nutritional balance,

Reprinted with permission of *Nutrition Today.* Copyright July/August 1972 by Nutrition Today Inc.

* Dr. Fineberg is Chief of the Diabetes and Obesity-Diabetes Clinics at the Metropolitan Hospital in New York, Assistant Clinical Professor of Medicine at the New York Medical College and Flower and Fifth Avenue Hospitals, and Chief of the Department of Medicine, Prospect Hospital, Bronx, N. Y.

they are all that medical science has to offer for the management of obesity at this time. No wonder so many patients seek a way out of this harsh and difficult-to-accept reality and turn to some "magic" diet formula instead, which offers a welcome escape. That the balanced, calorically restricted regimen has a high rate of failure is not surprising because it demands so much of patient and physician alike. The extent and duration of success seem to be directly related to the degree of personal effort applied by the physician. But sometimes the best that an enlightened and conscientious physican can do will fail in cases of very pronounced obesity because the patient sooner or later concludes that the treatment is worse than the disease or his fear of the consequences. This is true especially in massive obesity, a state in which the unfortunate individual's weight is two, three or four times the desirable level. It is extremely rare for such a person to achieve and maintain satisfactory control of his affliction.

INVISIBLE FACTOR

Before considering the fallacies and inadequacies of fad and crash diets, the composition and requirements of a nutritionally sound, balanced diet which will produce a significant rate of weight loss in the vast majority of cases should be reviewed in more detail. A sensible reducing diet should accomplish its purpose, the loss of fat from the body stores, with a minimum of risk to the individual and the least variance from a diet of commonly used foods. Caloric restriction is the essential prerequisite if the patient is to lose weight. The daily caloric deficit should be great enough to cause a loss of at least 2 to 3 lbs. per week during the early weeks of dieting. Most experienced therapists in the field are convinced that a majority of severely obese people, owing to an error or errors in their metabolism, have a daily caloric requirement for maintenance of ideal weight that is far below the levels set forth in the 1968 revision of the Recommended Dietary Allowances of the National Research Council's Food and Nutrition Board: 2800 calories for men and 2000 for women. This inherently lower caloric requirement, combined of course in most instances with ingestion of calories in excess of the average requirement, is the root cause of severe obesity. Without such errors in body chemistry these severely obese individuals would still have grown fat but probably to a lesser degree. Far too frequently, this totally invisible underlying factor is disbelieved or ignored by the physician, and all the blame for massive obesity is placed on an unmeasured and perhaps only moderately excessive caloric intake.

The traditionally prescribed 1000-calorie diet was most likely chosen originally by trial and error since its long-term application does produce satisfactory weight loss in practically all individuals. The actual degree of restriction may be varied according to individual response between 800 and 1400 calories daily.

However, such a calorically restricted diet should be a balanced diet, including a maximum of the required nutrients. It should comprise one or more servings a day from the Four Basic Food Groups, the milk, meat, vegetable-fruit and bread-cereal groups, and include a small amount of fat. These, in fine, are the bare elements of a balanced diet, often mentioned but seldom described. This simple regimen will provide a mixed nutrient intake of carbohydrates, proteins, fats, vitamins and minerals; the only drastic change is in the amount of calories. Much of the caloric reduction is in fat and some in carbohydrate, while protein intake is reduced least and remains entirely adequate. Proportionately, of course, this means a higher intake of protein. Even this sensible diet should very soon be supplemented, as an added precaution, by a multiple vitamin-mineral preparation to guard against the possible development of subclinical or borderline deficiencies.

This weight-reducing diet is the only suitable one for the treatment of obesity because all that is needed to make it a proper balanced diet for maintenance—as opposed to reduction—of weight is an increase in the size of portions. In this manner it prepares the patient for continued dietary control of his obesity for the rest of his life.

Anyone who has ever become seriously obese will always be a prime candidate—even after successful weight reduction—for rapid reversion to his previous overweight state. Even after attainment of the ideal or desirable weight, therefore, obesity should be considered to be controlled but never cured. The obese individual should be a permanent diet watcher! Like the diabetic or the hypertensive patient, he should remain under treatment at all times. The sensible diet I have described teaches him how to eat and what to eat for the rest of what may possibly be closer to a normal life span. The physician's major contribution to the program is his success in persuading the patient to accept and adhere to this new way of life.

The greatest obstacle to the proper medical management of obesity is posed by reducing diets that have been concocted by a combination of faulty reasoning and wishful thinking. Adherence to such ill-advised diets may upset the obese individual's nutritional equilibrium and produce a state of malnutrition. This condition can develop in a number of ways.

WISHFUL THINKING

All diets, balanced or unbalanced, "fad" or "crash," will produce weight loss if the total calories they provide in twenty-four hours amount to less than the individual's caloric requirement for weight maintenance at the start of dieting. At an equal—or slightly greater—intake of calories, weight loss will appear to be somewhat faster on some diets than on others. But no diet will result in loss of fat if it ignores the principle of the conservation of energy and the first law of thermodynamics by not providing for significant caloric restriction.

Probably the most misleading type of fad diet is derived from the school of thought that permits unlimited consumption of certain high-protein foods. Examples of such "Eat-All-You-Want" diets that are being widely promoted are the "Calories-Don't-Count" diet, which adds safflower oil to unlimited proteins and fats with very little carbohydrate; the "All-the-Meat-You-Want" diet; and "The Doctor's Quick Weight Loss Diet" allowing unlimited amounts of certain meats, fish, eggs and cheeses and requiring ingestion of at least 8 glasses of water daily. The life span of each of these diets is brief because it takes at most a few days or weeks for the people misled into following them to discover that they cannot continue to follow them. In desperation, these individuals then turn from one fad diet to another, unable to find a way out of their adipose predicament. The reason for the failure of these diets is simple enough: they run counter to the basic principles of balance, minimal change, and the teaching of good dietary habits for permanent control.

After a short time on one of these diets the patient is only able to choke down a limited amount of calories. He usually becomes repelled or satiated and winds up with an unplanned reduction in calories which does cause loss of weight. If he tolerates the diet better than most, he will not lose weight and may even gain. These diets may spring from an unconscious delusion but as a rule they are a deliberate ploy on the part of the "expert" prescribing them. Belief in them is self-delusion on the part of the victim. The dieter neither finds the diet satisfactory nor does he achieve anything approaching a lasting loss of weight.

Another type of fad diet may require some caloric restriction but demands either a sharp reduction of carbohydrate intake or no carbohydrate at all. An example is "The Drinking Man's Diet," which substitutes alcohol for carbohydrates. As Dr. Frank L. Iber of Tufts University pointed out in NUTRITION TODAY (January/February 1971), alcohol calories are not only nutritionally empty but are devoid of the type of energy that muscle tissue can utilize. Other diets of this type have been cloaked in a mantle of respectability by such names as "Mayo Clinic Diet"—a name that has been applied over the years to more than a dozen diets, none of which of course had the frailest connection with this renowned institution—or "Air Force Diet." This last, needless to say, has been emphatically disowned by the Air Force. In these diets, carbohydrate intake is reduced to 60 grams or much less, while fat and protein are usually unlimited. The "scientific" explanation being offered for the alleged effectiveness of low-carbohydrate diets is that in the fat person carbohydrate is rapidly converted to adipose tissue rather than being used for energy, whereas calories from fat and protein are burned up in the metabolic processes and are not stored as body fat. This is simply not true. What does appear to be true to some extent is that excess calories from whatever source, carbohydrate, protein, or fat, are less readily utilized and more readily stored in the fat person, in whom the process of lipogenesis is enhanced. *The initially greater weight loss resulting from a low-carbohydrate diet providing the same number of calories as a balanced, mixed-nutrient diet is actually due to an additional loss of body water, not fat.* Ignorance of this scientifically proven fact has probably led to more confusion in the dietary treatment of obesity than any other single factor. To understand this, a strong differentiation must be made between fat loss and scale-weight loss. The scale measures total weight only—and cannot distinguish fat loss from water loss or loss of vital lean tissue. It can never indicate what portion of a weight increase or decrease is due to change in fat content and what portion to a change in water content. A diet that contains carbohydrates but is well below the individual's caloric requirement in total caloric content will produce a reduction in scale weight which will parallel fat loss for only a few weeks in most individuals. Then, although the body fat of these persons continues to decrease, retention of

---

740-calorie "normal protein diet"

Breakfast   Calories
    4 oz. orange or grapefruit juice or
    5 oz. tomato juice 50
    Portion of cooked cereal 100
    Coffee with artificial sweetener
                                    150

10:00 A.M.
    4 oz. buttermilk or fat-free milk 50

Lunch
    4 tablespoons cottage cheese 60
    Lettuce and tomato salad 40
    Canned fruit—unsweetened, or gelatin 50
    Tea or coffee
                                    150

3:00 P.M.
    4 oz. buttermilk or fat-free milk 50

Dinner
    4 oz. chopped lean steak or
    3 oz. hamburger meat or
    6 oz. chicken or fish 260
    1 leafy vegetable 30
                                    290

10:00 P.M.
    4 oz. buttermilk or fat-free milk 50

                  Total calories   740

water will set in and mask or counter-balance the fat loss. The patient's weight as measured on the scale may show little or no change. This metabolic abnormality of water balance, the cause of which remains unknown, has been conclusively demonstrated to be due to the carbohydrate portion of the diet. It is not uncommon to see extreme examples of this in which patients will actually begin to gain weight on the scale while in negative caloric balance. If the diet contains little or no carbohydrate, this apparently disturbing and obstructive phenomenon does not occur, hence the greater effectiveness of such diets. It is of extreme practical importance to recognize that uncorrected salt and water retention is often responsible for the failure of obese patients to lose weight on a low-calorie diet of mixed nutrients to which they actually adhere. Failure to recognize and correct this retention by the judicious use of diuretics is probably the most important single reason for lack of response to the treatment of obesity in patients who are properly motivated and cooperative. This can be a very frustrating experience for them.

ENERGY FOR THE BRAIN

Yet carbohydrate must be furnished in the diet, despite this disadvantage, for a number of compelling reasons. First of all, if lifetime calorie control is to be acceptable to the patient, the diet must have some palatability and appeal. Much of the variety and taste in foods is furnished by carbohydrates. In addition, carbohydrate is an essential nutrient although not quite as indispensable as certain of the amino acid constituents of protein. The body has a specific need for carbohydrate as a source of energy for the brain and for other specialized functions. The Food and Nutrition Board of the National Research Council has suggested that the normal adult requires approximately 500 carbohydrate calories daily. If these are not provided in the diet, they will be derived from the breakdown of protein and fat, by the process of gluconeogenesis. Glucose is synthesized from protein only in certain body tissues and at a rate insufficient to meet specific demands. Carbohydrate is required so that fat, either endogenous or exogenous, may be completely oxidized in the body. In the absence of a sufficient amount of carbohydrate, an intermediary product of fat metabolism, acetylcoenzyme A, is formed, which condenses to form ketones. When the ability of the kidneys to excrete ketone bodies is exceeded, they accumulate in the blood, producing ketosis. This is an abnormal and undesirable metabolic state which occurs in starvation and in individuals on unbalanced, carbohydrate-deficient diets.

Another category of fad diets are those which are low or inadequate in protein. An example is the greatest crash "diet" of all time, "total fasting"! This is a recent fad of medical origin. The victim is given noncaloric liquids only and of course no protein. Other examples are the experimental low-protein "Rockefeller Diet," the Grapefruit Diet, the Water-melon Diet, the Skimmed Milk and Banana Diet, and the "Doctor's Quick Inches-Off Diet." An adequate protein intake is a basic requirement for health. A reducing diet, just like a normal diet, must contain sufficient protein to maintain the body structure. The recommended daily minimum is almost a gram of protein per kilogram of desirable body weight. If this amount is not furnished in the reducing diet, the vital need has to be filled by the breakdown of the individual's own lean, non-fat, protein tissue. Most of this will come from muscle and some of it from organ tissue. Instead of mobilizing and reducing only the excessive and harmful stores of body fat, there is actual catabolism of healthy, vital body structure. Metabolic studies of nitrogen balance performed in obese individuals undergoing total fasting revealed that 65% of their weight loss was due to loss of lean body tissue and only 35% was due to loss of adipose tissue. These studies have shown that fasting and diets with insufficient protein cause rapid weight reduction, but at the expense of lean tissue. To put it mildly, this is physiologically undesirable! A low-calorie weight-reducing diet must provide for a sufficient intake of essential amino acids to prevent any breakdown of body protein and insure that the weight loss produced is entirely due to the mobilization and utilization of fat.

ILLUSIONARY LOSS

Because of the constant metabolic need of the body for protein replacement, the total eventual weight lost on a diet of no calories, or total starvation, will not be greater—paradoxical as this may seem—than that resulting from adherence to a 700 to 900-calorie diet providing adequate protein! It has been observed repeatedly that the weight lost owing to catabolism of lean tissue is rapidly regained upon resumption of even a very low-caloric intake which includes protein. This is due to the rapid replenishment of the stores depleted during the period of negative protein balance. For every pound of protein replaced, there will be an increase of four pounds of body weight; apparently, three pounds of water are incorporated into the intracellular portion of each pound of actual protein mass. Even though the individual is still in negative caloric balance on the refeeding diet, he will thus continue to gain weight until the protein has been completely restored. In the long run, therefore, only the weight lost from fat depots can be prevented from returning. A reducing diet which contains no protein or insufficient protein not only causes weight to be lost from the wrong storehouse but much of the total weight loss is an illusion created by loss of water. Worst of all, this type of weight loss is completely futile because even with careful refeeding recovery of the lost weight cannot be prevented! This can have a serious, traumatic psychological effect on the actively cooperating fat person who has starved or half-starved himself for a prolonged period of time. He cannot understand why his weight should rapidly increase again with very little increase in calories. Many such victims of crash or unbalanced dieting or "dieting with malnutrition" have only slightly less understanding of this phenomenon than their physicans. At this point they may even conclude that thy are hopeless "glandular" or metabolic freaks whom no doctor understands or can help and become totally discouraged from further efforts to control their obesity.

In order to realize fully the fallacies, pitfalls and dangers of all fad diets, past, present and future, we should keep in mind the basic principles of the sensible approach to long-term dieting and good nutrition. Some of these are axiomatic in the light of our medical knowledge of nutrition and may be summarized as follows:

1.   A diet must produce a negative caloric balance if any weight loss is to occur.

2.   No weight will be lost through any conceivable change in proportion, combination, or omission of certain nutrients unless the caloric intake falls below the caloric requirement.

3.   An estimated average daily allowance of calories derived from a diet of mixed nutrients is the fundamental basis for lifetime control of obesity.

4.   Obesity of the common type should be considered to be controllable but not curable.

5.   Any individual who has ever developed a serious or massive degree of obesity must watch his diet for the rest of his life.

6.   Even reaching a "normal" or "desirable" weight is futile and possibly harmful if this weight is maintained for a relatively short time only.

7.   The loss of fat weight must be accomplished by a method whose major tool is a diet which, once weight reduction has been achieved, can be easily adapted for permanent control and is not detrimental to health.

8.   Diets very low in carbohydrate or protein may seem more efficient in that they produce some added weight loss for a given amount of caloric deficit, but this is a transient illusion attributable to water loss or changes in water balance. Actually, no added loss of fat is produced.

9.   A diet based on such an unbalanced "magic formula" is plainly injurious to health if the patient adheres to it for any length of time because he is then, in reality, "dieting with malnutrition."

There seems little doubt that the penalty of obesity is fewer years of life. Not only is life shortened by undue overweight, but death is usually preceded by a host of acute and chronic illnesses.

1000-calorie balanced diet (balance of carbohydrate, protein, fat plus vitamins and minerals)

Breakfast (160 calories)
1 serving of fruit juice
1 egg or substitute
½ slice of bread
Coffee or tea

> **Egg substitutions:**
> A.   4 tablespoons cottage cheese
> B.   1-inch cube American cheese
> C.   3 crisp bacon strips
> D.   1½ oz. meat
> E.   ½ cup oatmeal without cream or sugar **or** cornflakes with 4 oz. skim milk.

Lunch (260 calories)
A.   1 cup vegetable soup (can)
    1 hard-boiled egg
    ½ slice of bread
    1 cup (6 oz.) fat-free milk
or
B.   1 cup vegetable soup (can)
    4 tablespoons cottage cheese
    ½ slice of bread
    1 medium tomato and ¼ head lettuce
    1 serving of fruit
    Coffee or tea (no cream or sugar)
or
C.   3 oz. lean hamburger
    ½ slice of bread
    1 serving of fruit
    Coffee or tea (no cream or sugar)

3:00 P.M. (50 calories)
½ glass fortified, fat-free milk (4 oz.)

Dinner (500 calories)
2 cubes bouillon
1 serving of meat, 4 oz.
2 servings of vegetables (with a pat of butter or margarine)
1 slice of bread
1 serving of fruit
Coffee or tea (no cream or sugar)

Evening or bedtime (50 calories)
½ glass fortified, fat-free milk (4 oz.)

It is, therefore, all the more distressing that there are a great many people and not a few physicians and dietitians who continue to believe that the demand for people to do everything possible to keep from becoming or remaining obese is based entirely on some sort of vain pursuit of the "slim look." If many people continue to look upon slimness of figure as a fad, then, to the degree that they do so, our efforts to get at the root of the malady are vitiated.

At present, medical science is not trying as hard as it should to come to grips with the causes of obesity, and there seems little doubt that the failure to accept obesity as a disease or at least as the prodromal condition for other diseases is abetted by the frustrations most physicians experience when they try to do something about it.

FACTS OF OBESITY

The advice to slim down is based on sound medical thinking, and it may well be accepted even more widely in the future. Medical advice about eating habits and food selection in all states of health, including obesity, is in fact taken more and more seriously. Physicians should therefore not allow themselves to be discouraged when an obese patient says he cannot or will not follow his advice.

Regrettably, scientific half-truths, unproven and unsubstantiated conclusions, and just plain bunk about obesity and its treatment are still being welcomed by many as the ultimate truth and are often enthusiastically espoused. Inasmuch as medical knowledge in the entire field of nutrition is still hazy and incomplete, the patient is faced with the impossible chore of trying to separate fact from fiction. The trouble with most popular books about obesity and reducing diets is that only half of what they say is accurate but the reader does not know which half! This is not surprising since there are as yet few ironclad and immutable facts in any branch of medicine. Medicine is a "practice" and appropriately so called. It is based on valid conclusions drawn from an accumulation of data and experience, and these conclusions are continually being subjected to review and amendment as additional experience is gained. Nutrition is a relatively new science, and only in the last few decades have we assembled sufficient data to incriminate obesity as the forerunner of many diseases. No wonder, therefore, that the doctor often finds himself in a dilemma where obesity is concerned.

These, to this physician, are the facts of obesity. It seems inescapable to conclude that if the obese patient will abjure fads, ignore gossip, and be deaf to rumor and all the other cajolements that prey upon our natural human weakness in seeking shortcuts to health, he will realize that he cannot escape the torturous path leading to weight reduction, and he will finally be motivated to face up to the reality that weight can be lost only through serious, hard work. Not many are able to work so hard on themselves. But many more could if they would only learn from the repeated disappointments they have suffered by swallowing nutritional half-truths and trying fad diets.

32

A CRITIQUE OF
LOW–CARBOHYDRATE KETOGENIC
WEIGHT REDUCTION REGIMENS

a review of Dr. Atkins' diet revolution

Council on Foods and Nutrition

There has been a rekindling of public interest in the low-carbohydrate ketogenic diet touted as a "miraculous" and "revolutionary" approach to weight reduction. A recent example is the publication and extensive promotion of a book, *Dr. Atkins' Diet Revolution*.[1] The Council on Foods and Nutrition of the American Medical Association evaluated the claims made by Dr. Atkins and considered certain general questions concerning the "low-carbohydrate diet."

HISTORY OF LOW–CARBOHYDRATE DIETS

The low-carbohydrate diet approach to weight reduction is neither new nor innovative. About a century ago, an English surgeon, William Harvey[2] devised a diet for obesity that specifically interdicted sweet and starchy foods, while permitting meat ad libitum. One of his portly patients, William Banting[3] attested to the efficacy of Harvey's diet in *A Letter on Corpulence, Addressed to the Public*. During the last 20 years, there has been a cyclical recrudescence of similar diets having in common the following major features: (*a*) a low to very low carbohydrate con-

Reprinted from the *Journal of the American Medical Association*, June 4, 1973, Vol. 224, No. 10. (c) 1973 American Medical Association. Reprinted by permission.

tent, (*b*) no restriction of protein and fat, and (*c*) "unrestricted calories." Variants of the diet have been described in 1953 by Pennington [4, 5] ("Treatment of Obesity with Calorically Unrestricted Diets"), in 1960 as the Air Force diet,[6] in 1961 by Taller [7] (*Calories Don't Count*), in 1964 as *The Drinking Man's Diet*,[8] in 1967 by Stillman,[9] and, most recently, by Atkins [1] (*Dr. Atkins' Diet Revolution*).

Over the years, starting with the "Banting Diet," such regimens have been awarded a succession of eponyms and, from the very beginning, have been proclaimed to the public in glowing terms. If such diets are truly successful, why then, do they fade into obscurity within a relatively short period only to be resurrected some years later in slightly different guise and under new sponsorship. Moreover, despite the claims of universal and painless success for such diets, no nationwide decrease in obesity has been reported.

PHYSIOLOGICAL EFFECTS

An examination of the claims associated with advocacy of low-carbohydrate diets suggests that, in some instances, the authors found a way of circumventing the first law of thermodynamics, namely: "The energy of an isolated system is constant and any exchange of energy between a system and its surroundings must occur without the creation or destruction of energy." [10] For example, claims have been made that an unlimited calorie intake (excluding carbohydrate) is associated with a consistent and physiologically advantageous loss of weight (which presumably continues as long as the diet is maintained).

Most of the diets focus on diet composition, placing special emphasis on carbohydrate restriction while ignoring the calorie content of the diet. Some of the authors appear to believe that low-carbohydrate diets generate sufficient ketone bodies (eg, "incompletely burned" fat) to cause urinary losses of ketones in amounts sufficient to account for remarkable rates of weight loss in the face of high caloric intake. Dietary carbohydrate, particularly sugar, is considered by some advocates to be a nutritional "poison" that promotes "hypoglycemia," diabetes, atherosclerosis, and, of course, obesity.

To understand how diets induce changes in body weight, it is necessary to consider their effect on body composition—notably, fat, lean tissue, and water. Obesity is defined as an accumulation of fat in undesirable excess. Such fat can be lost only when calorie expenditure exceeds calorie intake. When water is retained in the body, weight may remain stable or increase even though fat is being lost. When lean tissue is broken down, weight loss may be rapid; however, this kind of weight loss is generally thought to be undesirable. Thus, short-term changes in weight on any diet have little meaning unless the composition of the weight loss is known.

While it is widely understood that calories are obtained from food, it is not as well comprehended that calories (energy) are lost from the body as heat, as excreta and detritus (urine, stools, sweat, etc), in the breath, and as metabolic and mechanical work (the body's metabolic processes and physical activity).   There are no other significant pathways of energy loss and no weight reducing regimen can operate without utilizing these channels.   No weight reducing diet, including the low-carbohydrate ketogenic diet, can be effective unless it provides for a decrease in energy intake or somehow increases energy losses.

Some observers have suggested that the excretion of large quantities of ketones in the urine might account for the extra weight loss alleged to occur in association with low-carbohydrate ketogenic diets.   However, when ketone excretion incident to such diets actually has been measured, it has been found to range between 0.5 and 10 gm/24 hr.[11, 12]   Studies carried out on starving nondiabetic persons indicate that at most about 20 gm of ketones per day may be excreted in the urine.[13, 14]   And, as Folin and Denis [15] have shown, the total acetone excretion with the breath is quantitatively insignificant; at most, 1 gm/day.   Since the caloric value of ketones is about 4.5 kcal/gm, it is clear that, in subjects on ketogenic diets, ketone losses in the urine rarely, if ever, exceed 100 kcal/day, a quantity that could not possibly account for the dramatic results claimed for such diets.

Another claim made by proponents of the low-carbohydrate high-fat diet has been based on observations by Kekwick and Pawan [16] in 1956 that obese patients on extremely high-fat diets of 1,000 kcal (90% of calories from fat) lost weight more rapidly over an eight- to ten-day period than when they were on an isocaloric diet containing a similar proportion of carbohydrate.   To explain their findings, these authors suggested that "obese patients must alter their metabolism in response to the contents of the diet."   However, when Pilkington and associates [17] studied the effect of similar diets for periods of 18 to 24 days, rate of weight loss was the same for both diets.

During the first few days of their study, Pilkington et al did observe differences in rate of weight loss similar to those reported by Kekwick and Pawan; however, they concluded that these temporary differences were due chiefly to changes in water balance.   Olesen and Quaade,[18] conducting similar studies, reported observations and conclusions similar to those of Pilkington et al.   Finally, it should be mentioned that some years earlier, Werner [19] studied subjects on the Pennington version of the low-carbohydrate diet and found that, apart from transient changes in water balance, the rate of weight loss in obese subjects on the low-carbohydrate diet that restricted calories was similar to that of a "balanced" diet of equal caloric value.

The excretion of sodium and water from the body can be inhibited by dietary carbohydrate.[20, 21]   Bloom [22] has shown that the weight loss of fasting can be decreased or abolished by the sodium and water retention that occur after ingestion of 600 kcal of carbohydrate. This effect on weight occurs even while the subject remains in negative caloric balance. It should also be pointed out that diets devoid of or very low in carbohydrate tend to promote a temporary sodium loss from the body. In addition a diet very high in protein content places an extra solute load on the kidneys necessitating an increase in excretion of urinary water: thus a low-carbohydrate diet, by several mechanisms, may cause dehydration, if suitable precautions are not taken. Patients whose renal function is already compromised may have difficulty in handling the extra burden placed on their kidneys by such a diet.

BASIS FOR WEIGHT LOSS

No scientific evidence exists to suggest that the low-carbohydrate ketogenic diet has a metabolic advantage over more conventional diets for weight reduction. The fact remains, however, that some patients have lost weight on the low-carbohydrate diet "unrestricted in calories." Why is this so? Yudkin and Carey [23] have reported experiments that provide an adequate explanation of the long-term weight loss that can occur when a "ketogenic" diet is consumed. These workers studied six obese adults who were carefully instructed in the weighing and recording of their complete diets. They were told to eat their usual food for two weeks. At the end of this time, they were asked to reduce the carbohydrate in their diets to about 50 gm/day for an additional two weeks and to eat as much protein and fat as they liked. Specifically, the subjects were told that they could eat unlimited amounts of such foods as meat, fish, eggs, cheese, butter, margarine, and cream. The intake of calories, protein, fat, and carbohydrate from the daily dietary records was then calculated.

In all subjects there was a reduction in calories ranging from 13% to 55% during the time they were consuming the low-carbohydrate diet. Interestingly, none of the six subjects ate more fat, and three of them showed a significant reduction of fat intake, ranging from 22 to 35 gm/day. It was concluded that weight lost on such diets was principally due to the consumption of fewer calories.

When obese patients reduce their carbohydrate intake drastically, they are apparently unable to make up the ensuing deficit by means of an appreciable increase in protein and fat. This is especially noteworthy when one considers the fact that carbohydrates comprise 45% or more of the average American's diet.[24] It is difficult to unbalance a diet to this extent and continue to consume the same calories as before. However, for persons who are adapted to a diet virtually devoid of carbohydrate it is not hard to maintain body weight. Tolstoi [25] and McClellan and DuBois [26] studied two normal men who maintained their usual weight for one year on a diet that consisted exclusively of lean and fat meat. The two men consumed about 120 to 130 gm of protein and enough fat to provide a total intake of 2,000 to 3,000 kcal/day. Thus, the weight reduction that occurs in obese subjects who are shifted to a low-carbohydrate diet seems to reflect their inability to adapt rapidly to the marked change in dietary composition. There appears to be no inherent reason why body weight cannot be maintained on a diet devoid of carbohydrate if the other essential nutrients are provided.

At the other extreme, a majority of human beings, particularly those in Asia and Africa, remain lean on diets extremely high in carbohydrate (by American standards) and correspondingly low in fat.[27, 28]   Thus, there is equally no inherent reason to associate a diet rich in carbohydrate with obesity.

POTENTIAL HAZARDS

What are the potential hazards of a diet very low in carbohydrate and rich in fat? Perhaps the greatest danger is related to hyperlipidemia, which may be induced by such a regimen. Hypercholesterolemia and hyper-triglyceridemia are associated with an increased risk of developing coronary heart disease.[29, 30]   A diet rich in cholestrol and saturated fat could be responsible for accelerating artherosclerosis, particularly in susceptible persons. The two subjects reported on by Tolstoi [25] developed a visible lipemia on their all-meat (low-carbohydrate) diets, and their plasma cholesterol rose to high levels (in one subject up to 800 mg/100ml).

Ketogenic diets also may cause a significant increase in the blood uric acid concentration. It appears that, by competing with uric acid for renal tubular excretion, elevated blood ketones can promote hyperuricemia. In patients with a gouty diathesis, the increment in hyperuricemia induced by such a regimen could exacerbate the underlying disease.

Bloom and Azar [31] have reported that all of the subjects whom they studied on "carbohydrate-free diets" complained of fatigue after two days on the diet. "This complaint was characterized by a feeling of physical lack of energy [and] was brought on by physical activity. The subjects all felt that they did not have sufficient energy to continue normal activity after the third day. This fatigue promptly disappeared after the addition of carbohydrate to the diet."

Another observation made by Bloom and Azar was that the subjects on the low-carbohydrate diets developed postural hypotension. The average systolic pressure fell 30 mm Hg and the diastolic 15 mm Hg when the subjects assumed an upright position after being supine.

EVALUATION OF DR. ATKINS' DIET REVOLUTION

In light of these facts, some of the claims in *Dr. Atkins' Diet Revolution* can be examined. It is alleged that ". . . carbohydrates—not fat—are the principal elements in food that fatten fat people. They do this by preventing you from burning up your own fat and by stimulating your body to make more fat. . . . Protein and fat combinations alone do not do this." [1(p 7)]

How does this thermodynamic miracle take place? It is stated that the diet promotes the production of "fat mobilizing hormone" (FMH) ". . . and the production of FMH is the whole purpose of this diet—and the reason it works when all other diets fail." [1(p 16)] But, according to Dr. Atkins, "FMH releases energy into your bloodstream by causing the stored fat to convert to carbohydrate. Thus, the fatigue clears without having to call upon the defective insulin mechanism." [1(p 73)] Accordingly, ". . . this is the diet revolution; the new chemical situation in which ketones are being thrown off—and so are those unwanted pounds, all without hunger." [1(p 13)]

As for a "fat mobilizing hormone" (FMH), no such hormone has been unequivocally identified in man. Fat is mobilized when insulin secretion diminishes.[32] Also, it is recognized that growth hormone and catecholamines stimulate fatty acid mobilization from the fat depots; however, neither of these substances is known to physicians and scientists as "FMH." Thus, the existence and physiological role of a putative FMH in man remain to be established.

The assertion that carbohydrates are the principal elements in food that fatten is, at best, a half-truth. In point of fact human subjects can gain weight by increasing their intake of fat, the most concentrated source of calories available. This was the rationale for the successful use of oral fat emulsions in the treatment of underweight persons.[33] Also, obesity is prevalent in North America, where the proportion of fat in the diet is higher than that in most other countries,[34] whereas obesity is relatively rare in large areas of the world where the "hidden sugar" of rice starch comprises a very high proportion of the total daily food intake.[35]

Body fat is burned in increasing quantity when total calorie intake is inadequate—regardless of the quantity of carbohydrate in the inadequate diet. Body fat is made from dietary fat as well as from dietary carbohydrate. This fact is obvious when one considers that the linoleic acid in the body's fat depots (usually 10% to 12%) cannot be made in the body but is derived entirely from the diet. Indeed, the fatty acid pattern of fat in the body's adipose stores tends to reflect the pattern of fatty acids in the diet.[36]

The notion that sedentary persons, without malabsorption or hyperthyroidism, can lose weight on a diet containing 5,000 kcal/day is incredible. No reliable nutritional studies have been reported to support such a claim. Nor is it possible to explain the alleged weight loss in the presence of a high calorie intake on the basis of ketonuria.[11-13]

With respect to ketosis, it is of particular interest to consider the experience of the Canadian Army during World War II with pemmican (dehydrated prime beef with added suet) as an emergency ration for infantry troops. In the Canadian study,[37] the pemmican derived 70% of its calories from fat and 30% from muscle. Thus, the ration was essentially free of carbohydrate.

The performance of the troops using pemmican and tea as the sole components of their ration deteriorated so rapidly as to incapacitate them in three days. When carbohydrate was added to the ration the men recuperated to a reasonably high level of performance.

While on the carbohydrate-free diet, the men complained of nausea and several of them vomited. Pathologic fatigue was evident. On the morning of the fourth day of the diet, physical examination disclosed a group of listless, dehydrated men with drawn faces and sunken eyes, whose breath smelled strongly of acetone. Because of anorexia and water loss the men had lost weight rapidly.

Throughout Dr. Atkins' book, the statement is made that fat is readily converted to carbohydrate; this is biochemically incorrect. Available biochemical evidence indicates that the even-numbered carbon chain fatty acids stored in adipose tissue triglycerides cannot be used for appreciable net synthesis of carbohydrate.[38] Essentially all stored fat is composed of even-numbered carbon acids. The glycerol released during hydrolysis of triglyceride is potentially available for carbohydrate synthesis; however, glycerol is not a fat. In addition, glycerol in adipose tissue is derived entirely from circulating glucose. It comprises about 10% of the calories available when triglycerides are broken down and their components oxidized. There is no evidence that the fatty acid released from stored triglyceride ". . . stabilizes the gyrations in your blood sugar level." [1(p 73)]

The book vigorously condemns carbohydrates as being nutritionally pernicious. Dr. Atkins states that "It is important, then, to understand that sugar has antinutrient properties. . . . Starch is the major source of hidden sugar." [1(p 57)] To describe starch as the major source of hidden sugar is naive. All carbohydrates in the diet must be converted to "sugar" by the digestive processes prior to their absorption by the intestine. To refer to sugar as having "antinutrient properties" is inaccurate. Although the thiamin (vitamin B_1) requirement increases somewhat when dietary carbohydrate increases, this does not mean that sugar is an "antinutrient" any more than is linoleic acid, a dietary constituent that may increase the body's requirement for vitamin E.

The book also puts great stress on "hypoglycemia" and its alleged relationship to obesity: "Hypoglycemia is undersuspected and underdiagnosed to an extent without parallel in medicine." [1(p 71)] Dr. Atkins' position on hypoglycemia should be considered in the light of the following statement [39] recently published Feb. 5 (223:682, 1973) in THE JOURNAL.

> Recent publicity in the popular press has led the public to believe that the occurrence of hypoglycemia is widespread in this country and that many of the symptoms that affect the American population are not recognized as being caused by this condition. These claims are not supported by medical evidence. Because of the possible misunderstanding about the matter, three organizations of physicians and scientists (the American Diabetes Association, the Endocrine Society, and the American Medical Association) have issued the following statement for the public concerning the diagnosis and treatment of hypoglycemia:
>
> "Hypoglycemia means a low level of blood sugar. When it occurs, it is often attended by symptoms of sweating, shakiness, trembling, anxiety, fast heart action, headache, hunger sensations, brief feelings of weakness, and, occasionally, seizures and coma. However, the majority of people with these kinds of symptoms do not have hypoglycemia; a great many patients with anxiety reactions present with similar symptoms. Furthermore, there is no good evidence that hypoglycemia causes depression, chronic fatigue, allergies, nervous breakdowns, alcoholism, juvenile delinquency, childhood behavior problems, drug addiction or inadequate sexual performance. . . ."

It is curious that hypoglycemia does not appear to be a problem in parts of the world where carbohydrate provides up to 80% of dietary calories. Indeed, it is of interest that in those same high-carbohydrate areas diabetes mellitus is less common than in the United States.[27] Also, it has been shown [40] that diabetic patients consuming a diet low in cholesterol (100 mg/24 hr), high in carbohydrate (64% of total calories), and low in fat (20% of total calories) maintained good to excellent regulation without an increase in insulin requirements and with a decrease in plasma cholesterol levels. Plasma triglycerides did not increase.

According to Dr. Atkins, most overweight people are hypoglycemic. A majority of physicians probably would not agree with this statement since it is well known that obese patients tend to be resistant to their own insulin. Moreover, there is no sound evidence to suggest that Dr. Atkins' recommendations of ". . . megadoses of B-complex, C, and especially E vitamins" [1(p 153)] will help keep blood sugar at an even level. The blood sugar remains remarkably stable without the help of unphysiologic doses of vitamins.

The diet encourages a high intake of saturated fats and cholesterol. The possible hazards of this practice are shrugged off with statements such as: "Studies have shown that you cannot absorb more cholesterol than is in two eggs each day." [1(p 282)] This is not entirely correct. It is not impossible to increase the plasma cholesterol level somewhat further by increasing the intake of egg cholesterol beyond this quantity.[41-44] More to the point, when they are added to a low cholesterol diet, two egg yolks per day can cause an undesirable increase in the plasma cholesterol concentration. Moreover, a rise in plasma cholesterol is not necessarily "compensated for" by a concurrent decrease in triglycerides. Indeed the most ominous type of hyperlipidemia, from the standpoint of coronary heart disease, is the form in which the plasma cholesterol concentration is elevated while the triglyceride level is normal (Type II).[45]

When a person consumes a diet very high in fat, he tends to develop an exaggerated alimentary lipemia.[46, 47] Some persons may already suffer from an inability to clear fat properly. There is also preliminary evidence to suggest that elevated levels of free fatty acids (such as would occur in patients consuming a low-carbohydrate ketogenic diet) may promote both vascular thrombosis and cardiac arrhythmias.[48-55]

An elevation of the plasma uric acid level is a frequent, if not invariable, concomitant of the low-carbohydrate ketogenic diet. If it becomes necessary to prescribe a drug like allopurinol to counteract such diet-induced hyperuricemia, then the risk of untoward side effects from the drug[56] is added to the nausea, anorexia, and fatigue that so often occur during adaptation to a diet virtually devoid of carbohydrate.

In summary, the approach to treatment of obesity recommended by Dr. Atkins is to restrict carbohydrate intake to less than 40 gm/day thus inducing a state of ketonuria as measured by means of a dipstick.

SUMMARY OF CRITIQUE OF DR. ATKINS' DIET REVOLUTION

The material cited appears to be more than sufficient to make the following points clear:

1. The "diet revolution" is neither new nor revolutionary. It is a variant of the "familiar" low carbohydrate diet that has been promulgated for many years.

2. The rationale advanced to justify the diet is, for the most part, without scientific merit. Furthermore, no evidence is advanced that controlled studies were ever carried out to validate the observation that weight can be lost by sedentary subjects who consume a carbohydrate-poor diet providing 5,000 kcal/day.

3. The Council is deeply concerned about any diet that advocates an "unlimited" intake of saturated fats and cholesterol-rich foods. In persons who respond to such a diet with an elevation of plasma lipids and an exaggerated ailmentary hyperlipemia, the risk of coronary artery disease and other clinical manifestations of atherosclerosis may well be increased—particularly if the diet is maintained over a prolonged period.

4. Any grossly unbalanced diet, particularly one which interdicts the 45% of calories that is usually consumed as carbohydrates, is likely to

induce some anorexia and weight reduction if the subject is willing to persevere in following such a bizarre regimen. However, it is unlikely that such a diet can provide a practicable basis for long-term weight reduction or maintenance, i. e., a life-time change in eating and exercise habits.

5. It is unfortunate that no reliable mechanism exists to help the public evaluate and put into proper perspective the great volume of nutritional information and misinformation with which it is constantly being bombarded. The Council believes that, in the absence of such a mechanism, members of the media and publishers as well as authors of books and articles advising the public on diet and nutrition have a unique responsibility to ensure that such information and advice are based on scientific facts established by responsible research. Bizarre concepts of nutrition and dieting should not be promoted to the public as if they were established scientific principles. If appropriate precautions are not taken, information about nutrition and diet that is not only misleading but potentially dangerous to health will continue to be conveyed to the public.

6. Physicians should counsel their patients as to the potentially harmful results that might occur because of adherence to the "ketogenic diet." Observations on patients who suffer adverse effects from this regimen should be reported in the medical literature or elsewhere, just as in the case of an adverse drug reaction.

REFERENCES

1. Atkins RC: *Dr. Atkins' Diet Revolution: The High Calorie Way to Stay Thin Forever.* New York, David McKay Inc Publishers, 1972.

2. Harvey W: *On Corpulence in Relation to Disease.* London, Henry Renshaw, 1827, pp 109, 122.

3. Banting W: *Letter on Corpulence, Addressed to the Public* (London, 1863) ed 2. London, Harrison, 1863, p 22.

4. Pennington AW: An alternate approach to the problem of obesity. *J Clin Nutr* 1:100–106, 1953.

5. Pennington AW: Treatment of obesity with calorically unrestricted diets. *J Clin Nutr* 1:343–348, 1953.

6. *Air Force Diet.* Toronto, Canada, Air Force Diet Publishers, 1960.

7. Taller H: *Calories Don't Count.* New York, Simon and Schuster Inc Publishers, 1961.

8. Jameson G, Williams E: *The Drinking Man's Diet.* San Francisco, Cameron and Co, 1964.

9. Stillman IM, Baker SS: *The Doctor's Quick Weight Loss Diet.* Englewood Cliffs, NJ, Prentice-Hall Inc, 1967.

10. White A, et al: *Principles of Biochemistry.* New York, McGraw-Hill Book Co Inc, 1954, p 9.

11. Grande F: Energy balance and body composition changes: A critical study of three recent publications. *Ann Intern Med* 68:467–480, 1968.

12. Azar GJ, Bloom WL: Similarities of carbohydrate deficiency and fasting. II. Ketones, nonesterified fatty acids, and nitrogen excretion. *Arch Intern Med* 112:338–343, 1963.

13. Lusk G: *The Elements of the Science of Nutrition.* New York, W. B. Saunders Co, 1906, p 63.

14. Deuel HJ Jr, Gulick M: Studies on ketosis. 1. The sexual variation in starvation ketosis. *J Biol Chem* 96:25–34, 1932.

15. Folin O, Denis W: On starvation and obesity, with special reference to acidosis. *J Biol Chem* 21:183–192, 1915.

16. Kekwick A, Pawan GLS: Calorie intake in relation to body weight changes in the obese. *Lancet* 2:155–161, 1956.

17. Pilkington TRE, et al: Diet and weight reduction in the obese. *Lancet* 1:856–858, 1960.

18. Olesen ES, Quaade F: Fatty foods and obesity. *Lancet* 1:1048–1051, 1960.

19. Werner SC: Comparison between weight reduction on a high-calorie, high-fat diet and on an isocaloric regimen high in carbohydrate. *N Engl J Med* 252:661–665, 1955.

20. Gamble JL, Ross GS, Tisdall FF: The metabolism of fixed base during fasting. *J Biol Chem* 57:633–695, 1923.

21. Hervey GR, McCance RA: The effects of carbohydrate and sea water on the metabolism of men without food or sufficient water. *Proc R Soc (Biol)* 139:527–545, 1952.

22. Bloom WL: Inhibition of salt excretion by carbohydrate. *Arch Intern Med* 109:26–32, 1962.

23. Yudkin J, Carey M: The treatment of obesity by the "high-fat" diet. The inevitability of calories. *Lancet* 2:939–941, 1960.

24. *Recommended Dietary Allowances,* 7th ed. publication 1964. National Academy of Sciences. Washington, DC, 1968, pp 9–10.

25. Tolstoi E: The effect of an exclusive meat diet on the chemical constituents of the blood. *J Biol Chem* 83:753–758, 1929.

26. McClellan WS, DuBois EF: Prolonged meat diets with a study of kidney function and ketosis. *J Biol Chem* 87:651–668, 1930.

27. West KM, Kalblfleisch JM: Glucose tolerance nutrition, and diabetes in Uruguay, Venezuela, Malaya and East Pakistan. *Diabetes* 15:9–18, 1966.

28. McLaren DS, Pellet PL: Nutrition in the Middle East, in Bourne GJ (ed): *World Review of Nutrition and Dietetics,* vol 12. Basel, Switzerland, S. Karger, 1970, pp 43–127.

29. Kannel WB, et al: Serum cholesterol, lipo-proteins, and the risk of coronary heart disease: The Framingham Study. *Ann Intern Med* 74:1–12, 1971.

30. Brown DF, Kinch SH, Doyle JT: Serum triglycerides in health and in ischemic heart disease. *N Engl J Med* 273:947–952, 1965.

31. Bloom WL, Azar GJ: Similarities of carbohydrate deficiency and fasting. I. Weight loss, electrolyte excretion, and fatigue. *Arch Intern Med* 112:333–337, 1963.

32. Cahill GF Jr: Physiology of insulin in man. *Diabetes* 20:785, 1971.

33. Shoshkes M, et al: Fat emulsions for oral nutrition; use of orally administered fat emulsions as caloric supplements in man. *J Am Diet Assoc* 27:197–208, 1951.

34. *Obesity and Health. A Source Book of Current Information for Professional Health Personnel,* publication 1485. Washington, DC, US Public Health Service, Division of Chronic Diseases, 1966.

35. Insull W, Oiso T, Tsuchiya K: Diet and nutritional status of Japanese. *Am J Clin Nutr* 21:753–777, 1968.

36. Christakis G, et al: Effect of a cholesterol-lowering diet on fatty acid composition of subcutaneous fat in man. *Circ* 26:648, 1962.

37. Kark RM, Johnson RE, Lewis JS: Defects of pemmican as an emergency ration for infantry troops. *War Medicine* 7:345–352, 1945.

38. West ES, et al: *Textbook of Biochemistry,* ed 4. New York, The Macmillan Co Publishers, 1967, pp 1050–1052.

39. Statement on hypoglycemia, editorial. *JAMA* 223:682, 1973.

40. Stone DB, Connor WE: The prolonged effects of a low cholesterol, high carbohydrate diet upon the serum lipids in diabetic patients. *Diabetes* 12:127–132, 1963.

41. Beveridge JMR, et al: Dietary cholesterol and plasma cholesterol levels in man. *Canad J Biochem Physiol* 37:575, 1959.

42. Bronte-Stewart B: Lipids and atherosclerosis. *Fed Proc* 20 (pt III, suppl 7): 127–134, 1961.

43. Connor WE, Hodges RE, Bleiler RE: The serum lipids in men receiving high cholesterol and cholesterol-free diets. *J Clin Invest* 40:894–901, 1961.

44. Inter-Society Commission for Heart Disease Resources, Atherosclerosis and Epidemiology Study Groups. Primary prevention of the atherosclerotic disease. *Circ* 42:A–55–A–95. 1970.

45. Fredrickson DS, Levy RI, Lees RS: Fat transport in lipoproteins—An integrated approach to mechanisms and disorders. *N Engl J Med* 276:34–42, 94–103, 148–156, 215–225, 273–281, 1967.

46. Brunzell JD, Porte D Jr, Bierman EL: Evidence for a common saturable removal system for removal of dietary and endogenous triglyceride in man. *J Clin Invest* 50:15a, abstract #48, 1971.

47. Connor WE: Effect of dietary lipids upon chylomicron composition in man. *Fed Proc* 18:473, abstract #1861, 1959.

48. Greig EBW: Inhibition of fibrinolysis by alimentary lipaemia. *Lancet* 2:16–18, 1956.

49. Merigan TC, et al: Effect of chylomicrons on fibrinolytic activity of normal human plasma in vitro. *Circ Res* 7:205–209, 1959.

50. Philip RB, Wright HP: Effect of adenosine on platelet adhesiveness in fasting and lipaemic bloods. *Lancet* 2:208–209, 1965.

51. Farbiszewski R, Worowski K: Enhancement of platelet aggregation and adhesiveness by beta lipoprotein. *J Atheroscler Res* 8:988–990, 1968.

52. Oliver MT, Yates PA: Induction of ventricular arrhythmias by elevation of arterial free fatty acids in experimental myocardial infarction, in Moret P, Feifar Z, (eds): *Metabolism of the Hyparic and Ischaemic Heart.* Basel, Switzerland, S. Karger, 1972, p. 359.

53. Oliver MF, Kurien VA, Greenwood TW: Relation between serum-free fatty acids and arrhythmias and death after acute myocardial infarction. *Lancet* 1:710–714, 1968.

54. Hoak JC, Warner ED, Connor WE: Effects of acute free fatty acid mobilization on the heart, in Bajusz E. Rona G (eds): *Myocardiology: Recent Advances in Studies of Cardiac Structure and Metabolism.* Baltimore, University Park Press, 1972, vol 1, pp 127–135.

55. Hoak JC, Connor WE, Warner ED: Toxic effects of glucagon-induced acute lipid mobilization in geese. *J Clin Invest* 47:2701–2710, 1968.

56. *AMA Drug Evaluations,* ed 1. Chicago, American Medical Association, 1971, pp 196–197.

F

**The nutrition crisis
in heart disease and atherosclerosis**

F The nutrition crisis in heart disease

PROBABLY the most controversial and pervasive area of the nutrition crisis is the effect of diet on coronary heart disease (CHD). Dr. H. Hurt reviews the history of the relationship of diet to heart disease, including the development of the American Heart Association's recommendations to reduce cholesterol and animal fats in the diet. Hurt points out that the cholesterol ban is based on experiments that may not relate to man. He also suggests that bias was introduced into many of the human studies. His analysis of the data indicates that one should not link CHD to any one factor. He shows that butter, egg and dairy food consumption patterns do not correlate to heart disease death patterns, as we have been told. Hurt concludes by warning against a drastic change in the U. S. diet unless more conclusive evidence is found.

Dr. George Mann corroborates Hurt's findings in the next article on animal fats. Mann shows how scientists sometimes fail to interpret data properly and consequently, their conclusions are misinterpreted by the media. Mann believes that CHD is the result of a lack of physical exercise. His work with the Masai tribe of Africa supports his hypothsis, as do other studies.

In strong disagreement with Hurt and Mann is Dr. Kannel, who tries to demonstrate that cholesterol causes CHD. He contends that while the evidence is not direct, it is indisputable. He responds to many of the questions Mann raised. Dr. H. Schroeder expands on the controversy in the following article on the relationship of trace metals to CHD and atherosclerosis. He cites epidemiological evidence showing less incidence of such deaths in hard water areas. It almost seems as though a relationship could be found between CHD and any food.

Other factors associated with high blood pressure, CHD and atherosclerosis are the genetic makeup of an individual and the effects of the daily environment. Dr. F. T. Hatch concludes that genetics may be the most important risk factor, overriding diet and environment. Dr. P. Peacock examines the environmental factors and writes that although extremes of temperature certainly increase CHD-related deaths the resulting stress involved is not the major cause of those deaths. Similarly, stress from light, noise, some pollutants and physical endurance factors has no major effect on CHD. He believes, as do others, that cigarette smoking is a major risk factor.

33

HEART DISEASE—IS DIET A FACTOR?

H. D. Hurt *

Data derived from extensive population surveys and animal experiments have provided indirect evidence associating elevated blood cholesterol levels with the increased incidences of atherosclerotic heart disease. As a result of this apparent relationship, recommendations have been made regarding the kind and amount of fatty acids and cholesterol which should be consumed for optimal health. Before massive changes are made in the eating habits of our population, the actual causal relationship between dietary fat and cholesterol to subsequent blood cholesterol levels and atherosclerotic heart disease should be determined. Although several risk factors have been characterized which will possibly aid in identification of those individuals most prone to development of atherosclerotic heart disease, the potential benefit from reducing a single risk factor in the prevention of the disease has not yet been conclusively demonstrated. The relative importance of dairy products as contributors of dietary saturated fatty acids and cholesterol is discussed in relationship to their association to heart disease.

Recently there has been an increased interest among the medical, scientific and lay communities regarding the relationship between our dietary habits and this nation's number one killer—coronary heart disease. This

Reprinted from *Journal of Milk and Food Technology*, June 1972, Vol. 35, No. 6 (P. 340–348).

Presented at the 58th Annual Meeting of the International Association of Milk, Food, and Environmental Sanitarians, San Diego, California, August 15–19, 1971.

* National Dairy Council, 111 North Canal Street, Chicago, Illinois, 60606.

renewal of interest concerning a problem which has existed since the beginning of mankind is primarily a result of the latest reports from the Framingham Study on heart disease and the recent recommendations which have been made to the public by the federally-financed Inter-Society Commission for Heart Disease Resources.

HEART DISORDERS

There are many different types of disorders of the heart such as congenital heart disease, angina pectoris, hypertensive heart disease, and atherosclerotic heart disease. The basic characteristic of atherosclerotic heart disease is the formation of obstructions or atheroma in the major blood vessels of the heart. In the simplest of terms, atheroma formation is believed to begin by the buildup of fat and other lipid-soluble materials in the inner linings of the walls of the blood vessels. Early stages of this disease are noted by the appearance of yellow fatty streaks in isolated areas. As the disease progresses, the fatty streaks become hardened and more obstructive. Eventually, the blood vessel will become completely obstructed, causing the flow of blood which is carrying oxygen and other nutrients to a particular area of the heart to stop. The affected tissues then die, resulting in a sudden and unpredictable heart attack. A fact often overlooked is that almost everyone in the world over the age of 12 has atherosclerosis to some degree (13). The National Health Examination Survey of 1960–62 estimated that 3.1 million Americans between the ages of 18–79 had definite coronary heart disease and 2.4 million had suspected coronary disease which represented approximately 5% of the population at that time (4).

ATHEROSCLEROTIC HEART DISEASE

Atherosclerotic heart disease is unquestionably the most important health problem facing this country today. Last year, of the 850,000-plus people who died of causes other than accidents, more than 165,000 of the deaths were a direct result of a coronary heart attack occurring in individuals under 65 years old. Today, it has been estimated that one man in every five will suffer some degree of disability before the age of 60 as a result of a coronary attack, and one in every 15 will meet an early death. Because of the magnitude of this health problem, not only should every attempt be made to learn its real causes through science and research but individuals should reappraise what is already known and take steps to implement programs which may provide some degree of protection from this disease.

Causes

Research studies to date have been unable to clearly define the causes for the buildup of atheroma which eventually leads to atherosclerotic heart disease. The countless numbers of surveys and laboratory studies with man and lower animals suggest there are a multiplicity of factors which may increase a person's "risk" of developing a coronary condition (29). The most comprehensive study conducted in this country to date which attempted to characterize the factors associated with heart disease was the well-known population survey commonly referred to as the Framingham Study (16). This investigation of 5,127 men and women living in Framingham, Massachusetts, was initiated in 1949. No attempt was made to modify the normal habits of this free-living population, for the study attempted to characterize every-day conditions existing in individuals who were eventually afflicted with coronary attacks. Based upon the results, it was anticipated that some clues regarding the cause of this disease would be obtained. During the ensuing 20 years, extensive clinical evaluation of the subjects and statistical correlation of the information gathered clearly identified several parameters that could be associated with the increased incidence of heart disease. Based upon a composite of the results from this and similar studies, the likelihood of having a coronary heart attack appears to be associated with: *age*—older people are more susceptible; *sex*—men have a higher incidence of heart attacks than women, until the late 40's; *genetics*—those who come from a family with a history of coronary problems are more susceptible; *stress*—the status conscious young man living under constant deadlines and tension may be more prone to coronary attack; *smoking*—heavy cigarette smokers appear to be more susceptible; *lack of exercise and obesity commonly associated with one's physical condition,* may lead to early death; and the most discussed risk factor, *dietary habits,* especially the consumption of cholesterol and saturated fatty acids which are largely derived from animal products (7).

Cholesterol

More than a century ago cholesterol and other fatty materials were identified as major constituents of the atheroma blockages in the blood vessels. In 1913, the Russian scientist Anitschkow demonstrated that feeding cholesterol to rabbits could increase blood cholesterol concentrations and produce atherosclerotic lesions of the heart and major blood vessels. Numerous human population surveys, or epidemiological studies, conducted in various parts of the world have demonstrated that many populations having high incidences of coronary heart attacks also have high blood cholesterol levels. Animal and human studies conducted under carefully controlled laboratory conditions have shown that the type and amount of dietary fat consumed will have a significant effect on blood cholesterol concentration. Diets containing a large amount of polyunsaturated fatty acids tend to decrease blood cholesterol concentrations whereas diets high in saturated fatty acids tend to increase blood cholesterol. Thus the association between dietary fats, cholesterol, and coronary heart disease has come to be regarded as an irrefutable fact (1, 18).

GUIDELINES FOR PREVENTION AND CARE OF HEART DISEASE

In 1965, a contract was negotiated between the Federal Division of Regional Medical Programs and the American Heart Association in an attempt to coordinate the efforts of several national professional organizations in developing guidelines for the care and prevention of cardiovascular disease. The American Heart Association created the Inter-Society Commission for Heart Disease Resources to accomplish this mission. The Commission is composed of 29 leading medical, nursing, and allied health organizations, and other experts selected for their special knowledge of heart disease (2).

Last December Commission members assigned to the epidemiology and atherosclerosis study groups issued a declaration for a national commitment to primary prevention as the principal means of controlling coronary heart disease. These Commission members expressed belief that hypertension, cigarette smoking, and high blood cholesterol levels were the three major "risk factors" associated with development of premature atherosclerotic heart disease.

In an attempt to reduce the incidence of coronary heart disease, the members of the two Inter-Society Commission study groups made the following recommendations regarding dietary changes:

(a) An individual's calorie intake should be adjusted to a level which would achieve and maintain optimal weight. For correction of obesity is known to be frequently associated with significant control of other related coronary heart disease risk factors such as diabetes.

(b) An individual should restrict dietary cholesterol intake to less than 300 mg per day. Currently, it is estimated that the average daily consumption of cholesterol is 600 mg per day. (An egg contains approximately 275 mg cholesterol and an 8-oz glass of whole milk 27 mg cholesterol.)

(c) An individual should substantially reduce dietary intake of saturated fatty acids in an attempt to lower blood cholesterol levels. It was recommended that the present 40% of total calories as fat which is now consumed be reduced to less than 35%, with no more than 10% coming from saturated fatty acids.

To accomplish these goals, it was further recommended:

(a) That the food industry make available products which would meet the specifications of lower saturated fatty acids and cholesterol necesary to lower blood cholesterol levels.

(b) That the dairy industry develop low-fat, low-cholesterol milk and milk products, and switch to cows that produce large amounts of high-protein, low-fat milk.

(c) That modified cheeses, containing lower saturated fatty acid and cholesterol content, be developed to aid in the reduction of dietary intake of saturated fatty acids and cholesterol.

(d) That industrial and governmental regulations which currently use butterfat content of milk as a pricing standard be modified to use protein content as the standard.

(e) That labeling and advertising be regulated in a manner allowing the consumer to know the actual fat composition of his diet.

The Inter-Society Report also recommended that the Government initiate massive public and professional education campaigns directed toward instructing consumers to decrease their intake of saturated fatty acids and cholesterol by reducing the amount of meat, dairy products, baked goods, eggs, and cooking fats consumed. It was also suggested that school lunch, food stamp, other supplementary food programs, and government-administered feeding programs in the armed forces and veteran hospitals be revised to encourage a low saturated fatty acid, low cholesterol diet.

The perspective of this report further stated that American agriculture and the food industry are already fully able to implement the changes necessary for this preventive program. With a decisive national commitment, there was reason to believe that significant progress toward reducing atherosclerotic heart disease could be made as early as 1975, according to the report.

If these Commission recommendations were to become national policy, the impact on the food industry is obvious. Eggs, with their high concentration of cholesterol, and dairy foods, such as whole milk, cheeses, and ice cream, which have been singled out as villains in the etiology of heart disease, would have even less appeal in the marketplace than they do today. Highly marbled beef would undoubtdly come into disfavor.

Before the dietary habits of the nation are overturned, a closer inspection of the evidence which has been used to associate diet and heart disease should be made.

DIET AND HEART DISEASE

Dr. D. S. Fredrickson, Director of Intramural Research, National Heart and Lung Institute, recently reviewed the Inter-Society Commission recommendations. In a lecture presented to the Royal College of Physicians of London, Dr. Fredrickson stated, (12), "In the light of what is actually known, the injunctions on consumption of cholesterol and fats seem too radical as they stand. What evidence do we have that an egg yolk a day spells jeopardy for *all* Americans? Do we have enough information about marginal hyperglyceridaemia or incipient diabetes to advise everyone to eat a diet which will tend to provide more than half of the calories as carbohydrates? What of sucklings and older infants? The Commission's report leads to an inference that a third of their calories from fat should also be polyunsaturated. Are we convinced of the safety of a diet containing 10% of polyunsaturates to the extent that we want to insist on this in baby's formula? Finally, are we certain enough of the efficacy of such sweeping changes that we, as physicians, can convincingly follow them ourselves?"

Cholesterol

The concept of dietary saturated fatty acids and cholesterol as a primary cause of atherosclerotic heart disease is not universally accepted in the medical and scientific communities (5, 24). Unfortunately, the research which has been conducted to date regarding the relationship between our dietary habits and the risk of having a coronary attack has given rise to a tremendous volume of conflicting data which has thrust the scientific and medical communities into deep controversy.

The original findings of Anitschkow, who demonstrated the atherogenic effect of feeding rabbits diets high in cholesterol, would never have occurred, had the studies been conducted on an animal other than the rabbit. The rabbit is by nature a herbivorous animal, living almost exclusively on green plants and vgetables low in cholesterol. Thus, it is hardly surprising that this species of animal would respond abnormally when fed an atypical diet containing a large amount of cholesterol. Other laboratory animals, such as the guinea pig, which have been used to confirm the dietary cholesterol-heart disease hypothesis, are also extremely intolerant to dietary cholesterol; relatively small amounts of dietary cholesterol will result in significant rises in blood cholesterol concentrations. By contrast, the dog, rat, and other carnivorous animals that normally consume diets containing cholesterol are extremely tolerant to dietary sources and rarely respond with elevated blood cholesterol levels. It is often necessary to interfere with normal thyroid activity before any changes in blood cholesterol can be seen in these latter species. The human diet normally contains both plant and animal foods. Thus, man should respond to dietary cholesterol somewhere between the two extremes (10).

It should be recognized that cholesterol is not a foreign or toxic substance to the living organism. The chicken egg, which carries the entire nutrient supply for a developing embryo, contains large quantities of cholesterol. All body cells have been shown able to manufacture cholesterol. A point often overlooked is that cholesterol actually plays a vital role in the normal metabolic processes of man. It is found in and may be required in large quantities for normal development and function of brain tissue and is part of the membranes surrounding every cell in the human body. Cholesterol is the building block for the manufacture of our sex hormones and it is an absolute requirement for the production of bile acids which are necessary for normal fat digestion. The human body is able to manufacture cholesterol in much greater amounts than dietary sources will provide and regardless of diet, cholesterol synthesis by the liver and other organs is controlled by the requirements of the body (28).

Epidemiological or population survey studies (17, 26, 27) have shown that considerable differences exist between serum cholesterol levels and deaths from coronary heart disease in different populations. Specifically, it has been found that people living in less technically developed populations tend to have lower blood cholesterol levels than those populations living in highly developed countries. The fact that the incidence of heart disease parallels the level of blood cholesterol has been accepted as evidence of a causal association between the two. It would, however, be preposterous to believe that diet was the only factor differing among the population groups studied and is thus responsible for differences in the incidence of heart disease.

Details of the following studies provide insight into the evidence cited in support of the causal association between cholesterol, saturated fatty acids and coronary heart disease. In a study conducted in New York City (8) as part of a total program to prevent heart disease, 814 men were assigned to an experimental low-cholesterol, high-polyunsaturated fatty acid diet and were given close and frequent medical and dietary supervision. The obese individuals in this group were placed on a low calorie diet until their desired body weight was attained. By contrast, the individuals serving as controls in this study remained on their customary normal diet and were examined only once a year, with little or no other supervision. Thus, it is evident that the experiment was inadequately controlled from the beginning. During the four-year follow-up period, there was significantly greater incidence of coronary heart disease in the control group which was not supervised than in the test group which had received diet and other therapy. The researchers themselves did not attribute the reduced incidence of heart attacks solely to the fat-modified diet since there were at least four other important variables involved in the program which had been initiated to prevent heart attacks. Nevertheless, proponents of fat-modified diets quote this study in support of their case. The results obtained in this study could have been attributed, just as soundly, to the correction of obesity and/or to the psychological effects of frequent medical and dietetic review as to the low cholesterol and polyunsaturated fatty acid content of the diet.

The study of Leren, often quoted in support of the relationship between diet and heart disease (23), involved 412 heart attack survivors under 64 years of age. The subjects were randomly allotted to one of two groups with different dietary treatments. One, an experimental group, was fed a low saturated fatty acid diet plus 70 ml of polyunsaturated soybean oil per day coupled with close dietary supervision. A control group remained on the normal diet with little dietary supervision. More individuals in the experimental group were initially underweight and fewer were overweight. Although there was no deliberate attempt to regulate weight in either group, there was a rapid weight loss of almost 6 lb. in the experimental group (thought to result from the diarrheic effect of the added soybean oil), which did not occur in the control. Therefore, although weight reduction was a persistent factor, it was not considered in this study. Lack of adequate control is once again evident in this experiment. During the five-year follow-up period, a higher relapse rate of heart attacks was reported in the control group than in the experimental group fed the low-fat, low-cholesterol diet. The author's conclusion that the cholesterol-lowering diet reduced the incidence of heart attacks is subject to serious question, for this difference in coronary attacks may just as likely have been attributed to differences in total caloric intake and weight reduction.

In another study (11), dietary saturated fatty acids were substituted with unsaturated fatty acids "to the maximal degree compatible with palatability." The diet fed to the subjects in the experimental group was also substantially lower in cholesterol content (365 mg cholesterol per day) than the diet fed the control group (653 mg cholesterol per day). Double-blind conditions were adhered to, so that the researchers were unaware of which people were in either group. Although both groups showed a gradual decline in serum cholesterol over the eight years of the study, the experimental group receiving the high polyunsaturated fatty acid diet exhibited a 13% reduction in blood cholesterol. Seventy deaths in the control group were attributed to acute atherosclerotic events, compared with only 48 such deaths in the experimental group. Deaths attributed to non-atherosclerotic and uncertain causes were more numerous in the experimental group than among control subjects so that total mortality was nearly identical. Thus, lifespan was not increased by diet therapy. Closer inspection of this study reveals that total over-all adherence to the diets was only about 50%. In addition, there were twice as many withdrawals from the experimental group as from the control group during the duration of the trial, and withdrawal status was disregarded in data analysis of the report. Although recruitment was carried on continuously during the eight-year experiment, most recruitment occurred during the first two years. As a result, some people were in the experiment for longer periods than others. In addition, the weight of many participants changed considerably during the trial period. There was also a significant difference in smoking habits between the groups; the control group had more smokers in the one-to-two or more packs per day category. The questionable aspects of this experiment are admitted by the researchers, but are scarcely mentioned by those who use the results as further "proof" of the beneficial effects of polyunsaturated fatty acids.

In the often-quoted National Diet-Heart Feasibility Study (3), subjects were voluntarily placed on a rigid low-cholesterol, high-polyunsaturated fatty acid diet in an attempt to reduce their blood cholesterol levels and thus prevent coronary heart disease. The results of the study were inconclusive for several reasons. Ten percent of the volunteers withdrew from the program during the first year. Only 50% of the subjects were classified as fair-to-good adherers to the programs initiated, with at least 25% classified as poor adherers. Of the men who finished the first year, 41% did not volunteer for a second year. Another 9% dropped out the second year. More noteworthy, however, was that the blood cholesterol levels of the population which adhered to the fat-modified diet were only 11 to 14% lower and less than 8% in those who lost no weight.

Thus, it can be seen that the large numbers of uncontrolled risk factors and the inherent complexities involved in intervening in free-living populations have seriously affected the interpretation of the results of many of these studies. Cornfield and Mitchell (9) have pointed out several other shortcomings of the often-cited clinical studies supporting the association between diet and heart disease. Inadequate sample sizes, inadequate randomization of experimental subjects and exclusion from final analyses of subjects who have withdrawn from the studies have seriously affected interpretations. Statistical procedures used to evaluate results have tended to cause misinterpretation of the results. Consequently, many studies report difference due to dietary manipulation when only differences by "chance" actually exist.

In the studies which purportedly support the relationship between diet and blood cholesterol, it is obvious that only modest achievement has been attained with volunteer participants, who are supposed to be keenly interested in the program. How, then, can a clinician be expected to prescribe therapeutic diets for his patients with any confidence of adequate lipid reduction? The studies just cited are in agreement that dietary treatment will decrease blood cholesterol levels approximately 10%. However, the Food and Drug Administration would surely not approve the marketing of a drug which showed so modest a therapeutic value (25).

It has recently been estimated that if elevated blood cholesterol levels could be completely removed as a risk factor, the total effect would be to reduce the rate of incidence of heart disease from 14 to 11 per 100 men in 10 years (29). This would occur providing that 100% cooperation was obtained, provided that the serum levels *could* indeed be lowered and maintained through dietary manipulation, and provided that lower serum cholesterol levels would, in fact, decrease the incidence of heart disease—*all points which are currently open to considerable speculation.*   Thus, the concept of heart disease prevention through dietary change—through removal of one risk factor which, at best, would have only a minimal effect —not only remains theoretically unproven, but is also, from a practical standpoint, an unrealistic solution for a complex society that loves an abundance of food.   The true decrease in coronary deaths which could realistically be expected as a result of dietary changes is important, especially those individuals who would have to sacrifice their customary lifestyles in order to adhere to dietary changes.

The public is frequently advised to reduced total fat intake by avoiding butter, whole milk, cheese made from whole milk, and cream, as a means of reducing the risk of developing heart disease.   Thus it would be of interest to examine more closely the direct relationship between the consumption of dairy foods and atherosclerotic heart disease.

Dairy foods

A causal relationship between dietary cholesterol and fat and the incidence of heart disease was not borne out by Kahn (14).   Nutrient composition of foods available for civilian consumption, or nutrient "disappearance" figures, were compiled from 1909 to 1965.   Cholesterol and dietary fat disappearance values were then calculated from these data. The study demonstrated that in the past 50 to 60 years in this country, serum cholesterol changes associated with changes in dietary fat and cholesterol have not been very great.   Dr. Kahn concluded that, "This, in turn, indicates that the increased risk of coronary heart disease reported to have occurred over this period is not related to dietary fat changes to a very important degree.   Changes in fat consumption may well be a means of lowering present-day risk of coronary disease, but other environmental factors are more probably associated with having raised the risk from that of 50 years ago to the present level."

Recent studies demonstrate that per capita consumption of butter and saturated fatty acids has continually declined since 1959 (19).   However, during the same period total fat consumption has risen slightly, primarily because of the increased consumption of vegetable oils.   This trend in substitution of polyunsaturated vegetable oils for saturated fatty acids has been accompanied by significant increases in numbers of deaths from atherosclerotic heart disease.   Why hasn't this association been realized? These figures show that the increased incidence of coronary heart disease occurred during a period when per capita consumption of dairy foods and other animal fats declined.   How *can* these products, therefore, be related to heart disease?   The rise in incidence of coronary heart disease is not consistent with trends in dietary fat and cholesterol consumption.

In addition, a comparison (based upon 1966 statistics) of longevity of life, and death from cardiovascular diseases, between countries with the highest consumption of whole milk equivalent (1. Finland-1513 lb.; 2. Ireland-1356 lb.; 3. New Zealand-1312 lb.; 4. Denmark-973 lb.; 5. Norway-969 lb.) and the United States (at 609 lb., 16th in consumption), reveals that, except for Finland, the countries with the highest consumption of whole milk equivalent had fewer male deaths and a lower death rate from cardiovascular diseases from birth to 64 years of age than the U. S. Except for Finland, average life span projections for the male are higher in countries consuming considerably more whole milk equivalents than the United States. Australia, Switzerland, and France also consume more whole milk equivalents than the United States (836 lb., 921 lb., and 923 lb. versus 582 lb., respectively), yet experience a lower death rate of males aged 45 to 54 years from coronary heart disease (325, 126, and 2 versus 352/100,000 population, respectively).

Another point to consider when attempting to put dairy product fats and cholesterol into proper perspective is just how much fat and cholesterol do dairy foods contribute to the American diet in relation to other foods? In 1965, the average American daily consumed 160 mg of cholesterol from meat; 270 mg from eggs; and only 70 mg from dairy products and 18 mg from butter (14). Also, two 8-oz glasses of milk, recommended daily for adults, contain only 17 gm fat and 54 mg cholesterol. Approximately 40% of our daily caloric intake comes from fat. Considering all fat sources, only 13.0% of the total fat calories and only 4.5% of the total daily calories are derived from dairy product fats (excluding butter). The majority of fat calories are contributed by meat and cooking oils. An important point to consider is that one-third of the fatty acids of milk-fat are monounsaturated fatty acids, which neither raise nor lower blood cholesterol levels. Milk contains 4% polyunsaturated fatty acids, which tend to lower serum cholesterol levels. Therefore, only about 63% of milk fatty acids are saturated fatty acids. Furthermore, nearly 10% of the fatty acids in milk are small, short-chain fatty acids which are known to be metabolized in a manner which has no effect on blood cholesterol levels. Only one-third or less of milk's fatty acids are of the kind suspected of elevating blood cholesterol, if indeed they affect serum cholesterol levels at all.

Framingham study

Many of the factors associated with increased heart attack "risk" have been based on the results of the Framingham Study on Heart Disease. Part of the Framingham Study was a critical evaluation of the dietary habits of a sample of the Study's subjects to determine normal consumption totals for fat, saturated and polyunsaturated fatty acids, and cholesterol.

Publication of the 24th Report from the Framingham Study (15) in April, 1970, revealed that consumption of these nutrients was relatively uniform in the population group tested. However, significant differences in blood cholesterol levels were noted. It was thus concluded: "With one exception, there was no discernible association between reported dietary intake and serum cholesterol level in the Framingham Diet Study Group." The one exception was a weak negative association between caloric intake and serum cholesterol level in men. The report also concluded that there was "no suggestion of any relation between diet and the subsequent development of coronary heart disease in the study group, despite a distinct elevation of serum cholesterol in men developing coronary heart disease." Thus, although the Framingham Study has achieved significance through its identification of the risk factors associated with the development of coronary heart disease, it has been unable to implicate diet as a risk factor in the development of coronary heart disease.

Clarity on what these findings actually mean is essential. They *do* mean that in the population tested in this study, normal dietary habits of a free-living individual did not appear to be related to the blood levels of cholesterol found in the subjects tested. In other words, within the range of dietary intakes covered by this study, intake of dietary cholesterol did not seem to affect blood cholesterol levels. These results do not imply, however, that serum cholesterol levels could not be influenced by diet under other circumstances. Yet it is evident from this study that something other than diet was responsible for the wide ranges in observed blood cholesterol values. And, although blood cholesterol values can regularly be manipulated in controlled or laboratory animal studies, a decrease in blood cholesterol levels in unrestricted, free-living humans would appear to be exceedingly difficult to produce. If the influence of diet on blood cholesterol levels and on concurrent heart disease were of major importance, the results of this and other studies would transcend the weaknesses and deficiencies of the experiments and a clear-cut effect of diet change would be seen. As stated previously, if dietary manipulation *could* actually lower serum cholesterol values and, in turn, decrease the incidence of coronary heart disease, its effect would be very small indeed.

Hazards from diet manipulation

In criticism of recommendations that consumption of polyunsaturated fatty acids be increased: there has been very little experience with the types of diets recommended by the Inter-Society Commission for Heart Disease Resources. The Inter-Society Report recommendations encourage consumption of polyunsaturated fatty acids up to 10% of total calories consumed. It is possible that diets high in polyunsaturated fatty acids may decrease blood cholesterol concentrations as a result of the redistribution of cholesterol into other tissue pools (28). The health significance of alterations in specific cholesterol pools when the total body cholesterol pool remains the same is unknown.

Many fats and oils currently available commercially have been subjected to the process of partial hydrogenation, which results in the production of geometric (trans) and positional (conjugated) isomers of the unsaturated fatty acids. It has been reported that margarines produced in the United States may contain as much as 46.9% trans fatty acids and that some commercial oils contain as much as 62% positional fatty acid isomers. Certain metabolic reactions are known to be affected by the configuration of the fatty acids. When incorporated into cell membranes, permeability characteristics and other biological functions may be seriously altered (20, 21).

HYPERLIPOPROTEINEMIA

Recently, scientists have become increasingly aware that individuals have specific blood lipid characteristics which respond differently to dietary therapy. Normally, cholesterol and other lipid substances are insoluble in the fluids of the body unless complexed with a protein molecule. The complexes of lipid material and protein referred to as lipoproteins are readily soluble. Based upon their relative composition of triglycerides, cholesterol, phospholipids, and protein, the various classes of lipoproteins can be separated and identified by electrophoretic and ultracentrifugation techniques.

These disorders, commonly referred to as Type I through Type V hyperlipoproteinemia, or high lipidprotein concentrations, have made it possible to identify the particular type of blood lipid disorder which an individual may have and then prescribe therapy tailored to the individual's specific needs. The increased plasma concentration of certain fractions of lipoproteins, in particular the *beta*-lipoprotein fraction, has been associated with increased risk of atherosclerotic heart disease because of its high cholesterol content.

Types I, III, and V are relatively uncommon and will not be considered further here. The blood lipid disorder termed Type II is very common and is believed to be expressed as a dominant genetically inherited trait. This disorder has been associated with premature death from atherosclerotic heart disease. The plasma from fasting patients with this condition is clear and the cholesterol value may be excessively high, as indicated by a distinctive *beta*-lipoprotein band. The recommended dietary treatment for the condition requires a reduction in cholesterol and saturated fatty acid intake accompanied by an increased uptake of polyunsaturated fatty acids. Changing the ratio of polyunsaturated to saturated fatty acids from the usual 0.2 ratio to 2.0 and reducing dietary cholesterol to less than 200 mg per day have been regarded as acceptable guidelines to follow in correcting this type of hyperlipoproteinemia.

The Type IV, or endogenous hyperlipidemia, is considered the most common blood lipid disorder. These patients will have normal cholesterol levels accompanied by grossly elevated plasma triglyceride concentrations. Patients with this condition commonly suffer from coronary artery disease. Dietary treatment in this instance is of importance since most of the patients are obese. It has been recommended that caloric intake be restricted, for weight reduction alone may effect complete regression of this condition (22).

DAIRY INDUSTRY AND HEART DISEASE

The dairy industry is contributing toward unraveling the mystery of the causes of heart disease through its membership in National Dairy Council (NDC). NDC maintains an active extramural research program designed to learn more about the relationship of our dietary habits and heart disease as well as supporting research directed toward ascertaining the importance of other possible causes. This organization continues to keep up-to-date regarding this issue and avails itself to the industry for interpretation and guidance relating to the diet/heart association.

NDC shares with many eminent scientists the view that much yet needs to be learned about the cause or causes of coronary heart disease. We also share the conviction that the alleged answer to the problem of coronary heart disease would, at this time, be far better applied on an individual, physician-patient basis, as depicted in the individuality of blood-lipid disorders. An individual at risk must be identified and given individual medical advice as to all the things he can do to reduce his chances of developing coronary heart disease. Unless otherwise directed by a physician, the best advice is to eat a balanced diet from each of the basic food groups in amounts which will maintain desirable body weight and to participate in a program of regular exercise. Thus, the future position of the dairy industry regarding the role of diet and blood cholesterol in relation to coronary heart disease should be:

(a) to continue to give strong support to research directed toward determining the cause or causes of coronary heart disease;

(b) to intensify its effort to tell the scientific community and the general public what is known in this highly controversial area and to keep them appraised of all new developments;

(c) to reject all efforts to bring about massive changes in the dietary habits of the American people, especially with regard to the consumption of dairy foods, on the basis of the inconclusive evidence to date;

(d) to encourage, through a strong program of nutrition education at the national and community level, consumption of a balanced diet chosen from the four food groups, including the recommended two or more glasses of milk a day for adults, and three or more for children, at a caloric level to maintain ideal weight;

(e) and finally, to rely on the inter-dependence of a balanced diet, sensible weight control, regular exercise, and consultation with your physician on special problems as the wisest course to follow on the road to good health.

SUMMARY

In summary, it would thus appear that the relationship of dietary saturated fatty acids and cholesterol is not completely based upon well-established evidence; there are many loop-holes in the existing studies which implicate diet in the etiology of heart disease. Too little is known regarding the possible effects of dietary changes which have been recommended and finally it should be recognized that the effectiveness of such changes is only speculative.

Dr. Edward H. Ahrens, Jr., Chairman of the National Heart Institute Diet-Heart Review Panel, has stated that "available evidence supporting the proposition that the incidence of coronary heart disease might be reduced by dietary measures is suggestive but not convincing," and "that in the absence of conclusive proof on the diet-heart question, any dietary advice to the American public will always lack authenticity and authority, will be conducive to half-measures and will meet opposition which cannot be effectively countered."

Major scientific organizations such as the Food and Nutrition Board of the National Academy of Sciences-National Research Council; The Council on Foods and Nutrition of the American Medical Association, and the Committee on Nutrition of the American Academy of Pediatrics, apparently agree inasmuch as they have not issued specific dietary recommendations to the general public.

Dr. W. B. Kannel, Medical Director of the Framingham Study, stated, "The root cause of the increase in the prevalence of atherosclerotic disease that we see today may very well be laid on the doorstep of progress" (16). One medical man has even gone so far as to state that "the increased incidence of age-related atherosclerotic deaths should shine as a jewel in the crown of medical science. Our knowledge of medicine has eradicated other major causes of death such as tuberculosis and typhoid fever and, in turn, allowed us to live long enough to succumb to such a relatively painless death as atherosclerosis. No other disease in the history of mankind has been so considerate to allow so many to live so long a productive life" (6). This concept may certainly be kept in mind when evaluating the current status of our nation's population; however, regardless of the past successes of medical science, we would be discontent by our very own nature to be satisfied until this disease has been reduced to a minor health problem.

REFERENCES

1. Anonymous. 1970. Diet and coronary heart disease. Nutrah 1:1.

2. Anonymous. 1970. Report of Inter-Society Commission for Heart Disease Resources. I. Primary Prevention of the Atherosclerotic Diseases. Circulation 42:A-55.

3. Anonymous. 1968. National Diet-Heart Study Research Group, National Diet-Heart Study Final Report, American Heart Association Monograph No. 18. Circulation, Vol. 37 and 38.

4. Anonymous. 1965. Coronary heart disease in adults in the United States, 1960–1962. Data from the National Health Survey, Vital and Health Statistics. Series II, No. 10, U. S. Dept. of Health, Education and Welfare, Public Health Service, Washington, D.C.

5. Altschule, M. B. 1970. Can diet prevent atherosclerosis?—If so, what diet? Med. Counterpoint 2:13.

6. Barnes, B. O. 1971. The riddle of heart attacks. (*In preparation*).

7. Brown, H. B. 1970. Food patterns that lower blood lipids in man. J. Amer. Dietetic Ass. 58:303.

8. Christakis, G., S. H. Rinzler, M. Archer, and A. Kraus. 1966. Effect of anticoronary program on coronary heart disease risk factor status. J. Amer. Med. Ass. 198:597.

9. Cornfield, J., and S. Mitchell. 1969. Selected risk factors in coronary disease. Arch. Environ. Health 19:382.

10. Daly, M. J. 1970. Studies of the roles of animal fats in meat references in the diet-heart controversy. A. P. and R. S. 89, Penn. State Univ.

11. Dayton, S., M. L. Pearce, S. Hashimoto, W. J. Dixon, and U. Tomiyasu. 1969. A controlled clinical trial of a diet high in unsaturated fat in preventing complications of atherosclerosis. Circulation 40:Suppl. II.

12. Fredrickson, D. S. 1971. Mutants, hyperlipoproteinemia, and coronary artery disease. Brit. Med. J. 2:187.

13. Hartroft, W. S. 1965. Atheroma begins at birth. *In* F. A. Kummerow (ed.) Metabolism of lipids as related to atherosclerosis. Illinois.

14. Kahn, H. A. 1970. Change in serum cholesterol associated with changes in the United States civilian diet, 1909–1965. Amer. J. Clin. Nutr. 23:879.

15. Kannel, W. B. 1970. The Framingham study-Anepidemiological investigation of cardiovascular disease-Section 24-The Framingham diet study: diet and the regulation of serum cholesterol. National Heart and Lung Institute, Department of Health, Education and Welfare.

16. Kannel, W. B. 1971. The disease of living. Nutrition Today 6:2.

17. Keys, A. 1965. Serum cholesterol response to changes in the diet. Metab. Clin. Exp. 14:747.

18. Kritchevsky, D. 1967. Atherosclerosis and cholesterol. J. Dairy Sci. 50:776.

19. Kromer, G. W. 1971. Consumption patterns and trends for fats and oils in the United States. Paper presented at the 62nd Annual Meeting of the American Oil Chemists' Society, Houston, Texas, May 5.

20. Kummerow, F. A. 1967. Influence of fatty acids on the level of serum cholesterol. J. Dairy Sci. 50:787.

21. Kummerow, F. A. Personal communication.

22. Lees, R. S., and D. E. Wilson. 1971. The treatment of hyperlipidemia. New England J. Med. 284:186.

23. Leren, P. 1966. The effect of plasma cholesterol lowering diet in male survivors of myocardial infarction. Acta Medica Scand. Suppl. 466:1.

24. Mann, G. V. 1966. Causes of coronary heart disease—the tide turns. Food and Nutrition News 37:1.

25. Parsons, W. B. 1971. Treatment of hyperlipidemia: The rationale for combinations of lipid lowering drugs. Int. Med. Dig. 6:33.

26. Sharper, A. G. 1963. Serum lipids in three nomadic tribes of Northern Kenya. Amer. J. Clin. Nutr. 13:135.

27. Trulson, M. F. 1964. Comparison of siblings in Boston and Ireland. J. Amer. Dietetic Ass. 45:225.

28. Van Itallie, T. B., and S. A. Hashim. 1965. Avenues of control of cholesterol of serum cholesterol. *In* F. A. Kummerow (ed.) The metabolism of lipids as related to atherosclerosis. Illinois.

29. Werko, L. 1971. Can we prevent heart disease? Ann. Int. Med. 74:278.

34

THE SATURATED vs. UNSATURATED FAT CONTROVERSY

George V. Mann *

Last summer I was asked by the U. S. Senate Select Committee on Food, Nutrition and Health to give testimony on the "Diet-Heart" problem. This was to be heard in special Committee hearings in September. For reasons I do not fully comprehend, Committee Chairman Senator McGovern postponed the sessions on short notice. I had prepared a manuscript in preparation for the assignment which has been gathering moss since.

Because I feel intensely that the "other side" of the Diet-Heart controversy has not been either adequately or "officially" heard, I have elected to use the resumé which was prepared for the McGovern Hearings, for this occasion.

Drs. Stamler and Keys, among others, including the American Heart Association, have staged a relentless campaign including documentary programs on TV, over radio and in print damning meat, eggs and milk with puny evidence backed up by dramatic Madison Avenue techniques. The animal foods industries do not appear to me to have responded as they might—or should. I do not know who is responsible for the possum tactics of those assaulted industries, but I know as a nutritionist that the industry is allowing a few adventurists in science, and an aggressive vegetable food industry to sack the basis for the best diet in human history. One

Excerpted from "Proceedings of the Meat Industry Research Conference," 1972, American Meat Institute Foundation, Chicago, Illinois by permission of the National Live Stock and Meat Board.

* Department of Biochemistry, Vanderbilt University School of Medicine, Nashville, Tennessee 37232.

day—too late, I fear—this chapter in human absurdity will be written out.

With this preface I wish to present the material originally intended for the Senate Committee—and end with some practical, personal advice.

Those citizens who suppose that scientists are cool, shrewd, quiet recluses making infallible decisions based on all the evidence must be perplexed by the present dishevelled state of the Diet-Heart problem. Confusion and disagreement are rampant. The American Heart Association (1968) purports to know how to prevent and treat coronary heart disease (CHD) with diet; Keys (1968) advocates changing our national diet pattern as he has attempted to do in Scandinavia; Stamler (1966) proposes to revolutionize our life style, including our diet, in order to prevent CHD; Ahrens (1957) hopes to persist in his endless pursuit of the slippery polyunsaturates; and Frederickson (1967) would like us to believe that a quick and dirty phenotyping of serum lipoproteins will let every man choose an appropriate government dietary manual which will make the problem of CHD go away. And yet Cornfield, Dayton, Patterson, Morris and many others of us do not believe the evidence will support such a program to change the U. S. diet in order to control CHD.

After 20 years and several billion dollars in support how can scientists be so divided on the Diet-Heart question? I will review the events leading to the present position and propose a solution. However, that solution is a general one for such scientific dilemmas and not a specific one which guarantees a cure for CHD. No amount of money or effort can unequivocally guarantee cures, the cancer lobby notwithstanding.

In 1950 we knew four important facts about atherosclerosis.

(1) A similar disease could be produced in animals by feeding cholesterol.

(2) The vessel lesions are typically laden with lipids.

(3) There is a strong correlation between high levels of cholesterol in the blood and occurrence of clinical cardiovascular disease in human beings.

(4) There is an uneven distribution of coronary disease among different cultural groups, the disease tending to select those highly placed, socio-economically.

These facts led to a useful working hypothesis which can be summarized:

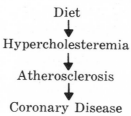

Diet
↓
Hypercholesteremia
↓
Atherosclerosis
↓
Coronary Disease

The research strategy followed was to test the validity of these hypothetical relationships and, of course, to try to interrupt the sequence. The National Institutes of Health and the American Heart Association began to fund intensive research in this area and within 2 years two important developments had occurred. Gofman *et al.* (1950) developed an elegant method for measuring serum lipoproteins and proposed these as the proper index of atherogenesis. Keys (1950) made some biometric and field observations and concluded that the causal agent in CHD is saturated animal fat in the diet. Unhappily, Gofman overextended his important findings to insist that lipoprotein patterns are both predictive and distinctive for particular kinds of disease. A great collaborative study was undertaken to examine that question and in 1956 it was concluded that the value of lipoprotein measurements for predicting disease had been overstated. Now 15 years later we have the spectacle of that very discredited hypothesis revived and aggressively promoted by Levy and Frederickson (1971), at the National Heart and Lung Institute, using far less efficient methods and far less interpretive restraint than Gofman used in 1950.

The Keysian hypothesis indicting saturated dietary fats as the cause of CHD became a classic example of the tyroepidemiologist's trap. Keys assumed that since A and B are found together then A must cause B. Being neither an epidemiologist nor a nutritionist it is understandable that he fell into this error. It is not so easy to see why after 20 years he remains entrapped unless it has proven to be a tender trap.

TeGroen *et al.* (1952) and Kinsell *et al.* (1952) showed small but real effects of dietary unsaturated fats in lowering serum cholesterol, and Ahrens has made a career of studying the relationship of lipid metabolism to CHD. But still we do not know the mechanism of this effect of polyunsaturates on cholesteremia. The importance of this lack is not our continuing ignorance but rather that the lipid diversion has usurped and blighted alternative work. The polyunsaturates have obscured and delayed solutions for 20 expensive years. And yet in 1969 the American Heart Association published as Monograph 28 the conclusions of the Diet-Heart Review Panel which plainly stated, "it is not proven that dietary modification can prevent arteriosclerotic heart disease in man." Why has the American Heart Association for 10 years used money given in good faith by a trusting public, to promote polyunsaturated food fats? It is indeed strange behavior.

By far the most useful research of the last 20 years in this field has been the Framingham Heart Program which began in 1948 in a community 30 miles west of Boston. Thanks to the patient efforts of a small group of persons in the U. S. Public Health Service, including Dr. Joe Mountain, Professor Felix Moore, Dr. Gilcin Meadors and Dr. Roy Dawber, this study of 5,000 citizens followed for 20 years, has been enormously productive. It has quantitated four risk factors which we are quite sure are antecedents of CHD. These are high blood pressure, hypercholesteremia, cigarette smoking and obesity. The Framingham Study could *not* show a relationship between diet and either cholesteremia or CHD. Careful dietary histories in a thousand of the subjects showed no relationship between dietary habits and health. But the Framingham Heart Program, a prospective study of free-living citizens, could never undertake the next crucial step and answer this practical question:

Will changing one of these risk factors, or all of them, change the behavior of coronary heart disease?

It is an academic exercise to identify predictors unless these can be changed in a way which will lessen the risk of disease. It is wrong to tell persons to avoid or to change those factors unless there is evidence that such changes have desirable effects. An intelligent man will immediately ask when advised to change his ways, "Is there evidence to show that if I correct these factors I can expect to diminish my risk of coronary heart disease?" He cannot be answered because this evidence for CHD does not exist. Even though it is often stated, or assumed to be so, such a claim is in fact an article of faith. In fact, as Table 1 shows, arteriosclerotic disease has increased since 1950, while the diet propaganda has flourished.

Now, we know how to treat high blood pressure effectively, almost everyone knows how to stop smoking cigarettes and we have, although we do not effectively practice, programs of weight reduction but we are not able effectively to lower serum cholesterol. Despite all the propaganda, the diets and drugs currently proposed achieve an average lowering of 10–15% of the initial level and this is only a tenth of our excess. Diet is indeed an important treatment for this disorder! In short, we don't know if treating risk factors will pay off, and hypercholesteremia, the risk factor second in importance in this array, is the least responsive to our treatments. It is apparent that scientists are in no position to defend the loud demands for dietary reform which we hear from Keys, Stamler and the American Heart Association. These people are confusing hypothesis with fact and that is a cardinal scientific sin.

Their error is compounded in other ways. When such unresolved scientific questions are taken to the people, as has been done, other scientists less familiar with the facts are bound to take sides and equitable peer review of scientific proposals becomes impossible. Alternative hypotheses are cast out. And so we have noted, 20 years of preoccupation with fatty acid metabolism as a hypothetical cause of coronary disease has created a stifling climate for competing hypotheses.

Table 1: The impact of cardiovascular research on mortality rates

Disease category	1955–65 change in mortality rate [a] Age-adjusted death rates to 1955 population	
	45–64 yr. of age	All ages
All cardiovascular disease	− 7.1	− 5.1
Arteriosclerotic heart disease	+ 5.5	+11.1
Hypertensive heart disease	−46.1	−45.8
Cerebrovascular disease	−19.7	−10.9
Congenital heart disease		− 5.4
Other cardiovascular diseases		− 3.8

[a] Age-adjusted death rates to 1955 U.S. population. Source: National Heart Institute–1969. Prepared by Heart Information Center, National Heart Institute, Bethesda, Maryland. Vital Statistics from National Center for Health Statistics, Department of Health, Education and Welfare, Rockville, Maryland.

Over the decade 1955–65, mortality rates declined in every major cardiovascular disease category except arteriosclerotic heart disease. Overall cardiovascular disease mortality fell by 5.1%: In most categories, total deaths increased despite declining mortality rate because of increases in the U.S. population.

Now what are these competing hypotheses? Here are five examples:

(1) Treating high blood pressure early, that is in youth when it often begins, will prevent CHD. This proposition has never been tested although at least 30 million Americans have high blood pressure.

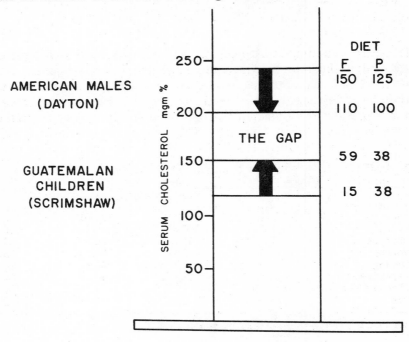

Figure 1: The level of cholesteremia in U.S. males treated with diet does not approach the low level found in other cultures free of CHD. Nor do Guatemalan children increase their low levels of cholesteremia to reach U.S. levels when fat and cholesterol are added to their diet. The unexplained gap is large.

(2)   Exposure to carbon monoxide causes atherosclerosis.   Astrup *et al.* (1970) have experimental evidence to support this proposition. There is evidence of widespread human exposure to carbon monoxide, some of it contributed by smoking, and methods are available for measuring the degree of this exposure in citizens, and yet this promising lead is not pursued, while great and expensive federal programs are undertaken to try to shore up the foolish lipoprotein, phenotyping scheme, tried and found wanting 20 years ago.

(3) Hard water supplies protect populations from coronary heart disease (Table 2).   Now water is easily hardened but would doing this make a difference in the behavior of the disease?   We cannot answer this.

Table 2: Water calcium and cardiovascular deaths in the U.K., 1958–64.   Age 45–64 years.   Expressed as deaths/100,000 [a]

Water Ca, ppm	Males	Females
10	751	355
10–39	721	330
40–69	636	306
70–99	633	281
100+	546	248

[a] Adapted from Crawford, Gardner and Morris.   1971.   Brit. Med. Bull. 27:21.

(4) Surface active materials, added to food by technologists for marketing advantages, cause hypercholesteremia in experimental animals (Table 3).   The safety of such food additives was not adequately tested when they were initiated several decades ago.   We each now receive over 3 pounds per year of food additive substances.   Are they contributing causes for coronary heart disease?   The answer is unknown.

Table 3: Additives in U.S. foods (millions of lb. added) [a]

	1955	1960	1963	1965
Surfactants	75.7	106.0	132.70	150.0
Acidulants	92.5	103.4	118.3	120.5
Thickeners	63.8	79.8	96.7	105.0
Flavoring	38.1	49.4	64.7	73.0
Leavening	64.5	67.1	64.3	64.0
Preservatives	21.9	31.1	44.4	50.0
Artificial sweeteners	0.25	3.54	6.30	10.0
Colors	1.69	2.34	2.55	2.6

[a] Adapted from H. J. Sanders, Chem. Eng. News, Oct. 10, 1966.

(5) Physical fitness protects from coronary heart disease.   I believe this is the most credible hypothesis we have.   There is much evidence to

support it.   There is very little evidence in opposition, and yet physical fitness is something of a joke.   The Federal machinery for the study of fitness has been abandoned.   The President's Commission on Physical Fitness wastes money on trivial but expensive advertisements.

The operational dilemma which existed in 1955 and continues now is this: When such a dietary hypothesis, or any hypothesis, purporting to explain the causation of a chronic disease in man is formulated it can only be evaluated by a great and expensive clinical trial (Schork and Remington, 1967), i. e., a test of the hypothesis in man.   Such trials are so tedious, so costly and so difficult that they cannot be undertaken without great circumspection and only when an unusually promising treatment is at hand (Table 4).

Table 4: Primary prevention, the numbers game [a]

Item		A	B	C	FN[b] D
Dropout	d	0.3	0.4	0.5	0.5
Effect	k	0.4	0.4	0.4	0.25
Incidence	P_c	0.05	0.05	0.05	0.05
Effect gradient	f	1	1	2	2
Confidence	α	0.05	0.05	0.05	0.05
	β	0.05	0.05	0.05	0.05
Sample	2N	7,830	9,080	12,640	35,000

[a] Adapted from Schork and Remington, (1968).   J. Chron. Dis. 21:13.

[b]FN   A–D are designs using different assumed values of the 6 statistical variables and giving the sample sizes shown in the last line for a 5-year study of the effectiveness of some treatment, say physical exercise, in the primary prevention of CHD.

The Diet-Heart question has been extensively examined since 1955 in what I would call preliminary trials.   Those investigators may pale at this designation because the trials ran up to 10 years, cost tens of millions of dollars and a major segment of the investigators' careers. The trials have been succinctly summarized by Cornfield and Mitchell (1969), professional biometricians.   Ten clinical trials involving 5,279 subjects in all and 36,000 or more man-years of observation in four nations were reviewed.   Six of those studies said yes, the dietary treatment seemed to work and four said no, it did not.   Cornfield and Mitchell concluded, "The better the experimental design, the less the effect of diet on CHD—there is no evidence here to change the Western diet."

In 1967 a sub-committee of the National Heart Foundation of Australia in a review entitled "Dietary Fat and Coronary Heart Disease" looked at seven prospective studies in three countries.   They concluded, "no conclusions about efficacy of diet are warranted."

Seymour Dayton with Dr. Lee Pearce (1969) and others conducted the monumental 10-year dietary trial with 812 men in the Veterans Administration facility at Los Angeles concluded, "the results of our own trial, even when buttressed by concordant observations in two other primary prevention studies, are not sufficient grounds for aggressive efforts to change the U. S. diet."

In 1961 the American Heart Association issued the first of three statements called "Diet and Heart Disease". This was leaked to the press and the oil industry prematurely began an intensive commercial promotion of unsaturated edible oils and fats. But despite all the misgivings and protests of those of us who doubted that the evidence supported the position taken by the Heart Association, and despite the aggressive exploitation of this stand by the food oil industry, the American Heart Association has continued, indeed enlarged its propaganda for oiling the U. S. diet as a means of preventing CHD. I judge the organization is trapped in its own public relations program. The facts show that this treatment doesn't work. Doctors know it. Scientists know it. Even Keys and Stamler know it. And yet, like a broken record the propaganda goes on. I am ashamed of this chapter in medical science, not because the diet hypothesis has been so long dying that it has delayed other useful research, but because of the mistrust, ill will and rejection it has brought to nutrition science and to the American Heart Association.

My own judgement in the Diet-Heart debate was strongly influenced by the following personal research. Experiments with primates showed that atherosclerosis was induced as readily with diets containing corn oil, an unsaturated fat, as with lard (Mann *et al.*, 1953). Studies with primitive groups of people including the Alaskan Eskimo, the Ibo people of Nigeria, the Congolese Pygmies and the Masai of Tanzania (Mann *et al.*, 1964) revealed thousands of carnivorous people who are taking more animal fat and cholesterol in their diet than do we but with low levels of blood cholesterol and essentially free from coronary heart disease (Figure 2).

We concluded that only two explanations were possible: either diet is not the determinant in CHD or some other circumstance of life protects against CHD.

Subsequently we have measured physical activity and fitness in the Masai (Mann *et al.*, 1965). Their fitness is superb. They are physically active (see Figure 3). With some difficulty, over a period of 5 years, we have collected the hearts of 50 Masai men. Surprisingly, these show atherosclerosis but only rarely coronary occlusions (Mann *et al.*, 1972). We believe this means that while the Masai do have atherosclerosis, habitual exercise and fitness make their vessels enlarge and so their atheromata are innocuous (Figure 5). The implication is clear enough. The Western epidemic of CHD is indeed caused by atherosclerosis, but all men have this, wherever examined (McGill, 1968). The saving trait which prevents the lethal complications of atherosclerosis is physical fitness. The way to cut off the epidemic of CHD is with a program of exercise.

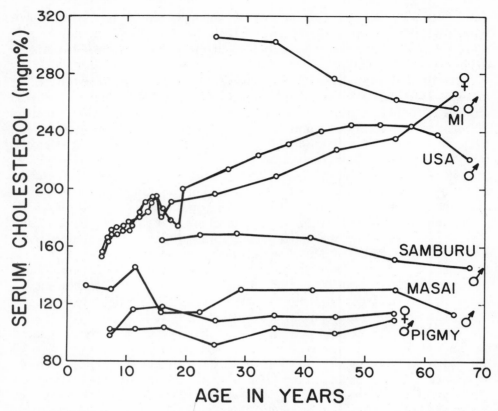

Figure 2: Cholesteremia by age in diverse cultures. The Samburu and Masai of East Africa subsist on camel's and cow's milk and meat and so have higher animal fat intakes than do Americans. The Pygmy is omnivorous.

Now I have just formulated an hypothesis, not a proven fact. This is not the time for a national rush to the gymnasium or the park to prevent CHD because that is the kind of error the diet protagonists are making. What is needed is a test of this fitness hypothesis. The difficulty is that neither I nor any other single scientist can do the test alone. I have tried (Mann *et al.*, 1969). The necessary design is too large, too expensive, too demanding for any but a collaborative effort, directed by some kind of a National study center. But in the last 5 years the National Institutes of Health have moved away from this function. They have dismantled the Chronic Heart Disease and Stroke Control Program. The President's Commission on Physical Fitness, managed often by ex-coaches, fritters away money on magazine and television advertising while adult Americans are uninformed about methods and goals in physical fitness. There is no national fitness program beyond the industrial efforts of the bicycle people and there is very little promise.

With limited funds, my colleagues and I have developed experience and methods for re-training middle-aged men (Garrett *et al.*, 1966); we have measured the amount of exercise necessary to re-train and to maintain fitness (Mann *et al.*, 1971); we have shown that fitness can be measured in a highly reproducible fashion thus making adherence to the treatment in a clinical trial quite a simple measurement. We have

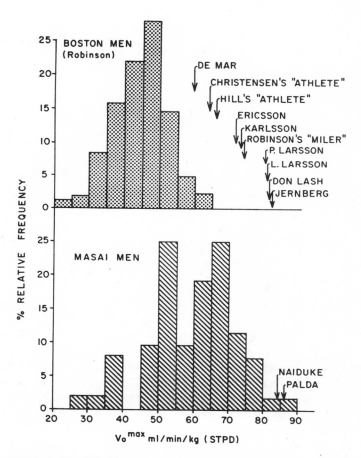

Figure 3: Physical fitness is expressed here as the $V_{O_2}^{max}$, the maximal amount of oxygen a man can consume per minute per kilogram of body weight. The workload was progressively increased by increasing the walking angle of a treadmill. The upper frame shows data for U.S. men and international class athletes, collected by Sid Robinson, then at the Harvard Fatigue Laboratory. The lower frame shows our data for Masai men, recruited from the bunda, measured under a tree in Tanzania. Note that two of these Masai men exceeded Jernberg's performance. Jim Ryun has recently surpassed them all.

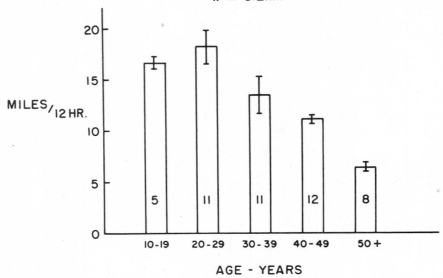

Figure 4: Pedometers were attached to Masai men at sunrise and removed at sundown. The calculation of distance adjusts stride length for height. The warriors are age 15–29 years. Men 30–49 oversee their herds while after 50 the main activity is attending committee meetings and hearings.

written a booklet for the Tennessee Heart Association (1970) to show physicians how to evaluate fitness and how to qualify men for undertaking a fitness program. But all of this is only preparatory for the day when the fitness hypothesis must be tested in a clinical trial.

How then do we resolve this dilemma? I propose the creation, or re-creation, of a National Center for Chronic Disease Control. This should be concerned with several chronic diseases. The need for studies of the management of diabetes is very great just now, but I focus here on its functions for coronary heart disease. I see three kinds of activity which might be undertaken:

(1) Sponsoring basic research in the mechanisms of atherogenesis. Work in this area is blighted by the preoccupation with fatty acid metabolism. Some hypotheses which need examination and go begging for support I have listed previously. They include carbon monoxide exposure as a cause of atherosclerosis, hard water as a protective agent against hypercholesteremia, and surfactants added to food as contributory to hypercholesteremia.

(2) Epidemiological surveillance. This needs to be done on an international scale. There are not now available efficient means for tabulat-

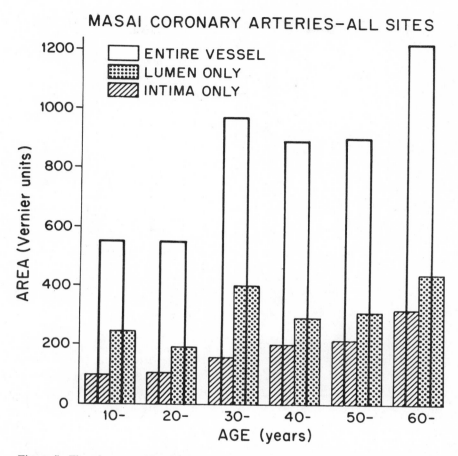

Figure 5: The changes with age in the caliber of the coronary arteries in 50 Masai men were measured at autopsy. Note that the vessels enlarge with age (open bars), so that the lumen increases (strippled bar) even while the intima (cross hatched) is thickening from atherosclerosis. We think exercise does this. Masai rarely have heart attacks.

ing the prevalence and incidence of cardiovascular disease. Out of this kind of information showing accurate regional differences of incidence are apt to come the clues for understanding mechanism and prevention. The Framingham Study started with subjects age 30–59 years. We know that the roots of CHD lie in the ages 15–30 when dramatic changes of blood cholesterol, blood pressure and physical activity are occurring, for unknown reasons. A cohort of young people should be selected and followed with the Framingham methods. Alas, when I proposed such a study to the National Heart and Lung Institute a few months ago, I was turned down. The proposal seems not to have been carefully read.

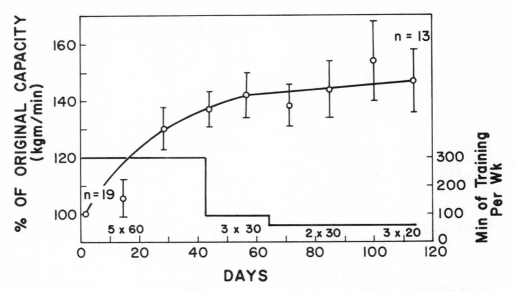

Figure 6: The amount of exercise necessary to maintain fitness in middle-aged Americans was titrated by successively diminishing the duration of weekly training sessions. Sixty minutes per week in two or three sessions were enough.

(3) The completion of clinical trials to test hypotheses. I have indicated that this task will always surpass the facilities of single institutions or individuals. It is, however, the only way that such hypotheses can be dealt with. Unless the trials are carefully chosen and designed, we are reduced to a perpetual argument, wasteful, delaying and indecisive.

In summary, my analysis indicates that our dilemma with the Diet-Heart question arises especially from the lack of suitable mechanisms for testing the prevailing hypotheses. If such a mechanism was created, I am not sure that the diet hypothesis would qualify for a test, with all the negative information we now have. But I am quite sure that other hypotheses are at hand and new ones will arise which will need testing. This is the mechanism we need to move ahead, scientifically and efficiently, toward the proper prevention of coronary heart disease.

Despite the rancor and division among us, I am confident that we are moving to a solution of the CHD problem. It is just that now we need the coordinating function of government and that is, I am quite sure, the very reason for the existence of government. I close with a quotation from Francis Bacon which I think is appropriate for all of us.

> I would address one general admonition to all; that they consider what
> are the true ends of knowledge, and that they seek it not either for
> pleasure of the mind, or for contention, or for superiority to others, or
> for profit, or fame, or power, or any of these inferior things; but for

the benefit and use of life; and that they perfect and govern it in charity. For it was from lust of power that the angels fell, from lust of knowledge that man fell; but of charity there can be no excess, neither did angel or man ever come in danger by it. [Francis Bacon, in preface to "The Great Instauration", 1618.]

LITERATURE CITED

1. Ahrens, E. H., Jr., *et al.* 1957. The influence of dietary fats on serum lipid levels in man. Lancet 1:943.

2. American Heart Association. 1961. Diet and Heart Disease.

3. American Heart Association. 1968. Diet and Heart Disease, EM379 RE 10–68. New York.

4. American Heart Association. 1969. Mass Field Trials of the Diet Heart Question, Monograph 28.

5. Astrup, P., *et al.* 1970. Effects of carbon monoxide exposure on the arterial walls. Ann. New York Acad. Sciences 174:294.

6. Cornfield, J. and S. Mitchell. 1969. Selected risk factors in coronary disease. Arch. Environ. Health 19:382.

7. Dayton, S. and M. L. Pearce. 1969. Prevention of coronary heart disease and other complications of atherosclerosis by modified diet. Am. Jour. Med. 46:751.

8. Fredrickson, D. S., R. I. Levy and R. S. Lees. 1967. Fat transport in lipoproteins, an integrated approach to mechanisms and disorders. N. Eng. J. Med. 276:34, 94, 148, 215 and 273.

9. Garrett, H. L., R. V. Pangle and G. V. Mann. 1966. Physical conditioning and coronary risk factors. J. Chron. Dis. 19:899.

10. Gofman, J. W., *et al.* 1950. The role of lipids and lipoproteins in atherosclerosis. Science 111:166.

11. Keys, A. 1968. Prevention of coronary heart disease: Official recommendations from Scandinavia. Circul. 38:227.

12. Keys, A., *et al.* 1950. The relationship in man between cholesterol levels in the diet and in the blood. Science 112:79.

13. Kinsell, L. W., *et al.* 1952. Dietary modification of serum cholesterol and phospholipid levels. J. Clin. Endocr. 12:909.

14. Levy, R. I. and D. S. Fredrickson. 1971. Dietary management of hyperlipoproteinemia. J. Am. Diet Assoc. 58:406.

15. Mann, G. V. 1970. Physician's handbook for evaluation of cardiovascular and physical fitness. Tennessee Heart Association.

16. Mann, G. V., S. B. Andrus, A. McNally and F. J. Stare. 1953. Experimental atherosclerosis in Cebus monkeys. J. Exper. Med. 98:195.

17. Mann, G. V., H. L. Garrett, A. Farhi, H. Murray and F. T. Billings. 1969. Exercise to prevent coronary heart disease: An experimental study of the

effects of training on risk factors for coronary disease in men. Am.J.Med. 46(1):12.

18. Mann, G. V., H. L. Garrett and A. Long. 1971. The amount of exercise necessary to achieve and maintain fitness in adult persons. Southern Med. J. 64:549.

19. Mann, G. V., R. D. Shaffer, R. S. Anderson and H. H. Sandstead. 1964. Cardiovascular disease in the Masai. J. Atherosclerosis Research 4:289.

20. Mann, G. V., R. D. Shaffer and A. Rich. 1965. Physical fitness and immunity to heart disease in Masai. Lancet 2(7426):1308.

21. Mann, G. V., A. Spoerry, M. Gray and D. Jarashow. Atherosclerosis in the Masai. Am. J. of Epidemiology 95:26 (Jan. 1972).

22. McGill, H. C., Jr. 1968. The geographic pathology of atherosclerosis. Lab. Invest. 18:463.

23. National Heart Foundation of Australia. 1967. Dietary fat and coronary heart disease, A Review. Med. J. Aust. 1(7):309.

24. Schork, M. A. and R. D. Remington. 1967. The determination of sample size in treatment control comparison for chronic disease studies in which dropout or non adherence is a problem. J. Chron. Dis. 20:233.

25. Stamler, J., *et al.* 1966. Coronary risk factors, their impact and their therapy in the prevention of coronary artery disease. Med. Clin. N. Amer. 50:229.

26. TeGroen, J., *et al.* 1952. The influence of nutrition, individuality and other factors on the serum cholesterol. Volding 13:556.

35

THE ROLE OF CHOLESTEROL IN CORONARY ATHEROGENESIS

William B. Kannel, M.D.*

Death as a consequence of a compromised circulation to the brain, heart, kidneys, and limbs is the most potent force of mortality operating in the world today, particularly in affluent societies. There is much to suggest that modification of life style by modern technology—which has replaced muscle power with machines and has provided a surfeit of rich food and drink while at the same time shrinking opportunities for physical exercise—has exacted an increased toll in cardiovascular mortality. The facts that atherosclerosis is the chief killer of mankind and that alteration of our ecology may be promoting it demand some kind of action.

Prevention of any disease requires at the very least some knowledge of the circumstances under which it arises, evolves, and terminates fatally in human populations. Such insight has accumulated in reasonably undistorted fashion from prospective epidemiologic studies such as the Framingham study. The characteristics of the potential coronary victim have been discerned and factors which increase risk identified. Based on estimates of the magnitude of the risk associated with some of these factors, singly and in combination, a profile of the potential coronary candidate can be derived which can predict disease over a wide range of probabilities—as much as 13-fold (Fig. 1). In short, a portrait of the

Reprinted from *Medical Clinics of North America*—Vol. 58, No. 2, March 1974, by permission of W. B. Saunders Company.

* Director, Framingham Heart Study, National Heart and Lung Institute; Lecturer, Harvard Medical School, Boston; Research Associate, Boston University, Boston, Massachusetts.

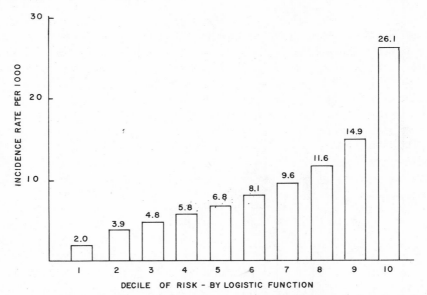

Figure 1: Average annual incidence of coronary heart disease according to decile of risk. 16-Year follow-up, men aged 45 to 54, Framingham Study. Note: The probability of coronary heart disease developing is defined by a logistic function using systolic and diastolic blood pressure, number of cigarettes per day, electrocardiographic signs of left ventricular hypertrophy, serum cholesterol, and glucose intolerance.

potential coronary candidate, at first hazy, but now increasingly sharp, has arisen.[12]

Atherosclerosis, and coronary heart disease in particular, is a disease that appears to evolve under the influence of multiple contributors and it is an oversimplification to focus on one factor to the exclusion of others. In fact, the concept of a single essential cause for any chronic disease has fallen into justified disrepute. Such a conceptualization is much too narrow. To date, no essential factor, without which the disease fails to occur, has been implicated in atherosclerotic disease. The disease appears to be ubiquitous in man beyond age 20 and can be looked upon as a concomitant of aging. Propensity to this vascular affliction can even be regarded solely as a function of the type of vasculature inherited. There is a good deal of evidence to support this pessimistic contention. While the general tendency to deposit lipid in the arterial intima may to a great extent be determined by the level of blood lipids and the blood pressure, dynamics of flow, arterial caliber, and the integrity of the vascular intima powerfully influence where atheromata will form.[6, 15, 20] The same lipid-laden blood bathes the intima of the veins and pulmonary arterial vasculature; yet atheromata do not develop in these unless turbulence or pressures such as those in the systemic arterial circulation are produced by abnormality. Failing this, veins and pulmonary arteries can be quite tortuous and still escape atheromatosis. Also, while almost everyone appears to have enough lipid to develop atheromata under the right circumstances, and local factors play a decisive role as to whether and where they will form, it is a fact that the rate of atheroma formation is proportional to the blood lipid and blood pressure values experimentally induced in animals [8, 10, 14] and spontaneously observed in man.[5]

To contend that the architecture of the vasculature is the sole or even the chief determinant of atheroma formation under these circumstances is as faulty in logic as to invoke cholesterol as the sole determinant of atheromatosis. Host susceptibility to any noxious influence, including cholesterol, varies over a wide range, and resistance to atherogenic precursors varies over a wide range.

A number of epidemiologic observations bear on the possibility of genetic influences including the sex ratio, racial variation, familial aggregation, familial hyperlipoproteinemias, and age trends, among others. Atherosclerotic disease may be looked upon basically as a concomitant of aging and can be regarded as preventable only to the extent that we can retard the "aging process." As in almost every other "chronic and degenerative disease," age is a powerful variable and the precocious occurrence of atherosclerosis in young persons can be regarded as simply the extreme or tail of the normal distribution. All of the known "risk factors" taken together, while related to age, cannot account for more than a fraction of the striking age trend in incidence of atheromatosis (Table 1).

Table 1: Risk factors in coronary heart disease. Linear discriminant function coefficients (standard units)*

Risk factors	Combined ages	30–39	40–49	50–62
Men				
Age	.5934	.2394	.3334	.2370
Cholesterol	.4444	.9613	.3207	.3790
Systolic blood pressure	.3334	.3427	.1669	.3809
Relative weight	.1890	.1941	.3619	.1036
Hemoglobin	—.1050	.0313	—.0134	—.2206
Cigarettes smoked	.4192	.6823	.5084	.3004
ECG abnormality	.2626	.2685	.2556	.2197
Women				
Age	.6259	.7325		.2600
Cholesterol	.2844	.7322		.1207
Systolic blood pressure	.5556	.1947		.4776
Relative weight	.0975	.0751		.1481
Hemoglobin	.0392	—.0304		.0734
Cigarettes smoked	.0625	—.0731		.1262
ECG abnormality	.3048	.2234		.2526

* From Kannel, W. B., and Gordon, T., eds.: The Framingham Study. An Epidemiological Investigation of Cardiovascular Disease. Section 27, Washington, D.C., U.S. Government Printing Office, 1971.

Whether this is simply a reflection of the biologic consequence of aging or a time-dose product of acquired "risk factors" is still unclear. Probably *both* altered tissue response and dosage of noxious influences are involved.

Families share more than genes and it is possible that those who sit and dine together may die together! It is clear that at any age in either sex some persons are distinctly more vulnerable than others to atherosclerotic disease outcomes depending on the number and intensity of "atherogenic" precursors in their makeup. Also, some persons manage to reach advanced age with little atherosclerosis suggesting that this "aging phenomenon" is not inevitable. We must learn what is responsible for this relative immunity and also those factors which, as regards atherosclerosis, make the potential victim of the process old beyond his years.

The ingredients of this "atherogenic profile" have been delineated from prospective epidemiologic studies in humans, at least in terms of the lethal clinical manifestations of atherosclerosis—coronary heart disease, brain infarction, occlusive peripheral arterial disease, and congestive heart failure. No essential factor—including lipid—has been identified as sufficient or absolutely necessary for the development of this disease. Abnormalities predisposing to atherosclerosis and to its clinical manifestations are at this point more a matter of degree than kind. Multiple contributors rather than a single etiologic "agent" appeared to be playing a role.[7, 11, 13] Biologic factors involved in atherogenesis—such as blood lipids, blood pressure, and glucose tolerance—are graded characteristics of normal body constituents, continuously distributed with no discernible bimodality to denote where normal leaves off and "abnormal" begins.

Some physicians may find it difficult to cope with the concept of multiple, interrelated continuous variables contributing to a disease process. What is the level of these normal body constituents which initiates and sustains the process of atherogenesis? An examination of either blood lipids or blood pressure—the commonest and most potent atherogenic precursors in the make-up of the potential coronary victim—in a general population sample, comparing those who remain free of clinical disease versus those who developed it, reveals Gaussian curves with long tails and no trace of bimodality (Fig. 2). There is a considerable overlap of values in diseased and well persons so that there is no value, however large or small, that lies distinctly in the distribution of one and not the other. Yet, risk of a coronary event is distinctly proportional to the antecedent level of either risk factor from the lowest to the highest values recorded in the population, the rate of increment accelerating around 200 mg. per 100 ml. for cholesterol (Fig. 3). Also, for blood pressure, risk is proportional to the level without any discernible critical "hypertensive" value where risk sharply rises. Even within the range generally conceded to be "normal" for these variables, risk varies over a fairly wide range (Fig. 4).

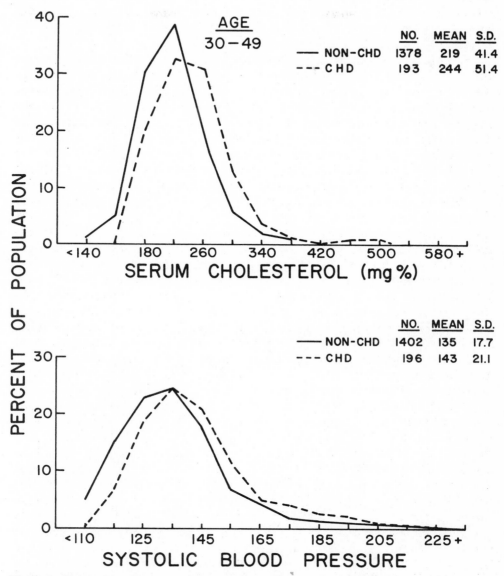

Figure 2: *Above.* Distribution of serum cholesterol in subjects free of coronary heart disease versus those developing coronary heart disease in 16 years. Men aged 30 to 62 at entry, Framingham Study. *Below.* Distribution of systolic blood pressure in subjects free of coronary heart disease versus those developing coronary heart disease in 16 years. Men aged 30 to 49 at entry, Framingham Study.

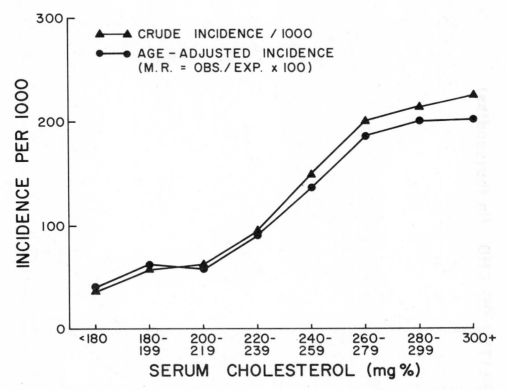

Figure 3: Risk of coronary heart disease (14 years) according to serum cholesterol concentration. Men aged 30 to 49 at entry, Framingham Study.

Thus, what is *typical* of apparently healthy persons in populations such as the United States may not in fact be "normal" or optimal at all. There is reason to believe, as judged by the values encountered in populations with low coronary mortality and little atherosclerosis at postmortem examination, that cholesterol values of Americans are far above optimal levels. Most Americans appear to have more than enough lipid to manufacture atheromata if given enough time. This may even be true for all human beings.

There apparently are pressures below which atheromata do not develop whatever the level of lipid in the blood—e. g., in the pulmonary arterial and venous circulation. Unfortunately such pressures within the systemic circulation are incompatible with life. Risk of all major atherosclerotic disease outcomes is proportional to the pressure in the systemic arterial circulation—systolic or diastolic, casual or basal—at all ages in both sexes. This is true even excluding persons with other risk attributes and, contrary to clinical folklore, there is no suggestion of a waning impact with advancing age (Fig. 4). However, its impact is profoundly influenced by the coexisting blood lipid value (Fig. 5).

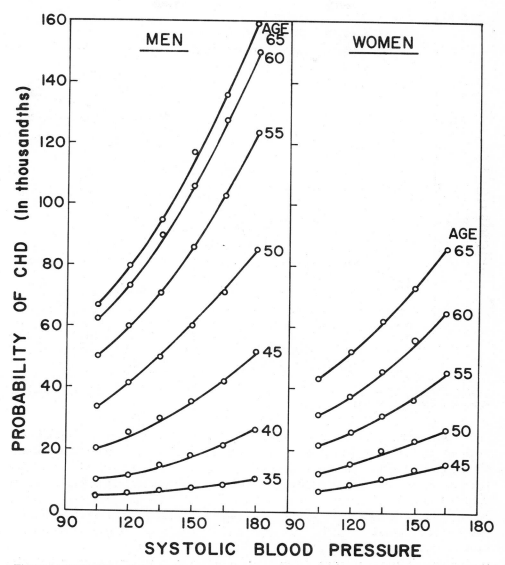

Figure 4: Probability of developing coronary heart disease in 8 years according to systolic blood pressure. Low risk persons aged 35 to 65, Framingham Study, 16 year follow-up. Persons with cholesterol 185, normal glucose tolerance, no left ventricular hypertrophy on electrocardiogram, nonsmoker. Source: Framingham Monograph No. 27.

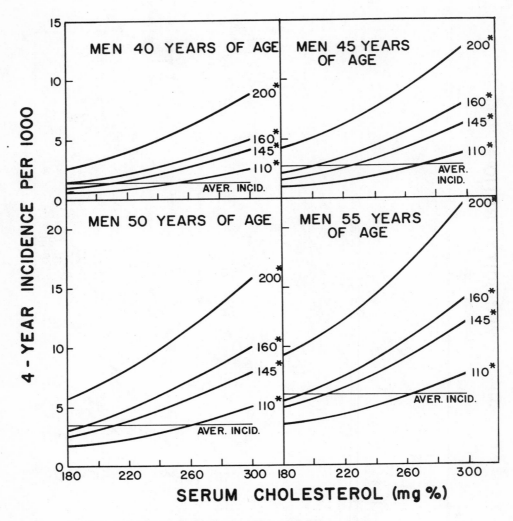

Figure 5: Four year incidence of coronary heart disease according to serum cholesterol concentration at specified levels of systolic blood pressure. Men aged 40 to 55, Framingham Study. Source: Framingham Monograph Section 23.

The relation of blood lipid to clinical atherosclerotic events is also no accidental association by virtue of its correlation with other major risk factors. Taking other known powerful contributors into account, either categorically (Fig. 6) or using discriminant analysis (which adjusts for the actual value of associated variables as a group, Table 1), reveals a significant residual effect of cholesterol as well as blood pressure. If one examines the regression of coronary incidence on the major contributors

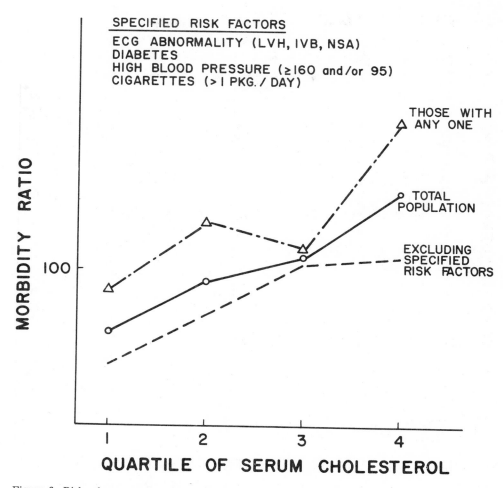

Figure 6: Risk of coronary heart disease (16 years) according to serum cholesterol concentration, excluding other factors. Men aged 30 to 62 at entry, Framingham Study.

to its occurrence, it becomes evident that overall the strongest of these factors is systolic blood pressure, followed in descending order by serum cholesterol, cigarette smoking, and blood sugar. The ranking is the same for women as for men with the exception of cigarette smoking which in women is quite weak. This is evident from a comparison of the size of computed regression coefficients suitably standardized for the different units and range of values of the variables under consideration (Table 2). It is also apparent from this table that both cholesterol and blood pressure contribute independently to risk of coronary events since the regression coefficients are only modestly reduced in the multivariate case which takes into account the effect of the other variables. Also, when adjustment is made for endogenous triglyceride carried in the pre-beta lipoprotein $S_f 20$–400 fraction) as well as other relevant factors, a risk gradient still persists

Table 2: Average regression coefficients of various contributors to incidence of coronary disease. 16 year follow-up in men and women aged 45 to 74 *

| | Standardized regression coefficients | | | |
| | Men | | Women | |
	Univariate	Multivariate	Univariate	Multivariate
Systolic blood pressure	.340	.264	.477	.408
Serum cholesterol	.257	.226	.296	.267
ECG–LVH	.234	.173	.262	.161
Cigarettes	.186	.246	−.024 †	.032 †
Glucose Intolerance	.172	.153	.124	.074 †

* *From* Kannel, W. B., and Gordon, T., eds.: The Framingham Study. An Epidemiological Investigation of Cardiovascular Disease. Section 27. Washington, D.C., U.S. Government Printing Office, 1971.

† Slope of CHD incidence on the variable is not significant at the 5 per cent level.

which is proportional to the serum cholesterol value (Fig. 7). The converse is not true. Evidently, as applied to the general population, serum lipid profiles are more useful for determining the cause of an elevated blood cholesterol and the best means to reduce it than for estimating the risk of coronary attacks.

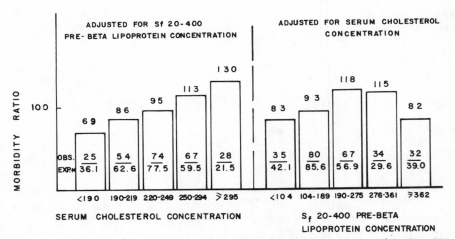

Figure 7: Risk of coronary heart disease (14 years) according to serum lipid, adjusted for associated variables. Men aged 38 to 69 years, Framingham Study. *Exp, Expected number of events obtained from "risk function" derived from: blood pressure, number of cigarettes, uric acid, glucose, relative weight, and other serum lipid under consideration.

Taking age and sex into account and assuming that the intrinsic architecture of the arterial vasculature is randomly distributed, serum lipids (cholesterol in particular), blood pressure, and carbohydrate tolerance appear to be the chief determinants of the rate of atherogenesis as it is clinically expressed. An examination of age-sex trends in blood lipid (Fig. 8) and in blood pressure (Fig. 9) reveals an intriguing similarity to

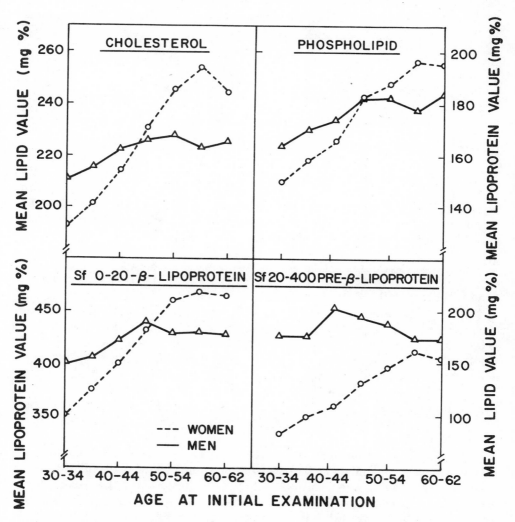

Figure 8: Mean value of serum lipids by age and sex at initial examination. Men and women aged 30 to 62 at entry, Framingham Study.

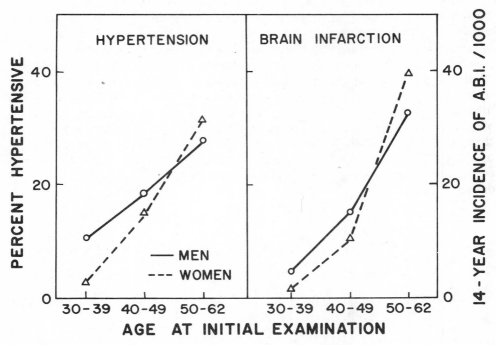

Figure 9: Prevalence of hypertension and incidence of atherothrombotic brain infarction by age and sex. Men and women aged 30 to 62 at entry, Framingham Study.

that in clinical atherosclerosis, where the relative immunity in women is lost with advancing age (Fig. 10). This raises the possibility that the closing gap in incidence in the sexes with advancing age derives to some extent from fact that pressures and lipid values in women rise to meet and finally exceed those in men. Epidemiologic studies such as the Framingham study can only provide clues to pathogenesis and not definitive answers. However, there is a considerable body of evidence to connect the blood cholesterol content with the development of atherosclerosis. The strengths and weaknesses of this information have been discussed at some length.[1, 2]

That an association exists between cholesterol and atherosclerosis is incontrovertible. That it is a *causal* association is more difficult to prove. We are currently in the position of having to prove guilt by association. An association is more likely to be "causal" if it precedes the disease by an appropriate incubation period, if it is strong, and, most important, if it makes sense. The association between cholesterol and atherosclerosis appears to meet all these criteria.

Prospective data show that blood cholesterol values long in advance of the disease are strongly related to the rate of development of its clinical manifestations consistent with the known insidious evolution of atherosclerosis. The risk varies in relation to the associated blood pressure, consistent with the filtration or perfusion hypothesis. Animal experiments in a variety of species have demonstrated unequivocally that lipid-induced atherogenesis is markedly accelerated by also producing hypertension.[8, 10, 14, 18] While the perfusion hypothesis is a gross oversimplification of this complex process, the data from epidemiologic clinical and post-mortem studies in man are quite consistent with it. It is likely that an alteration in the level or handling of blood lipids, augmented by the level of the blood pressure, is in most instances the final common pathway through which the multiple interrelated contributors to atherosclerosis operate. To argue that these are innocuous, nonsequitor concomitants of some more basic process seems overly iconoclastic in the face of the evidence.

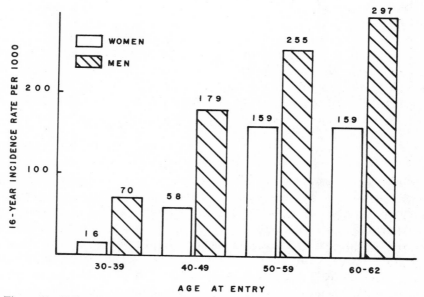

Figure 10: 16-Year incidence of coronary heart disease in men and women aged 30 to 62 at entry, Framingham Study.

That cholestrol is somehow associated with the atheroscierotic process and its evil consequences is incontrovertible. Whether it is etiologic in the sense of an essential factor or even the initiator of the process given the right substrate of circumstances is conjectural at this point, but not likely. Cholesterol seems to be the thread running through the web of circumstances culminating in a clinical atheroslerotic event. The conclusion that blood lipid (cholesterol in particular) makes some type of major contribution to the process of atherosclerosis and its lethal sequelae seems inescapable. The chain of evidence is too binding to be cast aside. Diseases associated with hypercholesterolemia are also associated with premature atherosclerosis.   Persons with inborn errors of cholesterol metabolism show extremely precocious development of atherosclerotic disease.   Persons with high cholesterol levels in epidemiologic study populations have been observed to develop coronary heart disease with greater frequency than those with lower values, the risk being proportional to the degree of elevation of blood cholesterol.   Countries with high average cholesterol values among their inhabitants report high coronary death rates, those with low values report low rates.   Atherosclerotic deposits are usually loaded with cholesterol and other lipids and the movement of cholesterol from the blood into deposits has been demonstrated.   Inducing high cholesterol values in animals produces atherosclerotic deposits that can be made to regress by lowering blood cholesterol.

There are problems with all of this evidence, [1, 2] but efforts are being made to further refine it, and thus far results have continued to confirm the findings in evermore convincing fashion.[3, 10, 19]   However, further clarification is still needed.   When or if the final link in the chain of evidence is forged, demonstrating that in man substantial lowering of cholesterol in fact reduces coronary morbidity and mortality in a controlled field trial, the need for this evidence will become less acute.   Such evidence is beginning to accumulate.[17] The problem is really largely a question of degree.   The contention that the deposition of cholesterol is only incidental to its availability in the circulation and that atheromata would probably form even in persons with low lipid values is valid.[1, 2]   However, the simple fact is that in animals and in man the process is unequivocally accelerated in proportion to the blood lipid level, and in persons with runaway cholesterol synthesis resulting from inborn errors of metabolism extremely precocious atherosclerosis occurs which has been known to strike down whole families of these unfortunates early in life, sometimes in the teens.   Further, while the fibrotic vascular lesions of atherosclerosis may develop in the face of seemingly innocuous lipid levels and the lesions may contain only modest amounts of lipid, possibly formed in situ, these are generally not the lesions that occlude vessels and precipitate thrombi.   It is the fatty atheromatous abscess that is especially likely to precipitate such vascular catastrophies.

The determinants of the generally high lipid values in the United States, the biologically optimal range of values, the details of its regulation, and the pathogenesis of the atherosclerotic lesion, however, require further clarification.   The reasons for incriminating diet as one of the chief determinants of lipid levels in a population are substantial but somewhat confusing.

It is paradoxical that in free-living affluent populations no one has convincingly demonstrated a difference in nutrient composition of the diet between persons who develop coronary heart disease and those who do not.   Nor has there been a demonstration, *within* such populations, of a connection between the nutrient content of the diet and serum cholesterol values from one person to the next. Yet, there is much to suggest that the nutrient composition of the diet may be an important if not the key determinant of the general level of cholesterol in a population.

The evidence linking blood cholesterol content to the nutrient composition of the diet is too substantial to dismiss. An impressive amount of evidence has accumulated from epidemiologic studies, animal investigation and manipulative studies in humans to incriminate the saturated fat, cholesterol and refined carbohydrate in the diet as promoting hyperlipidemia and being atherogenic. Areas in which the population exhibits high cholesterol values characteristically have diets different in composition and calories from those where low values are usual. Migrants from low to high cholesterol areas are found to have higher cholesterol values and to have changed, among other things, their dietary pattern. Manipulation of the diet can alter serum cholesterol values in a predictable fashion in humans, and in animals can produce atherosclerotic deposits or cause established lesions to regress.[3] Both have even been shown to occur in monkeys on American table diets.[19]

Again fault can be found with each one of these pieces of evidence but they too paint a rather consistent picture. Critics of the animal experiments correctly point out the "unnatural" dietary conditions employed to induce atherosclerosis, but the same indictment must be made concerning the unnaturalness of the zoo environment when findings in such animals are cited to refute animal experiments purporting to show diet-induced atherosclerosis.[1, 2] Also, there is reason to believe that the diet of the average American is far from "natural." Over the past century some rather profound changes have been made in the saturated fat, cholesterol, refined sugar, and salt content of the diet. It is highly unlikely that if man were returned to his "natural" primitive predatory state that he could obtain this much fat and salt in his diet. It takes a highly organized society to sustain this rich a diet without expending considerable calories of energy to acquire the foodstuffs.

The absence of a correlation between what people say they eat and their blood cholesterol values within free-living affluent populations on uniformly high intakes of all the incriminated nutrients has been taken by some to mean that diet plays no role in the evolution of atherosclerosis or its serum lipid precursors. However, it may be that the association does not reveal itself to casual observation, and diet may still constitute the chief factor determining the average blood cholesterol value of a population. Failure to demonstrate an association between diet and serum cholesterol values from person to persons *within* an affluent population may stem from the fact that there are not enough people who habitually consume the kind of diet characteristic of low cholesterol areas of the world, or that which must be fed in order to lower lipids on a metabolic ward. Evidently, at the high nutrient intakes characteristic of affluent populations, the variation in cholesterol values found *within* the population depends on factors other than the degree of overload of the incriminated nutrients. Good possibilities are innate ability to cope with the nutrient overload, energy balance, and state of health.

In free-living affluent populations there may simply not be a biologically correct range of nutrient intakes to allow a demonstration of the influence of diet on blood lipids *within* the population. For example, Connor has shown that in the range of dietary cholesterol intakes between 0 and 400 mg. per day, blood cholesterol levels achieved are proportional to intake. Beyond this range, there is little discernible association between the two.[4] The bulk of persons in affluent populations are above this range in their cholesterol intake and may also be above the threshold for saturated fat and refined carbohydrate.

While studies within free-living populations have not shown much relation of dietary practices to interindividual lipid values, there are some studies carried out in captive populations such as mental hospitals which have conclusively shown that when subjects actually adhere to diets low in cholesterol and saturated fat, substantial decreases in serum cholesterol occur and then revert on return to house diet.[17]

Also, the problem appears to be more complex than originally conceived to be. Recent evidence suggests that some persons with high cholesterol values may be more sensitive to the carbohydrate overload of their diet, while others are unable to cope with the saturated fat and cholesterol. They may be distinguishable by their lipoprotein pattern, serum triglyceride values, glucose tolerance, and serum turbidity. Such factors have not to date been adequately taken into account in diet studies. This may also explain why physicians attempting to lower serum cholesterol values by dietary manipulation are sometimes disappointed with the result. They may, in some instances, have failed to ascertain the type of hypercholesterolemia present and did not tailor the dietary modification to the lipoprotein pattern.

However, whether one subscribes to the hypothesis that diet is the chief determinant of acquired hypercholesterolemia or not, the evidence incriminating hypercholesterolemia in atherogenesis is too formidable to brush aside. Much remains to be learned. Perhaps the partition of cholesterol among the various lipoprotein fractions determines its atherogenicity or the way in which it becomes elevated is responsible, but one thing is clear, it is somehow intimately involved in the process of atherosclerosis.

While there are problems with some of the observations linking cholesterol to atherogenesis and some of the details are a bit hazy, there is too much that remains to be explained away. True, not everything that looks like a goat is in fact a goat. But, when it also smells, tastes, feels, and sounds like one, it seems reasonable to start thinking in terms of goat! There is ample precedent for the concept that a disease can be prevented long in advance of the elucidation of its etiology, provided one can determine the chain of events in its evolution within a population. By interrupting this chain the disease can often be prevented. Cholesterol appears to be a distinct link in this chain but at present a multifactorial approach, modifying as many of the precursors as possible, would appear to offer the greatest hope of success in avoiding atherosclerotic disease. To this end a coronary profile can be arrived at for the asymptomatic patient using ordinary office procedures and a simple laboratory test. From the determination of a blood cholesterol, blood pressure, glucose tolerance, cigarette habit, and electrocardiographic status with respect to left ventricular hypertrophy (or intraventricular block or nonspecific S-T and T-wave changes), the probability of a coronary attack can be estimated over a wide range (Table 3)—in this case 20-fold. It can also be seen that a 260 mg. cholesterol value may be associated with only a 4 per cent probability of a coronary event in 8 years if all other factors are favorable, or with an ominous 32 per cent probability if all others are not. Thus cholesterol, like any other contributor to coronary mortality, is best considered one ingredient of a coronary risk profile. Its impact is profoundly influenced by associated risk factors.

Evidence available from the Framingham study strongly suggests that there is a common set of precursors for all the major cardiovascular atherosclerotic diseases, whether manifest in the heart, brain, or limbs. The major risk factors for coronary heart disease taken jointly will predict brain infarction and occlusive peripheral arterial disease at least as well as coronary heart disease. This provides additional evidence that these cardiovascular diseases arise from a common substrate and very likely share a common cause. It also strongly suggests that successful prophylactic intervention against one of these atherosclerotic diseases, if successful, might well carry the considerable bonus of a reduced incidence of the others as well. And a prophylactic approach to the atherosclerotic diseases is imperative if substantial inroads against the appalling annual toll of mortality they exact is to be made. The bulk of coronary mortality occurs suddenly and unexpectedly out of reach of medical care no matter how sophisticated it is or may become.

Table 3: Probability * of developing coronary heart disease in 8 years by sex, age, systolic blood pressure, cholesterol, left ventricular hypertrophy by EKG, cigarette smoking and glucose intolerance.   The Framingham Study.   16-year follow-up **

45 year old man ***

Does not smoke cigarettes   **Smokes cigarettes**

LVH–EKG negative

Glucose intolerance absent — Does not smoke cigarettes

CHOL	SBP 105	120	135	150	165	180
185	20	24	29	35	42	51
210	25	30	36	44	53	64
235	31	38	45	55	66	79
260	39	47	56	68	81	97
285	48	58	70	84	100	119
310	60	72	87	104	123	146

Glucose intolerance absent — Smokes cigarettes

CHOL	SBP 105	120	135	150	165	180
185	32	39	46	56	67	81
210	40	48	58	69	83	99
235	50	60	72	85	103	122
260	62	74	89	105	126	149
285	76	92	109	130	153	181
310	94	113	134	158	186	217

Glucose intolerance present — Does not smoke cigarettes

CHOL	SBP 105	120	135	150	165	180
185	25	30	36	44	53	64
210	31	38	45	55	66	79
235	39	47	56	68	81	97
260	48	58	70	84	100	119
285	60	72	87	103	123	146
310	75	89	107	127	150	177

Glucose intolerance present — Smokes cigarettes

CHOL	SBP 105	120	135	150	165	180
185	40	48	58	69	83	99
210	50	60	72	86	102	122
235	62	74	89	106	126	149
260	76	91	109	130	153	181
285	94	112	134	158	186	217
310	116	138	163	191	223	259

LVH–EKG positive

Glucose intolerance absent — Does not smoke cigarettes

CHOL	SBP 105	120	135	150	165	180
185	41	50	60	72	86	102
210	51	62	74	89	106	126
235	64	76	91	109	130	153
260	79	94	112	134	158	186
285	97	116	138	163	191	223
310	120	142	167	196	229	266

Glucose intolerance absent — Smokes cigarettes

CHOL	SBP 105	120	135	150	165	180
185	65	78	93	111	132	157
210	81	95	115	136	161	189
235	100	118	141	166	195	227
260	122	145	171	200	234	270
285	149	176	206	240	277	318
310	181	212	246	284	326	370

Glucose intolerance present — Does not smoke cigarettes

CHOL	SBP 105	120	135	150	165	180
185	51	62	74	88	106	126
210	64	76	91	109	129	153
235	79	94	112	133	158	186
260	97	116	137	162	191	223
285	119	142	167	196	229	265
310	146	172	202	235	272	313

Glucose intolerance present — Smokes cigarettes

CHOL	SBP 105	120	135	150	165	180
185	81	96	115	136	161	189
210	99	118	140	166	195	227
235	122	145	171	200	233	270
260	149	176	206	240	277	318
285	181	211	246	284	325	370
310	217	252	291	333	378	425

* Probability is shown in thousandths.

** *From* Kannel, W. B., and Gordon, T., eds.: The Framingham Study. An Epidemiological Investigation of Cardiovascular Disease. Section 27. Washington, D. C., U. S. Government Printing Office, 1971.

*** Framingham men aged 45 years have an average systolic blood pressure of 131 mm. hg and an average serum CHOL of 235 mg. per 100 ml. 67 per cent smoke cigarettes, 1.3 per cent have definitive LVH and EKG and 3.8 per cent have glucose intolerance. At these average values the probability of developing coronary heart disease in 8 years is 60/1000.

REFERENCES

1. Altschule, M. D.: Can diet prevent atherogenesis? If so, what diet? Medical Counterpoint, *2*:13–27, 1970.

2. Altschule, M. D.: The cholesterol problem. Medical Counterpoint, *2*:11–20, 1970.

3. Armstrong, M. L., Warner, E. D., and Connor, W. E.: Regression of coronary atheromatosis in Rhesus monkeys. Circ. Res., *27*:59, 1970.

4. Connor, W. E., Hodges, R. E., and Bleiler, R.: Serum lipids in men receiving high cholesterol and cholesterol-free diets. Circulation, *22*:735, 1960.

5. Cornfield, J.: Joint dependence of risk of coronary heart disease on serum cholesterol and systolic blood pressure: A discriminant function analysis. Fed. Proc., *21* (No. 4) 58–61, 1962.

6. Cox, G. E., Trueheart, R. E., Kaplan, J., et al.: Atherosclerosis in Rhesus monkeys. IV. Repair of arterial injury—an important secondary atherogenic factor. Arch. Path., *76*:166, 1963.

7. Dawber, T. R., Kannel, W. B., and Lyell, L. P.: An approach to longitudinal studies in a community: The Framingham Study. Ann. N.Y. Acad. Sci., *107*:539–556, May, 1963.

8. Deming, Q. B., Mosback, E. H., Bevans, M., et al.: Blood pressure, cholesterol content of serum and tissues and atherogenesis in the rat. J. Exper. Med., *107*:581–598, 1958.

9. Gordon, T., and Kannel, W. B.: Premature mortality from coronary heart disease: The Framingham Study. J.A.M.A., *215*:1617–1625, 1971.

10. Hartroft, W. S., and Thomas, W. A.: Induction of experimental atherosclerosis in various animals. *In* Sandler, M., and Bourne, G. H., eds.: Atherosclerosis and Its Origin. New York, Academic Press, 1963.

11. Kannel, W. B.: The epidemiology of coronary heart disease: Methodologic considerations: The Framingham Study. *In* Sonderdruck aus Epidemiologie Kardiovaskularer Krankenheiten. Bern, Stuttgart, Wein, Verlag Hans Huber, 1970.

12. Kannel, W. B., Castelli, W. P., and McNamara, P. M.: Epidemiology of acute myocardial infarction: Medicine Today, *2*:56–71, Oct. 1968.

13. Kannel, W. B., and McNamara, P. M.: The evidence for excess risk in coronary disease. Minn. Med., *52*:1197–1201, 1969.

14. Moses, C.: Development of atherosclerosis in dogs with hypercholesterolemia and chronic hypertension. Circ. Res., *2*:243–247, May 1954.

15. Texon, M., Imparato, A. M., and Lord, J. W.: Hemodynamic concept of atherosclerosis; the experimental production of hemodynamic arterial disease. Arch. Surg., *80*:47, 1960.

16. Truett, J., Cornfield, J., and Kannel, W. B.: A multivariate analysis of the risk of coronary heart disease in Framingham. J. Chronic Dis., *20*:511–524, 1967.

17. Turpeinen, O.: Diet and coronary events. J. Amer. Dietetic Assoc., *52*:209, 1968.

18. Wakerlin, G. E., Moss, W. G., and Kiely, J. P.: Effect of experimental renal hypertension on experimental thiouracil-cholesterol atherosclerosis in dogs. Circ. Res., *5*:426–434, July 1957.

19. Wissler, R. W.: Recent progress in studies of experimental primate atherosclerosis. *In* Miras, C. J., Howard, A. N., and Pooletti, R., eds.: Progress in Biochemical Pharmacology, Vol. 4. New York, S. Karger, 1968.

20. Young, W., Gofman, J. W., Tandy, R., et al.: The quantitation of atherosclerosis. I. Relationship to artery size. Amer. J. Cardiol., *6*:288, 1960.

36

THE ROLE OF TRACE ELEMENTS IN CARDIOVASCULAR DISEASES

Henry A. Schroeder, M.D.*

Certain trace elements are essential for the life or health of mammals—as well as of other living things. Vanadium, chromium, manganese, iron, cobalt, copper, zinc, and molybdenum are metals having a definitive role in mammalian metabolism or having demonstrated effects on growth or survival. Selenium, fluorine, and iodine are nonmetals with biologic effects. In addition, strontium may play a role in the formation of bones and teeth.

So basic are the functions of many of these elements, especially the metals, that it would not be surprising to find alterations in their concentrations in a large number of conditions involving malfunction or destruction of tissue, with secondary changes in tissue components. Furthermore, because metallic cofactors of enzymes or activators of enzyme systems perform basic metabolic reactions, it would not be surprising to discover that certain chronic diseases result from tissue deficiency of one or another trace element.

The evolution of industry based on the use of metals which culminated in the Industrial Revolution had as one of its side effects contamination of the globe with certain metals found naturally in low concentrations. Some

Reprinted from *Medical Clinics of North America*—Vol. 58, No. 2, March 1974, by permission of W. B. Saunders Company.

Supported by National Institutes of Health Grant HE 05076–12, Cooper Laboratories, Inc., and the CIBA Pharamaceutical Company.

* Professor of Physiology, Emeritus, Dartmouth Medical School, Hanover, New Hampshire.

of these metals are innately toxic, a quality not found in low concentrations of the elements essential for life or health: cadmium, lead, mercury, antimony, beryllium. Living things have evolved in the presence of very low concentrations of these toxic elements, and the need for detoxifying systems has been relatively unnecessary—until the present. Now, as best can be ascertained, the body burdens of industrialized urban man are elevated with respect to three elements: lead, cadmium, and arsenic, certainly the result of modern industrial practices. Therefore, it would not be surprising if some chronic disease resulted from metabolic breakdown coming from accumulation of an abnormal toxic trace element during a lifetime.

The common chronic diseases of our civilization which are unusual in some other people are atherosclerosis, hypertension, arthritis, cancer, diabetes, and cirrhosis of the liver, which make up the leading causes of death and disability. Some of these disorders are at least partly affected by dietary factors. Therefore, a search must be made on the relation of trace elements—deficiencies of essential ones and excesses of toxic ones— to common chronic diseases.

A great deal of investigative work has been done on these problems. In fact, the World Health Organization is now conducting a large survey on cardiovascular disease and trace elements in tissues and in the environment.[18] Enough evidence, both indirect and direct, has now accumulated to involve trace elements as causal factors of two cardiovascular diseases, atherosclerosis and hypertension.

ATHEROSCLEROSIS

Background

The body burden of chromium in Americans was low, many tissues being deficient, and levels declining with age.[34, 44] This finding contrasted with body burdens of Africans, Near Easterners, and Orientals, which were much higher. In fact, tissues of Thai had more chromium than any other group, and the incidence of aortic atherosclerosis was very low.[28] Furthermore, there were few atherosclerotic complications, such as myocardial infarctions or cerebral vascular accidents. High tissue levels of chromium were generally found in areas where there was little atherosclerosis, but in advanced countries levels tended to be low—such as in England,[48] where it was seldom detected.

The disorder of carbohydrate and lipid metabolism which causes serum cholesterol to increase with age and which produces lipid deposits in sub-intimal areas of the arteries is characterized by (a) elevated blood lipid levels and (b) abnormal tolerance for glucose. Consequences of these lipid deposits plus clotting of blood results in thrombosis of coronary and cerebral arteries and sometimes of femoral arteries, with resultant death or disability. In myocardial infarction or coronary thrombosis without infarction, the atherosclerotic process is believed to be enhanced by the frequent presence of hypertension, another disease.

It is not the purpose of this discussion to consider effects, but only causes, and to separate diseases which often occur together. The frequent coexistence of mild or moderate hypertension and coronary accident, however, obscures much epidemiologic data and leads to erroneous interpretations based on them. Therefore, we will consider atherosclerosis per se, whether it involves disease or death, in brain, heart or extremities, and treat it as one disease.

Epidemiologic data—the water factor

The death rate from coronary heart disease has long been shown to vary significantly from one area to another. This variation was discovered to be inversely related to some quality of drinking water associated with its hardness.[30-32, 48] The relation held not only in countries such as Great Britain,[21] Sweden,[3] and Canada,[1] but even in small countries such as the Netherlands,[18] and in states such as Washington [18] (but not in Oklahoma); but not in Japan, where the first observations were made.[16] There, cerebral vascular accident is the first cause of death, most cases being due to hemorrhage, and the relationship was demonstrated between this disorder and the acidity of river water, directly. Almost all Japanese waters are soft. At this point, the case for hypertension being related to water quality was as good or better than for coronary disease to be so related. At any rate, some geochemical factor in water, presumably elemental, was involved in cardiovascular deaths.

All reports, except those of Kobayashi [16] and Schroeder [30, 31] considered coronary heart disease and factors in water. It was not until Masironi examined the problem that a dichotomy between hypertensive heart disease and coronary heart disease appeared in the data, to the exclusion of the latter.[17] Masironi went back to Kobayashi's original thesis, that river water was related to death rates, and found significant correlations of a number of elements in water and regional death rates from hypertensive, but not coronary, heart disease.

Death rates in white males aged 45 to 64 years in 42 states were inversely correlated with the following trace elements and qualities of water: hardness, α-radioactivity, cobalt, nickel, chromium, molybdenum, vanadium, zinc, manganese, fluorine, and boron; these correlations were significant at the 0.05 to 0.01 level of confidence. In addition, death rates were inversely related to the concentrations of the toxic trace elements antimony, bismuth, cadmium, lead, silver, tin, at the same level of confidence, but insignificantly to barium, beryllium, iron and copper.

The results of all of these surveys were to leave us with a variety of elements related to death rates from hypertensive heart disease, without a single outstanding one suspected of being causal (Table 1).

Table 1: Correlation coefficients (r) of some waterborne trace elements and death rates from hypertensive heart disease and atherosclerotic heart disease (United States data, white males aged 45–64 years)

Element	River water, hypertensive heart disease		Municipal water, atherosclerotic heart disease	
	r	P	r	P
Potassium	–	–	−0.48	<0.0005
Magnesium	–	–	−0.40	<0.0005
Hardness	0.44	<0.01	−0.41	<0.0005
Silicon	–	–	−0.34	<0.0005
Sodium	–	–	−0.27	<0.01
Calcium	–	–	−0.23	<0.02
Vanadium	−0.41	<0.05	−0.34	<0.0005
Barium	0.26	–	−0.34	<0.0005
Copper	+0.11	–	+0.29	<0.005
Strontium	–	–	−0.29	<0.005
Lithium	–	–	−0.28	<0.005
Manganese	−0.35	<0.05	+0.26	<0.01
α-radioactivity	−0.42	<0.01		
β-radioactivity	−0.52	<0.001	−0.21	<0.025
Boron	−0.34	<0.05		
Lead	−0.46	<0.01		
Nickel	−0.36	<0.05		
Molybdenum	0.36	<0.05		

Data from Masironi [17] and Schroeder.[30]
Essential elements in italics.

When one examines the data with a view to deciding whether or not an element occurs in water in sufficient amounts to negate a food deficiency of the element, one is left with the conclusion that, with few exceptions, water usually supplies minor and negligible increments to the total dietary intake of trace elements. These relationships are given in Table 2. The median values show that water provides less than 7 per cent of the essential elements, fluorine being an exception. The extreme values —for hard water—indicate significant increments of magnesium, chromium, manganese, and molybdenum, each of which has been implicated in cardiovascular disorders. Such large increments must be rare.

Of the non-essential elements, water provides several times more silicon than food, but silicon is not readily absorbed by the intestine. Water also provides sizable increments of barium, strontium, boron, titanium and uranium in hard water areas. These elements have very low orders of toxicity. Some cadmium, which is toxic and cumulative, is provided by water, especially soft water running through pipes. Very toxic metals, such as bismuth, beryllium, and antimony, are present in water only in traces.

Table 2: Increment of bulk and trace elements in water to total dietary intakes

Elements	Water Median mg.	Maximum mg.	Food mg.	Per cent from water Median	Maximum
Essential					
Calcium	52	290	800	6.5	36.3
Magnesium	12.5	240	210	5.9	114.3
Sodium	24	396	4,400	0.5	9.0
Potassium	3.2	60	3,300	0.09	1.8
Vanadium	<0.008	0.14	2	0.6	
Chromium	0.001	0.07	0.1	1.0	70.0
Manganese	0.01	2.2	3	0.3	73.3
Iron	0.09	3.4	15	0.6	22.7
Cobalt	0.006	0.01	0.3	2.0	3.3
Nickel *	0.005	0.07	0.4	1.3	17.5
Copper	0.02	0.5	2.5	0.8	20.0
Zinc	0.5	2.1	13	3.8	16.2
Selenium	<0.02	–	0.15	<13.3	–
Fluorine	0.4	14	1.8	22.2	777.8
Molybdenum	0.003	0.14	0.34	0.9	41.2
Non-Essential					
Silicon	14.2	144	3.5	405.7	4100
Aluminum	0.1	3.0	45	0.2	6.7
Barium	0.09	0.76	1.24	7.3	61.3
Strontium	0.22	2.4	2	11.0	120.0
Boron	0.06	1.2	1.0	6.0	120.0
Bismuth	trace		0.002		
Beryllium	trace		0.00001	–	–
Antimony	trace		<1.0	–	–
Lead	0.007	0.12	0.41	1.7	29.3
Lithium	0.004	0.34	2.0	0.2	17.0
Silver	0.005	0.014	0.07	7.1	20.0
Tin	0.002	0.005	4.0	0.05	0.1
Titanium	<0.003	0.1	0.3	0.1	33.3
Uranium	0.0003	0.5	1.4	0.02	35.7
Cadmium	0.005	0.02	0.07	7.1	28.6

Data from Durfor and Becker,[6] Howell,[13] and Schroeder [41] at 2 liters per day.
* Nickel is possibly essential for mammals, but unproven.

Therefore, of these many studies, we can implicate marginal intakes in soft water areas and luxus intakes in hard water areas of magnesium, chromium, manganese, and molybdenum, and the reverse situation for cadmium. The water factor offers indirect evidence that a trace metal or metals affect human death rates from hypertensive heart disease and so indirectly from arteriosclerotic heart disease.

For many years we have puzzled over the question as to whether hard water was protective or soft water lethal in hypertensive heart disease.[30, 31] The conclusion that soft water has some detrimental quality appears the logical one. As soft water is usually acid and usually corrosive to pipes, some metal coming from water pipes is probably involved. The only metal with the ability to cause hypertension in rats [26] shown to be dissolved by soft water from pipes [45] is cadmium. Therefore, cadmium is suggested as the water factor, entering the body via water from galvanized pipes and solders.[35]

Atherosclerosis, experimental

Although many people have investigated atherosclerosis in animals, both laboratory and zoo, the approach has generally been on the basis of exercise, lipids, or carbohydrates. Wild animals seldom show the disease, but animals in captivity often do.

A diet designed for rats, of whole rye flour, dry skim milk, and corn oil, was found fortuitively to be deficient in chromium and to cause aortic plaques, elevated serum cholesterol and elevated fasting blood sugar.[27, 37] In other words, this diet reproduced in rats the human atherosclerosis syndrome.[44] Diets even lower in chromium, using refined white sugar as the major carbohydrate, also produced the syndrome, which was prevented by substitution of raw or dark brown sugar which contained adequate chromium.[17, 40] To date, attempts to reverse the disease, once established, have not been made.

Human counterpart by analyses

Persons in the United States and abroad dying of coronary heart disease had virtually no chromium in their aortas, whereas those dying of accidents or other diseases had aortic chromium [44] (Table 3). There were virtually no differences in hepatic chromium in the two groups. In general, tissues of United States subjects were low or deficient in chromium, compared to tissues of foreign subjects.[34, 44] These differences were especially marked in the case of aortic chromium (Table 4). In all five areas of the world, there was more aortic chromium, and it was more prevalent in subjects dying of accident or other causes than in subjects dying of atherosclerotic heart disease. Aortic chromium in subjects dying of other cardiovascular or cerebrovascular diseases was intermediate in value.

Causes of chromium deficiency

The exact causes of aortic chromium deficiency are not known, although relative body deficiency is probably the result of two factors. Natural chromium occurs as an organic complex called the glucose tolerance factor, which is stable, readily absorbed by the intestine, and passes the placental barrier. It is present especially in wheat germ, bran, and probably molasses, as well as in brewer's yeast. Chromic salts or simple complexes olate (form long, hexa-aquo molecules) in alkaline media, are absorbed by the intestine only to a point of 0.5 per cent,[5] and do not pass

Table 3: Chromium in aortas of subjects dying from atherosclerotic heart disease, other cardiovascular diseases, and accidents

Location	No. of cases	Aortic Chromium μg/g	Prevalence per cent	P
San Francisco				
Atherosclerotic heart disease	15	0.05±0.009	13.3	–
Atherosclerotic heart disease moderate	3	0.03±0.003	0	–
Accidents	10	0.23±0.076	80	<0.005
United States—9 cities				
Atherosclerotic heart disease	13	0.05±0.088	46.2	–
Other cardiovascular disease	15	0.20±0.090	60	–
Accidents	103	0.26±0.067	87.4	<0.005
Africa				
Cardiovascular disease	2	0.12±0.026	100	–
Other	11	0.19±0.025	90.9	<0.025
Mid-East				
Cardiovascular disease	3	0.22±0.084	66.7	–
Other	11	1.28±0.831	100	–
Far East				
Atherosclerotic heart disease	5	0.25±0.132	100	–
Cardiovascular disease	20	0.31±0.073	85	–
Accidents	8	0.97±0.532	100	–

Data from Schroeder et al.[44]

the placental barrier.[19]   Refining of wheat to make white flour, of sugar to make white sugar, and of fats to make white or yellow fats and oils removes most of the chromium available for the body (Table 5).   The use of much chromium-poor glucose or sucrose would add little to body stores, and would probably mobilize chromium from body stores into the blood,[7] from whence part is excreted in the urine, producing a net loss. Whereas chromium-rich sugars would have the same effect, the net result would be a favorable chromium balance.   The rat requires the human equivalent of 0.5 to 0.7 mg. per day to be in adequate balance; man receives 0.05 to 0.1 mg. in his food and water.

Table 4: Aortic chromium from various geographic areas

	No. cases	Mean ± SEM μg/g ash
United States	64*	1.9
9 cities	150	4.4±0.5
San Francisco	27	2.6±1.1
Honolulu	12	14±4.3
Anchorage	2	13±9.7
Far East	35*	15†
Japan	28	15±2.9
Taipei	10	26±10
Manilla	10	37±11
Bangkok	10	44±24
Hongkong	10	7.6±1.9
Africa	13*	5.5
Caucasoid	13	4.3±1.4
Negroid	41	7.5±2.8
Addis Ababa	5	3.7±1.8
Lagos	17	3.7±1.1
Cairo	8	6.0±2.1
Welkom	5	25±6.5
Bern, Switzerland	9*	30±23
India	9*	11†
Delhi	8	6.0±1.9
Lucknow	4	22±11
Bombay	8	71±55

Data from Schroeder et al.[44]

* Males 20 to 59 years old, only.

† Differs from United States value, $P < 0.001$.

As chromium is necessary for glucose and lipid metabolism,[40] it is likely that the decreased or absent aortic chromium in atherosclerosis reflects the decreased or absent chromium in the coronary arteries, and that this leads to abnormal metabolism and plaque formation. The intermediary steps, however, have not been determined. Until the natural organic complex of chromium is obtained for therapeutic trials, it will not be possible to reverse this condition in man, if the condition is reversible.

Table 5: Losses of chromium and manganese in common foods (wet weight)

Food	Refined Cr, μg/g	Refined Mn, μg/g	Unrefined Cr, μg/g	Unrefined Mn, μg/g
Wheat	0.03	6.5	0.05	46.0
Sugar	0.0–0.11	0.13	0.19–0.42	1.75
Animal fats	0.07–0.10	0.98	0.21–0.23	–
Vegetable oils	0.03–0.07	1.47	0.23	2.52
Hospital diet	0.056–0.066	0.96	–	3.0

Data from Schroeder [38, 44]

Other metals

We can examine a number of other elements for differences in aortic concentrations from the United States, Africa, Near East, and Far East (Table 6), bearing in mind that atherosclerosis is widespread in the

Table 6: Significant differences in elemental content of aorta in five areas of world (males aged 20 to 59, ppm ash, median values)

Element	United States	Africa	Near East	Far East	Switzerland
Essential					
Chromium	1.9	5.5	11*	15*	30*
Manganese	8	13*	18*	22*	9
Iron	2900	2800	4600	5600*	2300
Copper†	91	110	180*	160*	110
Non-Essential					
Aluminum	28	840*	1000*	450*	69
Barium	7	14*	19*	19*	17*
Nickel	<5	7	24	21*	13*
Silver	0.1	<0.1	1.4*	1.0*	<0.1
Titanium	<5	20*	59*	20*	12*
Bulk					
Calcium %‡	5.0	3.3	2.9	2.4*	6.6
Phosphorus %	7	6	13*	10*	8

* Differs from United States value, $P < 0.001$.

† Decreases with age, $P < 0.001$, $r = -0.51$.

‡ Increases with age, $P < 0.001$, $r = +0.43$.

Data from Tipton et al.[49]

United States but is less severe in the other areas and that differences in elemental content could reflect primary or secondary effects. Calcium and phosphorus levels declined as the presumed severity of atherosclerosis of the aorta decreased, from the United States to Africa to the Near East and to the Far East. Of 20 elements, 11 showed aortic concentrations significantly different from those in United States aortas; three of these were the essential trace metals chromium, manganese, and copper, which were higher in Near and Far Eastern samples than in those of United States subjects. Of the non-essential metals, five—aluminum, barium, nickel, silver, and titanium—had significantly higher concentrations in foreign than in United States aortas. From what is known of the innate toxicities of these metals, it is doubtful that aluminum, barium, silver, or titanium has other than a secondary nonspecific role in atherosclerosis. Therefore, from this indirect viewpoint, we must examine the possibility that deficiency of chromium, manganese, copper, or perhaps nickel could be a causal factor in the disease—chromium, copper, and manganese are listed as protective in Table 7. The elements which did

Table 7: Trace elements considered involved experimentally in cardiovascular diseases

	Protective	Inductive
Atherosclerosis	Cr, Mn, V, Co	Co (injected), Cu, Cr Deficiency
Hypertension	Zn	Cd, Zn Deficiency
Aortic calcification	F, Mg	F deficiency
Elasticity of arteries	Li, Cu	
Focal myocardial necrosis	Se	As

Adapted from Masironi [18]

not vary significantly in aorta from area to area are the essential: magnesium, vanadium, potassium, cobalt, zinc, molybdenum and non-essential cadmium, lead, strontium and tin.

The function of chromium has been discussed. Manganese inhibits experimental atherosclerosis in rabbits and influences lipid metabolism in atherosclerotic patients. The manganese content of the heart and aorta of atherosclerotic subjects is lower, and that of plasma is higher, than in healthy controls.[48]

Copper induces atherosclerosis in experimental animals.[11] Human subjects with a history of myocadial infarction had elevated serum copper concentrations.[10] Soft waters corrode copper pipes. Aortic copper in atherosclerosis is depressed, whereas myocardial copper is increased. Copper deficiency causes defective synthesis of aortic collagen and elastin, interfering with elasticity of blood vessels. In American aortas, ash and calcium increased with age, and presumably atherosclerosis (correlation coefficients, r, 0.43 to 0.51, $P < 0.001$) whereas copper and potassium decreased with age ($r = -0.51$ and -0.70 respectively, $P < 0.001$). Thus, copper may play a regulatory role.

Secondary changes of trace elements in atherosclerosis and myocardial infarction are shown in Table 8. Six metals are increased in aorta, 4

Table 8: Secondary changes in trace elements in atherosclerosis and myocardial infarction

	Increase	Decrease
Atherosclerosis		
Aorta	Fe, Mo, Co, Pb, Ag, Zn	Cu, Li, Mn, Cr
Heart	Co, Cu, Zn	Mn
Plasma, or blood	Mn	Zn
Myocardial Infarction		
Injured tissue, heart	Ba, Br, Sb	Mn, Mo, Al, Rb, Co, Cs, Zn
Serum	Cu, Ni, Mn, B, Mo, Ca	Zn, Fe
Urine	Cu	

Adapted from Masironi [18]

are decreased; the 4 may be etiologically involved. Six elements increase in serum; 3 are diagnostic of infarction. The injured myocardium collects 3 strange elements and loses 7, 4 of which are essential. Most of these changes reflect abnormal tissue.

HYPERTENSION

Excessive vasospasm leading to a permanent elevation of the blood pressure is a common phenomenon in civilized man. Whereas there are many factors in the genesis of hypertension—emotional, psychosomatic, nervous, endocrine, and renal—there is one common denominator in most cases, and that is altered arterial reactivity.

Successful treatment of hypertension is accomplished by two types of chemical agents, one of which acts on nerves and the other on blood vessels. The latter group are all chelating agents, complexing metals: hydralazine, EDTA, BAL, thiocyanate, nitroprusside, azide, and the like.[29] Thus, it appears that a metal is somehow involved in hypertension.

Experiments were conducted on rats fed for life small doses of each of 20 metals in drinking water, in a metal-free environment.[46] Blood pressures, heart weights, and microscopic sections were evaluated. The only trace metal causing hypertension was cadmium.[26] Cadmium accumulated in liver and kidney in concentrations common to civilized man,[42] and in blood vessels. When it was removed by injecting a zinc-loaded chelating agent, Na_2Zn CDTA, blood pressure became normal within a few minutes, and remained so.[39, 43] Zinc replaced some cadmium in liver and kidney. This agent is undergoing clinical trials.

Cadmium hypertension in rats duplicates moderate human hypertension in having elevated blood pressure, increased mortality, renal arteriolar sclerosis,[19] enlarged hearts, and increase in the severity of atherosclerosis.[37] Deaths from hemorrhage are common. The blood pressure of rats is extremely sensitive to dietary cadmium (Table 9) and when cadmium is virtually absent in the kidneys it is low. As our diet is deficient in cadmium (0.07 micrograms per gram) and as commercial diets contain sizable amounts (0.25 to 0.60 micrograms per gram) it is clear that all experiments which have been done on animal hypertension are complicated by renal cadmium, unless efforts at a cadmium-free environment were made. An intake of 1.0 ppm cadmium in rats is accompanied by demonstrable effects on fertility, viability of young, carbohydrate metabolism, and SGOT activity.[47]

Human deaths from hypertension were associated with more renal cadmium, or a higher ratio of cadmium to zinc, than were deaths from coronary heart disease or accidents. Likewise deaths from cerebral vascular disease were accompanied by more cadmium and a higher ratio than accidental deaths (Table 10). There was a good correlation of clini-

Table 9: Effects of cadmium in food and water on systolic blood pressure of rats

Age, months	0.1 PPM CD B.P. mm. Hg	0.62 PPM CD B.P. mm. Hg	5.1 PPM CD B.P. mm. Hg	P *
Females				
3	85±2.2	109±3.2	—	<0.001
4	87±4.4	110±3.7	—	<0.001
5	81±2.2	112±6.1	—	<0.001
7	—	115±4.0	—	<0.001
12	84±5.8	—	211±8.3	<0.001
13	82±3.4	—	—	—
17	92±4.9	—	182±12.6	<0.001
24	84±3.8	—	205±10.9	<0.001
30	99±4.2	—	229±12.9	<0.001
Males				
12	106±5.7	—	124±5.6	<0.025
17	94±3.8	—	122±4.5	<0.001
24	79±3.6	—	137±6.2	<0.001
30	93±5.1	—	198±7.9	<0.001
Females, 17				
Calcium in water			92 †	
No calcium			253 ‡	<0.001
Renal cadmium, ppm	0.03±0.002	2.0±0.21	54.7±4.82	<0.0001
Hepatic cadmium, ppm	0.03±0.008	1.2±0.18	20.9±3.91	<0.0001

* P is significance of difference between the 2 groups shown.

† 8 rats normotensive, 2 hypertensive (260 mm. Hg).

‡ All of 10 rats hypertensive

In all groups but three given calcium, there were 16 to 24 rats. In the third column, 5.0 ppm cadmium was given in water. Data from Kanisawa and Schroeder [15].

cal death rates from hypertension by country and renal cadmium.[25] Human hypertensive patients excreted 40 to 50 times as much cadmium in their urines as did normotensive controls, a phenomenon unrelated to proteinuria.[23]

These data indicate that cadmium is a causal factor in rat hypertension and probably in human hypertension. Against the latter hypothesis is the work of Morgan [20] who failed to confirm our observations on a group of negro subjects in Alabama. Negroes in the United States are peculiarly sensitive to hypertension, differing from whites in this respect.

There is a further paradox in this theory. Overdoses of cadmium do not cause hypertension, but induce renal damage and emphysema. Also, continuous ingestion of enough to cause osteomalacia—Milkman's syndrome—does not lead to hypertension. The overt toxicity of cadmium negates hypertension—recondite toxicity produces it. This situation also holds for industrial workers exposed to cadmium in air.

Air levels of cadmium were significantly and highly correlated with deaths from hypertensive heart disease in 28 urban areas of the United

States.[4] Cadmium occurs in cigarette smoke,[36] a known factor for coronary occlusion. The industrial consumption of cadmium has increased since 1940 at an exponential rate.[2] Cadmium alters vascular reactivity.

Table 10: Renal cadmium (ppm ash) and cadmium zinc ratios in human kidneys according to major cause of death

Cause of death	No. cases	CD mean μg/g	P *	CD/ZN mean μg/g	P *
United States Mainland					
Hypertension	17	4220	—	0.77	—
Accidents	117	2940	<0.0005	0.62	<0.01
Arteriosclerotic heart disease	27	2660	<0.0005	0.62	<0.01
Miscellaneous	26	3380	N.S.	0.58	<0.01
Foreign					
Hypertension	17	5080	—	0.94	—
Accidents	23	3170	<0.025	0.66	<0.005
Arteriosclerotic heart disease	12	2430	<0.01	0.49	<0.005
All cases					
Cerebral vascular accident	23	4266	—	0.80	—
Traumatic accident	140	2980	<0.0005	0.62	<0.005

* P is significance of differences of mean from hypertension or cerebral vascular accident. Data from Schroeder [25].

DISCUSSION

As one views the large amount of work on trace elements and cardiovascular diseases, it becomes clear that at least two metals are involved directly, and two others may act conjointly. In the first place, atherosclerosis is consistent with a deficiency disease of some function of carbohydrate and lipid metabolism. Two trace metals—chromium and manganese—are concerned with carbohydrate and lipid metabolism. Deficiency of chromium resulting from the use of refined foods is probably prevalent in this country. Deficiency of manganese in human diets consisting largely of refined foods is also possible. Although human requirements are not known, pigs need 40 ppm and cattle about the same amount, whereas human beings receive 2 to 5 mg. per day in a 2 kg. diet. Losses of 86 per cent from wheat by milling, 89 per cent from raw sugar by refining, and 75 per cent from rice by polishing could easily contribute to relative manganese deficiency. Manganese was low in Type A school lunches in this country.[22]

Manganese is involved in glucose utilization, and deficient animals showed reduced tolerance to ingested glucose, like chromium-deficient animals.[18] It is also involved in lipid metabolism, stimulating the hepatic synthesis of cholesterol and fatty acids. Manganous ion is a cofactor for mevalonic kinase, which synthesizes squalene and cholesterol. Whereas we do not know which of these two similarly acting metals is deficient (both could be), the weight of evidence favors chromium, for there is no manganese deficiency, either dietary or tissue, in rats exhibiting chromium deficiency and atherosclerosis.

The other trace metal believed causal in cardiovascular disease is cadmium as a factor in hypertension. Cadmium and zinc are intimately related, and are bound by the same protein—a high-cysteine, low-tyrosine molecule which is synthesized only in response to cadmium. They are metabolically antagonistic. Zinc is essential for many enzymatic reactions in all living things. Zinc has been found to have an increasing number of therapeutic actions on a variety of human disorders—anosmia, growth, sexual development, delayed wound healing, burns, ulcers of legs, postalcoholic cirrhosis of the liver, tolerance to ingested alcohol, and atherosclerotic ischemia of the legs, or peripheral vascular disease.[8, 9, 12, 14, 24, 50] Experimentally zinc has been found to be involved in DNA and RNA synthesis, learning behavior, protein metabolism, carbohydrate metabolism, reproduction, bone growth, integrity of skin, as well as in many enzymes. Analytical deficiency of plasma zinc is widespread,[9] found in pregnancy, women taking antifertility steroids, many older people, cases of burns, atherosclerotic complications, leg ulcers, atherosclerosis, and several chronic diseases, such as tuberculosis, infections, leukemia, some cancers, malnutrition, and uremia. Marginal zinc intakes come from the same sources as do marginal chromium and manganese intakes—refined grains, sugars, and fats.

Table 11: Experimental counterparts of human cardiovascular diseases. Trace metal imbalances

Abnormality	Rats	Human beings
Atherosclerosis, Cr deficiency		
Glucose tolerance	reduced	reduced
Response to Cr	normal	normal in 40–50%
Serum cholesterol	elevated	elevated
Response to Cr	reduced	moderately reduced in 40–50%
Aortic plaques	induced	? induced
Response to Cr	prevented	?
Status of tissue Cr	deficient	deficient, especially aorta
Hypertension, Cd excess		
Blood pressure	elevated	elevated
Response to Zn chelate	lowered	moderately lowered
Renal arteriolar sclerosis	present	present
Cardiac enlargement	present	present
Renal cadmium	40–60 ppm	40–80 ppm
Renal Cd:Zn ratio	>0.58	>0.70
Atherosclerosis	increased	increased

The most striking clinical effects of oral zinc are on peripheral vascular disease.[12] Doses of 150 mg. a day as the sulfate have caused improvement in the circulations of ischemic extremities, heart, and probably brains. Improved circulation is associated with no rise in blood pressure distal to an obstruction of an artery of a leg. This phenomenon indicates vasodilitation specifically in ischemic areas. The net results have been improvement in ischemic pain and dysfunction, healing of early gangrene, return of pulses to normal, and improvement of angina pectoris and cerebral ischemia. We have observed favorable effects with 30 mg. a day as the acetate, about double the usual adequate dietary intake.

The mechanism of action is not known, but it may involve the displacement of cadmium from ischemic arterial wall by zinc in excess.

That chromium and cadmium may not be the whole story in respect to trace elements and cardiac disease is suggested by microscopic findings on sections of hearts from rats fed 8 trace elements for life. Focal myocardial fibrosis—scars visible grossly which resemble healed myocardial infarcts microscopically—were found in a variable proportion of rats (Table 12). There were significantly more in rats given niobium, zir-

Table 12: Interstitial focal myocardial fibrosis in rats fed various trace elements for life in drinking water

| Element | Dose ppm | No. rats | Fibrosis | | P | Mycarditis, focal |
			No.	Per cent		
Controls	—	44	1	2.3	—	—
Selenate	3	64	1	1.6	N.S.	—
Tellurite	2	35	2	5.7	N.S.	—
Nickel	5	30	4	13.3	N.S.	—
Niobium	5	58	11	18.9	<0.25	1
Zirconium	5	54	12	22.2	<0.025	1
Lead * †	25	29	7	24.1	<0.025	—
Vanadium	5	27	7	25.9	<0.01	—
Antimony †	5	42	12	28.6	<0.01	—

P is difference from controls by Chi-square analysis.

* Males only.

† Recondite toxicity in terms of longevity.

Note: These sections of heart were all read by J. B. Blennerhasset, M.D., of the Department of Pathology, Massachusetts General Hospital, Boston.

conium, lead, vanadium, and antimony than in those fed nickel, tellurium, selenium and in the controls. Myocarditis, or recent infarcts, were seen in 2 animals. Possible significance of these chance findings lies in the ability of niobium to displace vanadium, zirconium to displace chromium, and in the recondite toxicity of lead and antimony, which shorten life span and longevity of rats.

CONCLUSIONS

Imbalances of trace metals may influence cardiovascular diseases causally, or may be involved secondarily. Chromium deficiency is a causal factor in atherosclerosis; manganese may also be deficient in this disease. The experimental evidence supports this theory, in that a replica of the human disease was developed in rats and prevented by chromium fed or in foods (Table 11).

Cadmium is a causal factor in hypertension. A replica of the human disease was developed in rats and cured by removing the causal factor by chelation. Zinc deficiency could also play a part in hypertension (Table 11).

Zinc given orally is a useful therapeutic agent in peripheral vascular disease even with gangrene, and also has favorable effects on ischemic hearts and brains.

The definitive roles of trace elements in the two major cardiovascular diseases deserves further study.

REFERENCES

1. Anderson, T. W., leRiche, W. H., and MacKay, J. S.: Sudden death: Correlation with hardness of water supply. New Eng. J. Med., *280*:805, 1969.

2. Athanassiadis, Y. C.: Air Pollution Aspects of Cadmium and Its Compounds. Tech. Report. Litton Systems, Inc., Environmental Systems Division, Bethesda, Maryland, 1969.

3. Biörck, G., Boström, H., and Widström, A.: On relationship between water hardness and death rate from cardiovascular disease. Acta Med. Scandinav., *178*:239, 1965.

4. Carroll, R. E.: The relationship of cadmium in the air to cardiovascular death rates. J.A.M.A., *198*:267, 1969.

5. Donaldson, R. M., and Barreras, R. F.: Intestinal absorption of trace quantities of chromium. J. Lab. Clin. Med., *68*:484, 1966.

6. Durfor, C. N., and Becker, E.: Public water supplies of the 100 largest cities in the United States, 1962. Geological Survey, Water-Supply Paper 1812, U.S. Govt. Printing Office, 1964.

7. Glinsmann, W. H., Feldman, F. J., and Mertz, W.: Plasma chromium after glucose administration. Science, *152*:1243, 1966.

8. Greaves, M. W., and Skillen, A. W.: Effects of long-continued ingestion of zinc sulfate in patients with venous leg ulceration. Lancet, *2*:889, 1970.

9. Halsted, J. A., and Smith, J. C.: Plasma-zinc in health and disease. Lancet, *1*:322, 1970.

10. Harman, D.: Atherogenesis in minipigs: Effect of dietary fat unsaturation and of copper. Circulation (Suppl. VI) *38*:8, 1968.

11. Harman, D.: Role of serum copper in coronary atherosclerosis. Circulation, *28*:658, 1963.

12. Henzel, J. H., Lichti, E., Keitzer, F. W., et al.: Efficacy of zinc medication as a therapeutic modality in atherosclerosis: Follow-up observations on patients medicated over long periods. *In* Proceedings of the Fourth Annual Conference on Trace Substances in Environmental Health, University of Missouri, Columbia, Missouri, June 23–24, 1970, p. 49.

13. Howell, G. P.: Elemental intake, output and balances of reference man. ICRP Report of Subcommittee II on Permissible Dose for Internal Radiation. Oxford, England, Pergamon Press (in press).

14. Husain, S. L.: Oral zinc sulphate in leg ulcers. Lancet, *2*:1069, 1969.

15. Kanisawa, M., and Schroeder, H. A.: Renal arteriolar changes in hypertensive rats given cadmium in drinking water. J. Exper. Molec. Path., *10*:81, 1969.

16. Kobayashi, J.: Geological relationship between chemical nature of river water and death-rate from apoplexy: preliminary report. Ber. d. Ohara Inst. f. landwirtsch. Biologie, *11*:12, 1957.

17. Masironi, R.: Cardiovascular mortality in relation to radioactivity and hardness of local water supplies in the USA. Bull. World Health Org., *43*:687, 1970.

18. Masironi, R.: Trace elements and cardiovascular diseases. Bull. World Health Org., *40*:305, 1969.

19. Mertz, W.: Chromium occurrence and function in biological systems. Physiol. Rev., *49*:163, 1969.

20. Morgan, J. M.: Tissue cadmium concentrations in man. Arch. Int. Med., *123*:405, 1969.

21. Morris, J. M., Crawford, M. D., and Heady, J. A.: Hardness of local water supplies and mortality from cardiovascular disease in county boroughs of England and Wales. Lancet, *1*:860, 1961.

22. Murphy, E. W., Page, L., and Watt, B. K.: Trace minerals in Type A school lunches. J. Amer. Dietet. Assoc., *58*:115, 1971.

23. Perry, H. M., Jr., and Schroeder, H. A.: Concentration of trace metals in urine of treated and untreated hypertensive patients compared with normal subjects. J. Lab. Clin. Med., *46*:936, 1955.

24. Pories, W. J., Henzel, J. H., Rob, C. G., et al.: Acceleration of wound healing in man with zinc sulfate given by mouth. Lancet, *1*:121, 1967.

25. Schroeder, H. A.: Cadmium as a factor in hypertension. J. Chron. Dis., *18*:647, 1965.

26. Schroeder, H. A.: Cadmium hypertension in rats. Amer. J. Physiol., *207*:62, 1964.

27. Schroeder, H. A.: Chromium deficiency in rats: A syndrome simulating diabetes mellitus with retarded growth. J. Nutr., *88*:439, 1966.

28. Schroeder, H. A.: Degenerative cardiovascular disease in the Orient. I. Atherosclerosis. J. Chron. Dis., *8*:287, 1958.

29. Schroeder, H. A.: Mechanisms of Hypertension, Springfield, Illinois, Charles C. Thomas, 1957.

30. Schroeder, H. A.: Municipal drinking water and cardiovascular death rates. J.A.M.A., *195*:81, 1966.

31. Schroeder, H. A.: Relation between mortality from cardiovascular disease and treated water supplies. Variations in states and 163 largest municipalities in the United States. J.A.M.A., *172*:1902, 1960.

32. Schroeder, H. A.: Relations between hardness of water and death rates from certain chronic and degenerative diseases in the U. S. J. Chron., Dis., *12*:586, 1960.

33. Schroeder, H. A.: Serum cholesterol and glucose levels in rats fed refined and less refined sugars and chromium. J. Nutr., *97*:237, 1969.

34. Schroeder, H. A.: The role of chromium in mammalian nutrition. Amer. J. Clin. Nutr., *21*:230, 1968.

35. Schroeder, H. A.: The water factor. New Eng. J. Med., *280*:836, 1969.

36. Schroeder, H. A., and Balassa, J. J.: Abnormal trace metals in man: Cadmium. J. Chron. Dis., *14*:236, 1961.

37. Schroeder, H. A., and Balassa, J. J.: Influence of chromium, cadmium and lead on rat aortic lipids and circulating cholesterol. Amer. J. Physiol., *209*:-433, 1965.

38. Schroeder, H. A., Balassa, J. J., and Tipton, I. H.: Essential trace metals in man: Manganese: A study in homeostasis. J. Chron. Dis., *19*:545, 1966.

39. Schroeder, H. A., and Buckman, J.: Cadmium hypertension. Its reversal in rats by zinc chelate. Arch. Environ. Health, *14*:693, 1967.

40. Schroeder, H. A., Mitchener, M., and Nason, A. P.: Influence of various sugars, chromium, and other trace metals on serum cholesterol and glucose of rats. J. Nutr., *101*:247, 1971.

41. Schroeder, H. A., and Nason, A. P.: Trace element analysis in clinical chemistry. Clin. Chem., *17*:461, 1971.

42. Schroeder, H. A., Nason, A. P., and Balassa, J. J.: Trace metals in rat tissues as influenced by calcium in water. J. Nutr., *93*:331, 1967.

43. Schroeder, H. A., Nason, A. P., and Mitchener, M.: Action of a chelate of zinc on trace metals in hypertensive rats. Amer. J. Physiol., *214*:796, 1968.

44. Schroeder, H. A., Nason, A. P., and Tipton, I. H.: Chromium deficiency as a factor in atherosclerosis. J. Chron. Dis., *23*:123, 1970.

45. Schroeder, H. A., Nason, A. P., Tipton, I. H., et al.: Essential trace metals in man: Zinc. Relation to environmental cadmium. J. Chron. Dis., *20*:179, 1967.

46. Schroeder, H. A., Vinton, W. H., Jr., and Balassa, J. J.: Effect of chromium, cadmium and other trace metals on the growth and survival of mice. J. Nutr., *80*:39, 1963.

47. Sporn, A., Cirstea, A., Ghizelea, G., et al.: Contributions to the study of the chronic toxicity of cadmium. Igiena *19* (No. 12):729, 1970.

48. Stitch, S. F.: Trace Elements in Human Tissue. A.E.R.E. MRC/R 1952, Harwell, Berks, 1956.

49. Tipton, I. H., Schroeder, H. A., Perry, H. M., Jr., et al.: Trace elements in human tissues. III. Subjects from Africa, the Near and Far East and Europe. Health Phys., *11*:403, 1965.

50. Vallee, B. L., Wacker, W. E. C., Bartholomay, A. F., et al.: Zinc metabolism in hepatic dysfunction: II. Correlation of metabolic patterns with biochemical findings. New Eng. J. Med., *257*:1055, 1957.

37

INTERACTIONS BETWEEN NUTRITION AND HEREDITY IN CORONARY HEART DISEASE

Frederick T. Hatch, M.D., Ph.D.*

Practically every family in the developed nations of the world has been afflicted with coronary heart disease (CHD). Despite the ubiquitous occurrence of the condition, heredity is known to contribute significantly in the pathogenesis (1–3). Strong genetic influences are exerted on several of the major "risk" or prognosticating factors. Likewise, it is known that some of the abnormal risk factors can be modified by alteration of nutrient intake and nutritional status.

This paper is an analytical essay oriented toward CHD in the general public, more specifically the male population of the United States and other

Reprinted from *The American Journal of Clinical Nutrition* 27: January 1974, pp. 80–90. Printed in U. S. A. The referenced article is U. S. Government sponsored work produced under Contract W-7405-Eng. 48 between the Regents of the University of California and U. S. Atomic Energy Commission and this permission does not in any way warrant title in the author.

The substance of this paper was presented in a Symposium on Nutrition and Its Relationship to Heart Disease at the 45th Annual Meeting of the American Heart Association, Dallas, Texas, November 19, 1972.

The author receives support from the U. S. Atomic Energy Commission. Previous work of the author reported herein was supported by the John A. Hartford Foundation and the American Heart Association.

* Senior Scientist, Biomedical Division, Lawrence Livermore Laboratory, University of California, Livermore, California 94550.

Helpful discussions and access to data prior to publication were provided by M. J. Albrink, T. B. Clarkson, W. E. Connor, J. L. Goldstein, W. B. Kannel, J. Slack, and M. P. Stern.

affluent nations, wherein the numerical incidence and social and economic burden of the disease are greatest (1, 4).

Demography of CHD

The first consideration is why atherosclerosis and CHD are so common in affluent populations in comparison with other nations. Figure 1

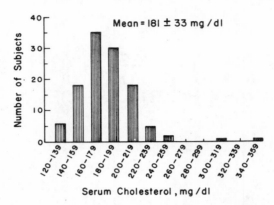

Figure 1: The frequency distribution of serum cholesterol levels among members of a freshman medical school class. Reproduced with permission of Academic Press (5).

illustrates the broad distribution of serum cholesterol levels in a class of freshman medical students, i. e., young adults with limited variation in environmental factors (5). Similar distributions at lower levels are seen in childhood or even in cord blood (6–8). Beginning in late adolescence and continuing through the middle decades of adult life, the mean levels of this distribution rise for both cholesterol and triglycerides (9) (Fig. 2). Similar changes occur in blood pressure, body weight related to height, and probably declining glucose tolerance. Thus, the affluent populations in middle life acquire distributions of several parameters that reach sufficient magnitude to contribute to the risk of developing CHD. However, the less affluent peoples tend to retain the more favorable distributions of earlier life (5). Confirmatory data exist on Irish (10) and Italian (11) men in their homeland and the United States.

The demography of CHD in our population is illustrated by calculations based on data from the prospective epidemiologic study at Framingham, Massachusetts. The risk of occurrence of CHD is calculated by a "multivariate analysis," which combines, with appropriate weighting, the effects of a half-dozen risk factors (12). In order of importance the major risk factors are: serum cholesterol, cigarette smoking, blood pressure, and for some age groups, body weight in relation to height. In the Framingham study, elevation of serum triglycerides or very low density lipopro-

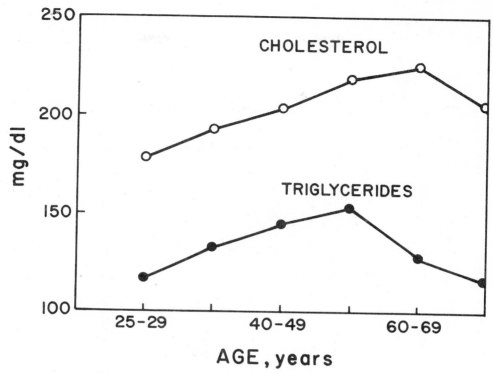

Figure 2: Age progression of mean levels of serum cholesterol and triglycerides in a series of 494 healthy adult men of Modesto, California. Calculated from data presented in (9).

teins did not appear to be a significant risk factor independent of serum cholesterol levels (13–15). However, recent data of Carlson and Bottiger (16) on Swedish males appear to indicate an independent additional contribution to risk by serum triglycerides. It is vital to realize that all these parameters were found to be continuous variables in the population; they did not at any arbitrary level suddenly become risk factors. In the multivariate analysis, two or three mild abnormalities can carry the same weight as one severe abnormality, and escalation of risk with increasing factors is not linear but exponential (12). Figure 3 presents the relationship between the magnitude of the multivariate risk factor, expressed in deciles, and percent of total cases of CHD (17).

Our model calculation encompasses the cohort of all men aged 30 to 39 years in the United States, which totals 11 million (18). Applying the risk pattern from the Framingham study (19), we follow these men through the three decades of middle life, until their average age is 65 years and calculate the incidence of new CHD plus sudden death related to CHD throughout each of the three decades (Table 1). Total incidence is the best single measure of the social burden of CHD; but it should be remembered that several studies have shown that the first manifestation is fatal more

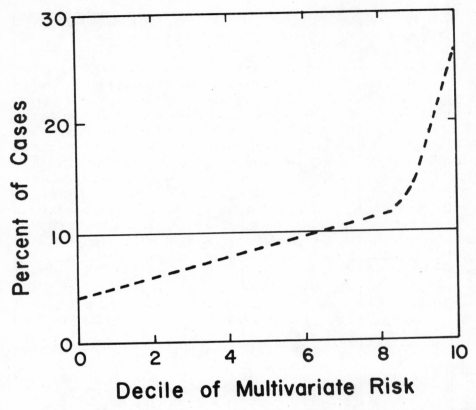

Figure 3: Exponential escalation of the fraction of CHD which develops at the upper end of the range of multivariate risk, calculated from a series of important risk factors (see text). Multivariate risk data from the prospective epidemiologic study at Framingham, Massachusetts. Redrawn from (17).

than one-half the time (20, 21), and that mortality is increased appreciably in those surviving an initial episode.

Table 1: Predicted incidence of CHD and sudden death in three decades of middle life in the cohort of all men (United States) aged 30–39 years (11 million subjects)

	Decile of risk							
	9–10		6–8		1–5		All	
Decade of followup	No. of men [a]	Incidence [a]	No. of men	Incidence	No. of men	Incidence	No. of men	Incidence
1	2.20	0.30	3.30	0.14	5.50	0.024	11.00	0.464
2	1.90	0.44	3.16	0.31	5.48	0.24	10.54	0.99
3	1.46	0.45	2.85	0.49	5.24	0.53	9.55	1.47
Total incidence	1.19		0.94		0.794		2.924	
Percent incidence	54		28		14		27	
Percent of total CHD	41		32		27		100	

[a] Data are in millions.

Note that the cohort of men is divided into three classes according to risk. First are those estimated to be in the highest two deciles for risk; this includes men with one of the defined syndromes of hyperlipoproteinemia, or severe hypertension, or a summation of multiple factors. Second are those in the sixth to eighth deciles, who are above average but not extreme in risk. Third are those in the lower five deciles, who are below average in calculated risk. Table 1 presents the number of men at risk and the incidence of CHD for each decade as well as a summary of the total 30-year incidence and its percentage distribution in the three classes of risk magnitude. The total incidence ranges from over one-half of those at highest risk to 14% of those at low risk, with more than one-quarter of the total cohort affected. Of particular interest is the prediction that the one-fifth at highest risk contribute 40% of the CHD, the one-third at next highest risk approximately one-third of the CHD, and the one-half at below-average risk nearly one-quarter of the total CHD. Even the latter subset represents over three-quarters of a million men affected.

Recent studies in London and in Seattle showed that 27 and 33% of the men surviving myocardial infarction exhibited major hyperlipoproteinemia (22, 23). The accelerated incidence of CHD in such cases is shown in Fig. 4, which compares data of J. Slack in London (24) with those for all Framingham males.

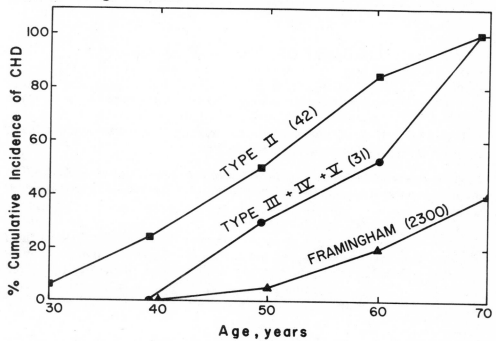

Figure 4: Accelerated incidence of CHD in the life histories of patients with various types of familial hyperlipoproteinemia. Calculated from the data of Slack (24) and compared with the experience of all men in the Framingham study. Numbers of subjects are given in parentheses.

Heredity and CHD

It is biologically inconceivable that abnormalities in the variety of major risk factors could originate from defects in any single gene. Thus, the pathogenesis of atherosclerosis has been termed multifactorial. In fact, the magnitude of most of the risk factors is also under multifactorial influences not only from the genotype but also from the environment, with varying contributions from each side (2, 25 (p. 259–265), 26, 27). Now let us consider how these influences interact and how they can be exploited for the prevention of CHD.

The science of biochemical genetics is demonstrating that many enzymes and plasma proteins are polymorphic; that is, within a given individual and within populations there are variations in the amino acid sequence, structure, and functional efficiency of molecules that serve a particular purpose (25, p. 225–242). These variations are considered to be under the control of the information carried in multiple allelic or corresponding genes, i. e., two or more genes having the same function and the same or slightly different base sequences. This polymorphism is the source of differences among humans in the efficiency of metabolic operations; it determines, for example, whether hyperlipoproteinemia develops in response to overnutrition.

Thus, for many biochemical and morphological traits of individuals, the inherited portion of their control is in the form of small increments from several different genes, each with a relatively small effect. In the case of serum cholesterol levels, the primary genetic determinant can be considered to be a number of genes affecting the synthesis, transport, and the removal of cholesterol in the body, many of these genes being subject to allelic variations in efficiency as described above. This complex mechanism, called "polygenic" control (28–34), results in a continuous distribution of magnitude of such traits in the population.

One trait classically used to illustrate polygenic inheritance is body height, which is predominantly under genetic control except in areas with serious problems of infection or malnutrition in childhood (30 (p. 186–188), 34 (p. 632–634). Figure 5 illustrates, from an epidemiological-genetic study at Tecumseh, Michigan, that both the heights and serum cholesterol levels of children are related to the heights and serum cholesterol levels of their parents, but not in the exact sense that would be dictated by simple Mendelian or single-gene inheritance (35). Thus, if the parents differ appreciably, the children tend to resemble the "mid-parent" value or average, with only a small fraction closely resembling either parent.

The Tecumseh study revealed similar behavior for relative weight, blood pressure, and glucose tolerance (35). This and much corroborative evidence suggest that all of these risk factors for CHD are under polygenic

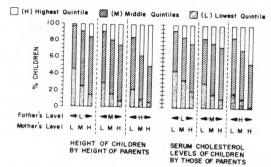

☐ (H) Highest Quintile   ▨ (M) Middle Quintiles   ▨ (L) Lowest Quintile

Figure 5: Patterns of resemblance between parents and children in body height and serum cholesterol level observed in the epidemiologic-genetic study at Tecumseh, Michigan. Height is generally considered to be a trait resulting from "polygenic inheritance"; the patterns shown do not conform to simple Mendelian inheritance. Note the similarity of the patterns for serum cholesterol to those for body height, particularly in the sets in which parents' values were disparate. Redrawn with permission from Circulation (35).

control. The mechanism of inheritance of serum triglyceride levels is less clear, but some data obtained by Slack suggests a similar mechanism (22, and J. Slack and D. Patterson, personal communication). The severest examples of hyperlipidemias, and possibly diabetes and hypertension, may sometimes exhibit single-gene inheritance, but this is controversial at present (22, 23, 30 (p. 196–208), 34 (p. 639), 36–41).

Nutrition and CHD

For the present discussion we consider diet and nutritional status, including exercise and energy balance, as a prime environmental influence on the risk factors for CHD. For example, in the Framingham study, the average relative weights of men who developed CHD during follow-up were somewhat greater than those of men who did not (42). In reality this relationship cannot be divorced from the influences of cigarette smoking and perhaps psychological stress and other items (1, 2). Thus, we have the familiar interaction of environmental factors such as diet, energy balance, and personal habits with particular genotypes to produce the phenotypes that are observed in terms of risk factor magnitude (25, p. 259–265).

Is diet really a risk factor for CHD? If so, why was diet found to correlate poorly with serum cholesterol levels and CHD incidence in the Framingham study (43)? Some have suggested that diet and nutritional status have little to do with the magnitude of risk factors, which is most unlikely as shown by worldwide epidemiology (5). Others have suggested that the American middle-class diet was too uniformly "bad" in terms of fat, cholesterol, and calorie intake for the observation of differences in risk, or that it always exceeded some mysterious thresholds beyond which risk was uniformly elevated (44). There may be some truth in these ideas, although the data do show quite wide individual differences in intake levels (Fig. 6) (43). The rational explanation in my opinion is that genetic con-

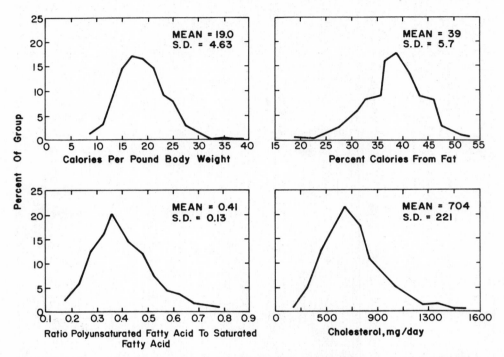

Figure 6: Significant features of the diet of 437 men of the Framingham study. Although few individuals consumed diets that were similar to those consumed in areas where CHD is uncommon, there was in fact a substantial range of variation in each of the parameters. Despite this variation a detailed statistical analysis failed to reveal clear-cut relationships between any diet parameter and the serum cholesterol level or the subsequent development of CHD. Redrawn from (43).

trol predominates in determining the magnitude of the risk factors; as dietary factors are only superimposed, we cannot expect to see clear-cut correlations that do not take differing genotypes into account.

The increases in serum cholesterol and triglyceride levels that occur during adult life in affluent populations seem to be predominantly influenced by the environmental factors, particularly nutritional ones (45). During the course of this increase there is a strong tendency for individuals to maintain the same relative position in the distribution that they displayed early in life. Figure 7 is a hypothetical representation of the genetically controlled and nutritionally modulated progression of serum

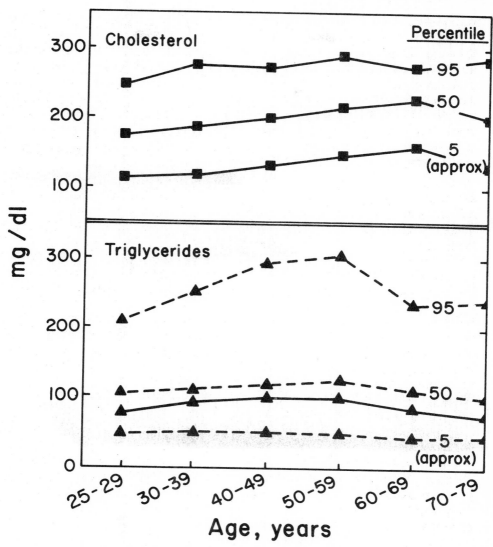

Figure 7: A hypothetical representation of the genetically controlled and nutritionally modulated age progression of serum lipid levels. The curve points were derived or estimated from data on 494 healthy adult men of Modesto, California (9). My hypothesis is that in general individuals will maintain their relative positions in the distribution, i. e., within the same shaded band, from early life throughout middle age despite trends in average levels that may depend on environmental factors. Hence the points for representative percentiles have been connected as if the individuals had been followed throughout the 45-year period, although the data were actually single observations on a population of men spanning the range from 25 to 70 years of age.

lipid levels with age. The relative position of individuals probably reflects their genotypes, and the increases with age are the result of modulations induced by nutritional and other environmental factors. Modulation of risk factors by external influence not only explains a number of puzzling

Labuza—Nutrition Crisis CTB—27

obsevations in epidemiological studies but also profoundly affects the strategy and expectations of preventive measures, which I shall discuss shortly. There is little documentation available to substantiate the foregoing speculation. Some evidence comes from a follow-up of serum lipid levels after nearly 30 years, which was recently carried out by Lavietes, Albrink and Man (46) in a small number of individuals who were originally studied as young adults. In males without major change in body weight, there was little change in the cholesterol and triglyceride levels; and in the case of cholesterol, there was a clear tendency for maintenance of similar relative positions or rank in the distribution after three decades. The few men who gained weight showed substantial increases in lipid levels. The Framingham data showed that in individual subjects cholesterol or blood pressure determinations repeated over two decades were highly correlated. When allowance is made for short-term and technical variation, the correlation between cholesterol values 18 years apart was 0.75, for systolic blood pressures 0.62. There is obviously a strong tendency for persons to retain their rank in the distribution of values (W. B. Kannel, personal communication). Serum triglycerides were not measured until late in the program; however, there was a moderately strong correlation between the concentrations of $S_{f20-400}$ or very low density lipoproteins determined initially and of triglycerides determined 18 years later.

Animal breeding studies confirming a strong genetic control of serum lipid concentrations have been reported for several species including mouse (47) and squirrel monkey (48, 49). The data were considered to be most compatible with a polygenic mechanism in the mouse and with a monogenic mechanism in the particular strain of monkey. Cholesterol feeding greatly enhanced the genotypic differences among monkeys, thus illustrating environmental modulation.

Overnutrition, whether it be in terms of intake of total calories, animal fats, or cholesterol, or simply large meals, exerts stress on the metabolic machinery (2, p. 698; 50). The resulting strain, or increase in the magnitude of risk factors, differs among individuals according to the relative efficiency of metabolic pathways dictated by polygenic inheritance. Thus, in the individual with all systems well-tuned there may be no increase in risk almost regardless of diet (39, p. 241), and there probably exists a spectrum of individuals who will be affected in greater and greater degree by overnutrition.

We are learning more about why overnutrition can unfavorably influence risk factors, at least in genetically prone individuals. Some of the possible reasons were illustrated in my studies of young men with CHD and their age-matched controls (2) and in a small series of patients with types IV and V hyperlipoproteinemia (51). In the pooled group of patients and controls there were significant positive correlations of relative body weight with serum triglycerides, free fatty acids, and glucose intolerance, and an inverse correlation with α-lipoprotein (Table 2) (50).

Table 2: Correlation coefficients between relative body weight and lipid metabolism parameters

		Relative body weight	Fasting serum trigly-cerides	Serum α -1-lipo-protein	Fasting serum NEFA
Relative body weight	n		52	52	41
	r		+0.44	−0.60	+0.43
	P		<0.01	<0.01	<0.01
Fasting serum triglycerides	n			52	41
	r			−0.36	+0.42
	P			<0.01	<0.01
Serum α-1-lipoprotein	n				41
	r				+0.05
	P				NS
Fasting serum NEFA	n				
	r				
	P				

NEFA = serum nonesterified fatty acids; n = number of subjects for which pairs of data items were available; r = linear correlation coefficient (Pearson product-moment method); P = probability that the observed r is due to chance; NS = not significant.

Additional correlations between overweight (not obesity) originating in adulthood and increased serum triglycerides have recently been found by M. P. Stern et al. (personal communication) in male populations in several California cities, and by García-Palmieri et al. in Puerto Rican men (52). Finally, the Framingham study data showed moderately large changes in serum cholesterol (53) and blood pressure (54) that were proportional to changes with time in relative body weight (Fig. 8).

Figure 9 shows diagrammatically some of the possible mechanisms of interaction between nutritional status and risk factors. It is known that protein subunits normally associated with α-lipoprotein are required for the functioning of the postheparin lipoprotein lipase (55, 56), which is implicated in the normal clearing of fat from the blood, and the lecithin-cholesterol acyltransferase (57, 58), which has another role, not clear as yet, in fat clearing. Resistance to insulin would also impair the activation of the postheparin lipase, and perhaps by indirect mechanisms cause increased synthesis of triglycerides in the liver (59–63). Both of these effects would be expected to result in increased serum triglycerides and very low density lipoproteins. Relative insulin deficiency may also hinder repair of minor injuries to the arterial wall (64).

Specific metabolic mechanisms for elevation of serum cholesterol and low density lipoprotein are not yet well understood (65–67). However, low density lipoprotein is believed to be an end product of the catabolism of the very low density lipoproteins, and thus the level of the former may in part reflect the rates of synthesis and release of the latter (68, 69).

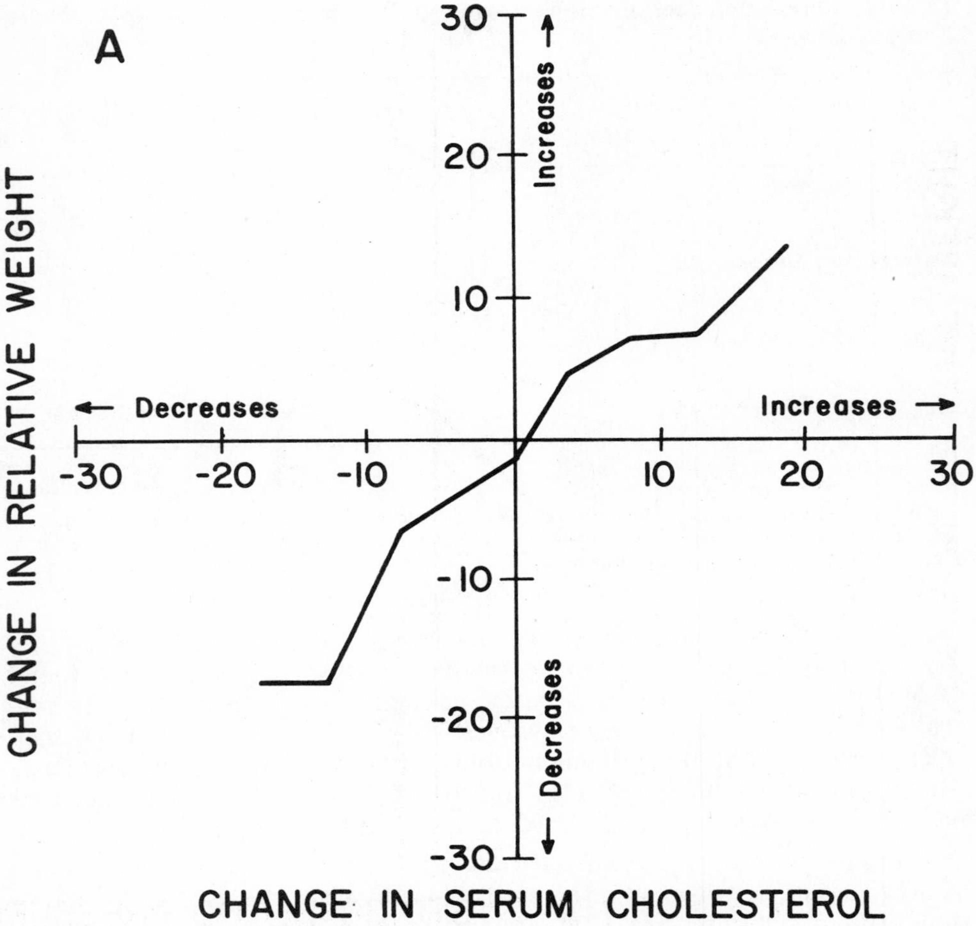

Figure 8: Changes in the serum cholesterol and blood pressure proportional to changes with time in relative body weight during follow-up of men in the Framingham study. Ordinates are changes in relative weight, viz., 100 times the ratio of subjects' body weight to the median weight for men of the same height at entry to the study. Abscissa in A is expressed in mg/dl; in B, in mm Hg. Reproduced from (53).

There seems to be a substantial, although speculative, basis for specific chemical and physiologic interactions between overnutrition and the polygenic systems controlling CHD risk. Indeed, energy balance appears to be the environmental factor exerting the strongest influence upon most of the major recognized risk factors for CHD.

Implications for prevention of CHD

Polygenic inheritance and its interactions with environmental factors have three important implications when we consider the possible means for prevention or lowering the risk of CHD. Firstly, the problem is complex

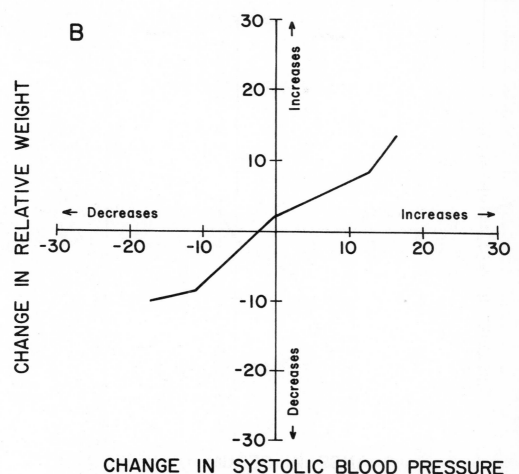

CHANGE IN SYSTOLIC BLOOD PRESSURE

and no simple solutions are foreseeable. Except possibly in a few rare instances, we shall not discover single-gene defects with a mechanism that we can determine. Thus, we are unlikely to find specific therapies based on gene functions, as is now becoming possible for some inherited diseases that do result from single-gene defects (40, 70). Secondly, we can apply measures that have modest effects on several risk factors as in the so-called "multiple intervention programs" (71). Because of the exponential nature of the relationship between the total magnitude of risk factors and the risk of CHD, a major reduction of risk can be anticipated (72). The polygenic complexity actually works in our favor because several small

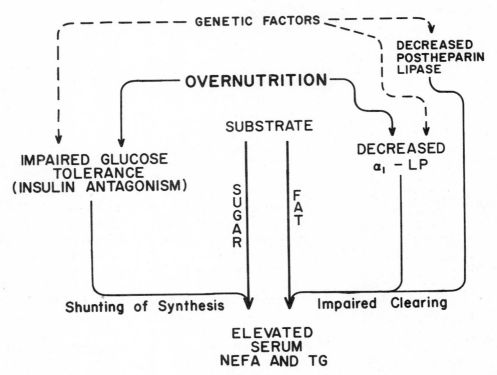

Figure 9: Schematic outline of some of the possible interactions between overnutrition and genetic factors that might contribute to disturbances of lipoprotein metabolism and to the risk of developing CHD.   NEFA = nonesterified fatty acids;   TG = triglycerides;   LP = lipoprotein. Reproduced from (50).

changes can be more than additive, and we need not understand the detailed mechanism to gain benefits.   Thirdly, the less the total magnitude of risk factors the easier it ought to be to modify them favorably.

It should now be clear that the most profitable intervention against CHD should consist of *individualized* preventive medicine (1, 73).   The measures to be applied should be tailored in vigor to the total risk estimate for each individual and should be tailored in specificity to affect those portions of the polygenic system that are showing strain, that is, the positive risk factors.   We cannot expect to be truly effective with "shotgun" measures directed at the public as a whole (74).   We must carry preventive medicine to the "grass roots" and survey as much of the public as possible.

I suggest as an approximation that those found to be in the top two deciles for risk will require vigorous dietary management and lipid-lowering or antihypertensive drugs and may thereby be moved into the range of deciles six to eight (Table 3).   The above average risks may require a moderately stringent diet to convert them into below average risks.   And the low risk population perhaps needs only admonitions against overnutrition, delivered as early in life as possible, to place their risk in the range of lowest decile.

Table 3: Individualized preventive medicine

Decile of risk	Preventive management	Treated decile
9–10	Strict diet and weight control Lipid-lowering drugs	6–8
6–8	Diet and weight control	1–5
1–5	Avoid overnutrition	1
All	Discourage cigarette smoking Treat hypertension when present	

Recently, several reports have indicated an affirmative answer to the crucial final question, i. e., that rates of incidence or recurrence of CHD can be reduced by lowering serum cholesterol levels and blood pressure by means of dietary treatment, drugs, and cessation of cigarette smoking (1, 75–78). The benefits cannot be regarded as fully proven, but encouragement is certainly given to the prosecution of the major intervention studies now underway.

If these changes could be accomplished, and if they truly resulted in lowering of risk to the new predicted values, we would expect the total 30-year incidence of CHD in our cohort of 11 million men to be lowered from 2.9 million to 1.4 million, approximately one-half the figure without intervention (Table 4). In deference to the role of heredity, however, the

Table 4: Treated cohort of all men aged 30–39 years equals 11 million

	Decile of risk			
	6–8	1–5	1	1–10
No. of men in decile (millions)	2.20	3.30	5.50	11.0
Total incidence (millions)	0.63	0.48	0.33	1.44
Percent incidence	29	16	6	13
Percent of total CHD	44	33	23	100

proportions of affected men in the higher, medium, and lower risk categories would remain as before, 40%, one-third, and one-quarter respectively. We can modulate the effects of the genotype, but at present we do not know how to override them.

SUMMARY

An analysis is presented of the demography of coronary heart disease (CHD) in the male population of the United States and of the nature of genetic and environmental (chiefly nutritional) factors contributing to the incidence in individual men. The estimation of risk is based on the "multivariate analysis" developed for the epidemiologic study at Framingham, Mass. A model calculation is made for all United States men initially 30 to 39 years of age over three decades of middle life. This reveals that CHD occurs in more than 50% of those at highest risk compared with only 14% of low risk men. Men above the 80th percentile in risk contribute 40% of the total CHD, whereas those below the 50th percentile in risk contribute only approximately 25%.

It is proposed that major risk factors are principally under "polygenic control," which is defined and illustrated with the principles of biochemical genetics. Nutritional status and other environmental factors are shown to modulate, but not to override, the expression of the genotype. Important implications of polygenic inheritance and its modulations are that CHD is not expected to be amenable to specific preventive measures, but that multiple interventions against risk factors, each of modest effect, will interact to achieve major reduction of risk. The concept of "individualized preventive medicine" is recommended to practitioners. A credible degree of success in preventive management would halve the total incidence of CHD; however, the fundamental genetic influence on risk would remain in evidence.

REFERENCES

1. Hatch, F. T. Atherosclerosis calls for a new kind of preventive medicine. Calif. Med. 109: 134, 1968.

2. Hatch, F. T., P. K. Reissell, T. M. W. Poon-King, G. P. Canellos, R. S. Lees and L. M. Hagopian. A study of coronary heart disease in young men. Circulation 33: 679, 1966.

3. Hammond, E. C., L. Garfinkel and H. Seidman. Longevity of parents and grandparents in relation to coronary heart disease and associated variables. Circulation 43: 31, 1971.

4. National Heart and Lung Institute Task Force on Arteriosclerosis. Arteriosclerosis. DHEW Publ. No. (NIH) 72–219. Washington, D. C.: U. S. Govt. Printing Office, 1971, vol. II.

5. Connor, W. E., and S. L. Connor. The key role of nutritional factors in the prevention of coronary heart disease. Preventive Med. 1: 49, 1972.

6. Glueck, C. J., F. Heckman, M. Schonfeld, P. Steiner and W. Pearce. Neonatal familial type II hyperlipoproteinemia: cord blood cholesterol in 1,660 births. Circulation 42: (Suppl. III) 11, 1970.

7. Noble, R. P. Abnormal lipoprotein patterns in young men. Circulation 38: (Suppl. VI) 18, 1968.

8. Friedman, G., and S. J. Goldberg. The effectiveness of a low cholesterol, low saturated fat diet in a free living pediatric population. Circulation 46: (Suppl. II) 152, 1972.

9. Wood, P. D. S., M. P. Stern, A. Silvers, G. M. Reaven and J. von der Groeben. Prevalence of plasma lipoprotein abnormalities in a free-living population of the Central Valley, California. Circulation 45: 114, 1972.

10. Trulson, M. F., R. E. Clancy, W. J. E. Jessop, R. W. Childers and F. J. Stare. Comparisons of siblings in Boston and Ireland. J. Am. Dietet. Assoc. 45: 225, 1964.

11. Miller, D. C., M. F. Trulson, M. B. McCann, P. D. White and F. J. Stare, Diet, blood lipids and health of Italian men in Boston. Ann. Internal Med. 49: 1178, 1958.

12. Truett, J., J. Cornfield and W. B. Kannel. A multivariate analysis of the risk of coronary heart disease in Framingham. J. Chronic Diseases 20: 511, 1967.

13. Kannel, W. B., W. P. Castelli, T. Gordon and P. M. McNamara. Serum cholesterol, lipoproteins, and the risk of coronary heart disease. The Framingham study. Ann. Internal Med. 74: 1, 1971.

14. Kannel, W. B., M. J. Garcia, P. M. McNamara and G. Pearson. Serum lipid precursors of coronary heart disease. Human Pathol. 2: 129, 1971.

15. Gofman, J. W., W. Young and R. Tandy. Ischemic heart disease and longevity. Circulation 34: 679, 1966.

16. Carlson, L. A., and L. E. Bottiger. Ischaemic heart-disease in relation to fasting values of plasma triglycerides and cholesterol. Stockholm prospective study. Lancet 1: 865, 1972.

17. Gordon, T., P. Sorlie and W. B. Kannel. The Framington study. An epidemiological investigation of cardiovascular disease. Section 27. DHEW Publ. Washington, D.C.: U.S. Govt. Printing Office, 1971.

18. World Health Organization. Demographic Yearbook. Geneva: World Health Organ., 1970.

19. Kannel, W. B. Handbook of coronary risk probability. Table unit. New York: Am. Heart Assoc., 1972.

20. Kuller, L., M. Cooper and J. Perper. Epidemiology of sudden death. Arch. Internal Med. 129: 714, 1972.

21. Gordon, T. and W. B. Kannel. Premature mortality from coronary heart disease. The Framingham study. J. Am. Med. Assoc. 215: 1617, 1971.

22. Patterson, D., and J. Slack. Lipid abnormalities in male and female survivors of myocardial infarction and their first degree relatives. Lancet 1: 393, 1972.

23. Goldstein, J. L., W. R. Hazzard, H. G. Schrott, E. L. Bierman and A. G. Motulsky. Genetics of hyperlipidemia in coronary heart disease. Trans. Assoc. Am. Physicians 85: 120, 1972.

24. Slack J. Risk of ischaemic heart disease in familial hyperlipoproteinemic states. Lancet 2: 1380, 1969.

25. Harris, H. The Principles of Human Biochemical Genetics. New York: Elsevier, 1970.

26. Harris, H., and D. A. Hopkinson. Average heterozygosity per locus in man: an estimate based on the incidence of enzyme polymorphisms. Ann. Human Genet. 36: 9, 1972.

27. Adlersberg, D., and L. E. Schaefer. Editorial. The interplay of heredity and environment in the regulation of circulating lipids and in atherogenesis. Am. J. Med. 26: 1, 1959.

28. Hamilton, M., G. W. Pickering, J. A. F. Roberts and G. S. C. Sowry. The aetiology of essential hypertension. 4. The role of inheritance. Clin. Sci. 13: 273, 1954.

29. Murphy, E. A. One cause? Many causes? The argument from the bimodal distribution. J. Chronic Diseases 17: 301, 1964.

30. Roberts, J. A. F. Multifactorial inheritance and human disease. Progr. Med. Genet. 3: 178, 1964.

31. Carter, C. O. Genetics of common disorders. Brit. Med. Bull. 25: 52, 1969.

32. Carter, C. O. An ABC of medical genetics. VI. Polygenic inheritance and common diseases. Lancet 1: 1252, 1969.

33. Stern, C. Principles of Human Genetics (2nd ed.). San Francisco: Freeman, 1960, p. 350.

34. Levitan, M., and A. Montagu. Textbook of Human Genetics. Fair Lawn, New Jersey: Oxford Univ. Press, 1971, p. 632.

35. Deutscher, S., F. H. Epstein and M. O. Kjelsberg. Familial aggregation of factors associated with coronary heart disease. Circulation 33: 911, 1966.

36. Nevin, N. C., and J. Slack. Hyperlipidaemic xanthomatosis. II. Mode of inheritance in 55 families with essential hyperlipidaemia and xanthomatosis. J. Med. Genet. 5: 9, 1968.

37. Carter, C. O., J. Slack and N. B. Myant. Genetics of hyperlipoproteinaemias. Lancet 1: 400, 1971.

38. Jensen, J., and D. H. Blankenhorn. The inheritance of familial hypercholesterolemia. Am. J. Med. 52: 499, 1972.

39. Dahl, L. K. Salt and hypertension. Am. J. Clin. Nutr. 25: 231, 1972.

40. Hatch, F. T., R. J. Havel, R. S. Lees, R. I. Levy and G. M. Reaven. Birth Defects Atlas and Compendium, edited by D. Bergsma. Baltimore: Williams & Wilkins, 1973, pp. 494, 495, 500, 504, 505.

41. Goldstein, J. L., H. G. Schrott, W. R. Hazzard, E. L. Bierman and A. G. Motulsky. Combined hyperlipidemia: genetic evidence for a distinct disorder. Circulation 46: (Suppl. II) 17, 1972.

42. Gordon, T., and J. Verter. The Framingham study. An epidemiological investigation of cardiovascular disease. Section 23. DHEW Publ. Washington, D.C.: U.S. Govt. Printing Office, 1970.

43. Kannel, W. B., and T. Gordon. The Framingham study. An epidemiological investigation of cardiovascular disease. Section 24. DHEW Publ. Washington, D.C.: U.S. Govt. Printing Office, 1970.

44. Medical World News, September 11, 1970, p. 15–17.

45. Heyden, S., C. G. Hames, A. Bartel, J. C. Cassel, H. A. Tyroler and J. C. Cornoni. Weight and weight history in relation to cerebrovascular and ischemic heart disease. J. Am. Med. Assoc. 128: 956, 1971.

46. Lavietes, P. H., M. J. Albrink and E. B. Man. Serum lipids of normal subjects with aging. Studies in a single cohort. Yale J. Biol. Med. 46: 134, 1973.

47. Yamamoto, R. S., L. B. Crittenden, L. Sokoloff and G. E. Jay, Jr. Genetic variations in plasma lipid content in mice. J. Lipid Res. 4: 413, 1963.

48. Clarkson, T. B., H. B. Lofland, Jr., B. C. Bullock and H. O. Goodman. Genetic control of plasma cholesterol. Studies on squirrel monkeys. Arch. Pathol. 92: 37, 1971.

49. Lofland, H. B., Jr., T. B. Clarkson, R. W. St. Clair and N. D. M. Lehner. Studies on the regulation of plasma cholesterol levels in squirrel monkeys of two genotypes. J. Lipid Res. 13: 39, 1972.

50. Hatch, F. T. Discussion in Proc. 1967 Deuel Conf. on Lipids. DHEW Publ. Washington, D.C.: U.S. Govt. Printing Office, 1967, p. 233.

51. Reissell, P. K., P. A. Mandella, T. M. W. Poon-King and F. T. Hatch. Treatment of hypertriglyceridemia. I. Total caloric restriction followed by refeeding a low carbohydrate, high fat diet in the carbohydrate-induced type (8 cases). II. Low fat diet plus medium-chain triglycerides in the fat-induced type (2 cases). Am. J. Clin. Nutr. 19: 84, 1966.

52. García-Palmieri, M. R., R. Costas, Jr., J. Schiffman, A. A. Colon, R. Torres and E. Nazario. Interrelationships of serum lipids with relative weight, blood glucose, and physical activity. Circulation 45: 829, 1972.

53. Kannel, W. B. Obesity and coronary heart disease. Nutrah (Am. Heart Assoc.) 1: 1, 1973.

54. Kannel, W. B., N. Brand, J. J. Skinner, T. R. Dawber and P. M. McNamara. The relation of adiposity to blood pressure and development of hypertension. Ann. Internal Med. 67: 48, 1967.

55. Havel, R. J., V. G. Shore, B. Shore and D. M. Bier. Role of specific glycopeptides of human serum lipoproteins in the activation of lipoprotein lipase. Circulation Res. 27: 595, 1970.

56. Havel, R. J. Mechanisms of hyperlipoproteinemia. Advan. Exptl. Med. Biol. 26: 57, 1971.

57. Fielding, C. J., V. G. Shore and P. E. Fielding. A protein cofactor of lecithin: cholesterol acyltransferase. Biochem. Biophys. Res. Commun. 46: 1493, 1972.

58. Schumaker, V. N., and G. H. Adams. Very low density lipoproteins: surface-volume changes during metabolism. J. Theoret. Biol. 26: 89, 1970.

59. Boyns, D. R., J. N. Crossley, M. E. Abrams, R. J. Jarrett and H. Keen. Oral glucose tolerance and related factors in a normal population sample. I. Blood sugar, plasma insulin, glyceride, and cholesterol measurements and the effects of age and sex. Brit. Med. J. 1: 595, 1969.

60. Abrams, M. E., R. J. Jarrett, H. Keen, D. R. Boyns and J. N. Crossley. Oral glucose tolerance and related factors in a normal population sample. II. Interrelationship of glycerides, cholesterol, and other factors with the glucose and insulin response. Brit. Med. J. 1: 599, 1969.

61. Nikkila, E. A. Control of plasma and liver triglyceride kinetics by carbohydrate metabolism and insulin. Advan. Lipid Res. 7: 63, 1969.

62. Salans, L. B., J. L. Knittle and J. Hirsch. The role of adipose cell size and adipose tissue insulin sensitivity in the carbohydrate intolerance of human obesity. J. Clin. Invest. 47: 153, 1968.

63. Sims, E. A., E. S. Horton and L. B. Salans. Inducible metabolic abnormalities during development of obesity. Ann. Rev. Med. 22: 235, 1971.

64. Kendall, F. E.   Editorial.   Does the pattern of carbohydrate nutrition hold a clue to atherosclerosis?   Circulation 36: 340, 1967.

65. Langer, T., W. Strober and R. I. Levy.   The metabolism of plasma lipoproteins.   In: Plasma Protein Metabolism, Regulation of Synthesis.   Distribution and Degradation, edited by M. A. Rothschild and T. Waldmann.   New York: Academic, 1970.

66. Quarfordt, S. H., A. Frank, D. M. Shames, M. Berman and D. Steinberg.   Very low density lipoprotein triglyceride transport in type IV hyperlipoproteinemia and the effects of carbohydrate-rich diets.   J. Clin. Invest. 49: 2281, 1970.

67. Langer, T., W. Strober and R. I. Levy.   The metabolism of low density lipoprotein in familial type II hyperlipoproteinemia.   J. Clin. Invest. 51: 1528, 1972.

68. Barter, P. J., and P. J. Nestel.   Precursor-product relationship between pools of very low density lipoprotein triglyceride.   J. Clin. Invest. 51: 174, 1972.

69. Schonfeld, G., C. L. Gulbrandsen, R. B. Wilson and R. S. Lees.   Catabolism of human very-low-density lipoproteins in monkeys: the appearance of human very-low-density lipoprotein peptides in monkey high-density lipoproteins.   Biochim. Biophys. Acta 270: 426, 1972.

70. Stanbury, J. B., J. B. Wyngaarden and D. S. Fredrickson (editors).   The Metabolic Basis of Inherited Disease (3rd ed.).   New York: McGraw-Hill, 1972.

71. Cooper, T. Arteriosclerosis.   Policy, polity and parity.   Circulation 45: 433, 1972.

72. Frantz, I. D., Jr., and P. L. Ashman.   Design of dietary experiments for preventing myocardial infarction.   J. Am. Dietet. Assoc. 52: 293, 1968.

73. Ostrander, L. D.   Alterations of factors predisposing to coronary heart disease.   Ann. Internal Med. 68: 1072, 1968.

74. Hatch, F. T.   Letter to editor.   Medical World News, October 9, 1970.

75. Miettinen, M., O. Turpeinen, M. J. Karvonen, R. Elosuo and E. Paavilainen.   Effect of cholesterol-lowering diet on mortality from coronary heart-disease and other causes.   A twelve-year clinical trial in men and women.   Lancet 2: 835, 1972.

76. Veterans Administration Cooperative Study Group on Antihypertensive Agents.   Effects of treatment on morbidity in hypertension.   Results in patients with diastolic blood pressures averaging 115 through 129 mm Hg. J. Am. Med. Assoc. 202: 1028, 1967.

77. Veterans Administration Cooperative Study Group on Antihypertensive Agents.   Effects of treatment on morbidity in hypertension.   II.   Results in patients with diastolic blood pressure averaging 90 through 114 mm Hg.   J. Am. Med. Assoc. 213: 1143, 1970.

78. Schuman, L. M.   The benefits of cessation of smoking.   Chest 59: 421, 1971.

38

ATHEROSCLEROTIC HEART DISEASE AND THE ENVIRONMENT

Peter B. Peacock *

Environmental factors associated with an increase in manifest coronary artery disease are temperature extremes, noise, soft water, exposure to sulfur dioxide and carbon monoxide, and constraints imposed by the living habits of the community concerned. The important constraints are the relative nonavailability of high-protein foods that are low in saturated fat and cholesterol, the general acceptance of cigarette smoking as permissible behavior, the lack of emphasis on preventive medicine and limitations on physical exercise.

The factors that determine the likelihood of developing atherosclerotic heart disease can be thought of as personal (e. g. sex, age, heredity), behavioral (smoking, diet, exercise), related to other disease (hypertension, diabetes), and environmental. One reason why the environmental factors are of interest is that they may be particularly susceptible to planned modification. These environmental factors include temperature, noise, air pollutants, too soft drinking water, the lack or excess of trace metals or vitamins in available food, the kind of food that is available to a given community, and living patterns imposed on a community by local custom or lack of planning.

Reprinted from *Transactions* of the New York Academy of Sciences, Vol. 35, No. 8, December 1973, pp. 631–635.

This paper was presented at a meeting of the Section of Environmental Sciences on February 21.

* American Health Foundation, New York, New York 10019 and Department of Public Health and Epidemiology, University of Alabama, Birmingham, Alabama 35233.

While the correlation between the amount of atherosclerosis found in the coronary arteries and the incidence rate of clinical attacks of acute myocardial infarction is reasonably high on a community basis, it should be remembered that on an individual basis extensive coronary atherosclerosis frequently exists without demonstrable clinical disease.   Conversely, many deaths clinically diagnosed as being due to acute myocardial infarction occur without coronary occlusion demonstrable at autopsy.   We should thus distinguish between those factors that increase the likelihood of developing atherosclerosis of the coronary vessels and those factors which increase the likelihood of dying when superimposed on the atherosclerotic process.

Statistical studies have repeatedly showed a clear seasonal periodicity in death rates from coronary artery disease, with up to 50% more deaths occurring during the winter months.[1]   In general, this increased death rate in winter is more marked in those parts of the world and this country where the winters are coldest,[2] and there is very little detectable seasonal effect in, for example, Alabama.   Since cold weather is associated with changes in the pattern of living, we cannot assume that the mechanism for this increase in the winter months is the environmental temperature alone.   A committee of the American Heart Association[3] considered the possible effects of violent physical activity, such as shoveling snow, and concluded that this was unlikely to be of any major importance, though exceptions did occur.   Canadian workers[4] have looked at the figures for Ontario, Australia, and Denmark and have suggested that the winter increase may be accounted for by more serious respiratory infections with a secondary effect on the heart.

At the other end of the temperature spectrum, a recent report from Finland reported 67 deaths in 1970 among persons taking sauna baths.[5] It was suggested that under these conditions the likelihood of abnormal heart rhythms is greatly increased, and this could well account for increased deaths among persons with already atherosclerotic coronary vessels.   On a community basis the effects of heat waves in increasing deaths from heart disease have been demonstrated on several occasions, with perhaps the most striking being that in St. Louis in 1966,[6] with over 300 excess deaths in six days and some one-third of those analyzed in detail being ascribed to atherosclerotic heart disease.

The new Occupational Health and Safety Act of 1970 has drawn attention to the possible importance of noise as a cause of increased deaths from heart disease.[7]   The evidence from experimental work on human beings that noise has a direct effect is shaky.[8]   The effect on the cardiovascular system of noise, if any, is interwoven with the whole complicated question of stress.   It has been shown on experimental animals[9] that noise, along with other forms of stress, can raise the blood pressure and increase the level of serum cholesterol.   These changes are known to be associated with an increased risk of coronary artery disease, but it is still unproved whether repeated insults can cause a permanent effect.

Perhaps because of difficulty in defining and measuring it, the better-known well-controlled prospective studies [10, 11] have not demonstrated a major role for stress in the causation of heart disease. Most investigators have been unable to identify an increased risk independent of such factors as cigarette smoking, coffee drinking,[12] and hypertension, though social conflicts have been related to myocardial infarction.[13]

Retrospectively, one will almost always find that persons who have had a coronary thrombosis give a history of preceding stress, but this can often be explained by selective recall. Occasional studies—like an old one by Russek and Zohman,[14] 91% of whose coronary cases gave a history of occupational stress and strain and only 20% of whose controls gave a similar history—are, however, difficult to explain if there is no relationship. In contrast; in Alabama the county with the highest age-adjusted death rate from coronary artery disease is a peaceful farming community where mechanization has largely eliminated the need for physical labor, a very large proportion of the population are cigarette smokers, and the diet is still abundant in amount and rich in dairy products and meat. In the psychological area there seems to be better evidence [15] linking the intrinsic so-called behavior pattern *A* to coronary artery disease [16] (though demonstration that this work is reproducible is still awaited) than that linking extrinsic stress to such disease.

Looking at other forms of radiant energy, we find no good evidence that exposure to ionizing radiation has increased death from coronary disease, and thus the Hiroshima survivors showed no excess of coronary artery disease.[17] The use of microwaves is extending rapidly in medical practice, and it might be as well to review more carefully any possible harmful effects of these waves before extending their clinical use further.

Air pollution episodes associated with high levels of sulfur oxides as occurred in London [18] and Donora [19] have been asociated with a marked increase in deaths from heart disease. While these episodes were unpleasant to experience, the deaths were largely limited to persons with preexistent chronic cardiopulmonary disease. The long term follow-up of persons who were incapacitated in the Donora episode [20] has not shown an increased long-term likelihood of developing heart disease, and the cardiac effects of chronic low-level exposures such as are found in New York are very questionable. Industrial workers exposed to CS_2 have, however, shown an increased death rate from heart disease.[21]

Of more importance from the point of view of heart disease is the question of exposure to carbon monoxide. Experimental animals fed cholesterol and exposed to low levels of carbon monoxide are known to develop atherosclerosis.[22] It is possible that this may be the mechanism accounting for the long-term effect of cigarette smoking on human beings. In Japanese populations living in *kakoi* (enclosed rooms) at high altitude and exposed to high levels of carbon monoxide over several months of the year, dramatically increased death rates from heart disease have been reported.[23] Despite this suggestive evidence, it has not been possible to show that such occupational groups as garage workers or tunnel employees show an increased risk of death from coronary artery disease, although some interesting and suggestive work has been done with municipal sanitation workers exposed to the exhaust fumes of their collection vehicles.[24] This population in New York definitely has an increased death rate from coronary artery disease—which may be due to this particular exposure, although other variables such as diet and cigarette smoking have not, perhaps, been fully accounted for. Undoubtedly the combination of driving in a closed automobile in heavy city traffic together with smoking cigarettes will expose the subjects to levels of carbon monoxide within the range that can be expected to produce atherosclerosis of the coronary arteries, and this may account for some of the usual excess of deaths from coronary artery disease found in our bigger cities.

Repeated studies from Europe (especially England) and this country have shown a positive relationship within a country (though not necessarily between countries [25]) linking soft water and coronary artery disease. This has been shown both by comparing communities at one time [26] and by looking at the effects of changing the water supply within or between communities.[27] Perhaps the most striking example of this comes from Monroe County, Fla.[28] (the Florida Keys) where the introduction of hard water from the mainland was associated with a marked drop in heart disease death rates followed by an increase when public demand coupled with the introduction of desalinization plants led to the water's being softened again. How hard water exercises its protective effect is unknown, although the element most closely associated with this protective effect is calcium.[29] It has been suggested from Canadian work [30] that the difference in death rates found between soft- and hard-water areas is accounted for by an excess of sudden deaths, with an increased susceptibility to lethal arrhythmias among residents of soft-water areas. One study [31] has suggested that in the United Kingdom the mortality from ischemic heart disease is closer associated with rainfall (more deaths with a higher rainfall) than with water softness.

Numerous studies have been published reporting apparent variations in death rates associated with differing elements in the water supply. Thus, high levels of cadmium have been associated with increased death rates from coronary artery disease.[32] Lack of lithium in municipal drinking water has also been associated with coronary artery disease,[33, 34] as have high levels of nitrate. Other metals that have been looked at include lead, chrome, and magnesium.[35] None of this work is very convincing, and none has been showed to be generally applicable. In the vitamin area attention has been concentrated [36] on vitamins C and D. The evidence for any major effect produced by the lack or excess of these vitamins is poor. Populations living on borderline or subliminal doses of these vitamins have extremely low death rates from coronary artery disease.

Perhaps more important than anything we have discussed to date is the problem created by established living patterns within a particular community. Even an individual who wishes to live sensibly may find this difficult. A visit to one of our supermarkets will show that available foods are usually high in cholesterol or saturated fat. Labeling of high-risk items is largely nonexistent. It is difficult to eat at one of our restaurants and stay within reasonable limits. Even if we wish it otherwise, the eating pattern to which our children will be exposed will be this standard American pattern.

Except for a few selected groups, such as physician groups, cigarette smoking is still entirely accepted, and this makes any control program just that much more difficult. The role of exercise in the prevention of heart disease is probably not large, but it does encourage sensible living, the avoidance of cigarette smoking, and the eating of sensible meals. In many of our cities it is not even possible to walk a few blocks because sidewalks have not been constructed.

The lack of emphasis on routine medical examinations makes it possible for up to half of all the hypertensives in this country to go undetected and hence untreated. When persons are known to be hypertensive, the medical code that regards it as unethical for a physician to call back patients who do not attend for treatment allows up to three quarters of these to go untreated. Despite dramatic known differences in risk, life insurance companies, with few exceptions, allow no rebate on premiums paid by persons who are nonsmokers and who live sensibly. The Seventh Day Adventists, who do not smoke, have a life expectancy among males at 35 that is six years longer than that for males in California.[37] If any community adjusted a living pattern based on what we know already about heart disease half the battle against coronary artery disease would be won.

REFERENCES

1. Rose, G. 1966. Cold weather and ischemic heart disease. Brit. J. Prev. Soc. Med. 20: 87.

2. Dunnigan, M. G., W. A. Harland and T. Fyfe. 1970. Seasonal incidence and mortality of ischemic heart disease. Lancet 2: 793.

3. American Heart Association. 1963. Report of the committee on the effect of strain and trauma on the heart and great vessels (Ch. P. D. White). Modern Concepts of Cardiovascular Disease 32: 793.

4. Anderson, T. W. and W. H. le Riche. 1970. Cold weather and myocardial infarction. Lancet 1: 291.

5. Taggart, P., P. Parkingson and M. Carruthers. 1972. Cardiac responses to thermal, physical and emotional stress. Brit. Med. J. 3: 71.

6. Henschel, A., Linda L. Burton, L. Margolies and J. E. Smith. 1969. An analysis of the heat deaths in St. Louis during July 1966. Amer. J. Public Health 59: 2232.

7. Medical News. 1970. Noise pollution can harm circulatory system. J. A. M. A. 211: 909.

8. Atherley, G. R. C., S. L. Gibbons and J. A. Powell. 1970. Moderate ascoustic stimuli: The interrelation of subjective importance and certain physiological changes. Ergonomics 13: 536.

9. Geber, W. F., T. A. Anderson and B. van Dyre. 1966. Physiologic responses of the albino rat to chronic noise stress. Arch. Environ. Health 12: 751.

10. Kannel, W. B., T. A. Dawber, A. Kagan, N. Revotskie and J. Stokes, 1901. Factors of risk in the development of coronary heart disease—Six years follow-up experience. The Framingham Study, Assoc. Intern. Med. 55: 33.

11. Keys, C. A., Aravanis, H. Blackburn, F. S. P. van Bucham, R. Bugina, B. S. Djordjevic, F. Fidanza, M. J. Karvonen, A. Menetti, V. Puddler and H. L. Taylor. 1972. Probability of middle aged men developing coronary heart disease in five years. Circulation 65: 815.

12. Boston Collaborative Drug Surveillance Program. 1972. Coffee drinking and acute myocardial infarction. Lancet 2: 1278.

13. Wardwell, W. I., M. Hyman and C. B. Bahnson. 1964. Stress and coronary disease in three field studies. J. Chron. Dis. 17: 73.

14. Russek, H. I. and B. L. Zohman, 1958. Relative significance of heredity, diet and occupational stress in coronary heart disease of young adults. Amer. J. Med. Sci. 235: 266.

15. Barron, C. I. and R. H. Rosenman. 1968. Coronary heart disease: a predictive study involving the aerospace manufacturing industry. Aerospace Med. 39: 1109.

16. Freidman, M., R. H. Rosenman, R. Straus, M. Wurm and R. Kositcheck. 1968. The relationship of behavior pattern A to the state of the coronary vasculature. Amer. J. Med. 44: 525.

17. Johnson, K. G., K. Yano and H. Kato. 1968. Coronary heart disease in Hiroshima, Japan: A report of a six-year period of surveillance, 1958–1964. Amer. J. Public Health 58: 1355.

18. Ministry of Health, London. 1954. Mortality and morbidity during London fog of December 1952. Report on public health and medical subjects. No. 95.

19. U.S.P.H.S. 1949. Air pollution in Donora, Pa., Preliminary report. Public Health Bulletin No. 306.

20. Ciocco, A. and D. J. Thompson. 1961. A follow-up of Donora ten years after: methodology and findings. Amer. J. Public Health 51: 155.

21. Tiller, J. R., R. S. F. Schiling and J. N. Morris. 1968. Occupational toxic factors in mortality from coronary heart disease. Brit. Med. J. 4: 407.

22. Goldsmith, J. R. 1970. Carbon monoxide research—recent and remote. Arch. Environ. Health 21: 118.

23. Astrup, P. 1967. Carbon monoxide and peripheral arterial disease. Scand. J. Clin. Lab. Investigation Suppl. 99: 193.

24. Cimino, J. 1972. Personal communication.

25. Strong, J. P., P. Correa and L. A. Solberg. 1968. Water hardness and atherosclerosis. Lab. Invest. 18: 620.

26. Neri, L. C., J. S. Mandel and D. Hewitt. 1972. Relation between mortality and water hardness in Canada. Lancet 1: 931.

27. Groover, M. E., G. E. Antell, J. E. Fulghum and O. H. Boorde. 1972. Death rates following a sudden change in hardness of drinking water. Presented at S.E.R. meeting (Feb. 28) Tampa, Fla.

28. Crawford, Margaret D., M. J. Gardner and J. N. Morris. 1971. Changes in water hardness and local death rates. Lancet 2:327.

29. Crawford, Margaret D., M. J. Gardner and J. N. Morris. 1968. Mortality and hardness of local water supplies. Lancet 1: 827.

30. Anderson, T. W., W. H. le Riche and J. S. MacKay. 1969. Sudden death and ischemic heart disease. New Eng. J. Med. 280: 805.

31. Roberts, C. J. & S. Lloyd. 1972. Association between mortality from ischemic heart disease and rainfall in South Wales and in the country boroughs of England and Wales. Lancet 1: 1091.

32. Schroeder, H. A. 1969. The water factor. New Eng. J. Med. 280: 836.

33. Voors, A. W. 1969. Does lithium depletion cause atherosclerotic heart disease? Lancet 2: 1337.

34. Blackly, P. H. 1969. Lithium content of drinking water and ischemic heart disease. New Eng. J. Med. 281: 682.

35. Bajaz, E. 1967. Heart disease and soft and hard water. Lancet 1: 726.

36. Shaffer, C. F. 1970. Ascorbic acid and atherosclerosis. Amer. J. Clin. Nutr. 23: 27.

37. Lemon, F. R. and J. W. Kuzma. 1969. A biologic cost of smoking. Arch. Environ. Health 18: 20.

G

The food-people-energy crisis

G The food-people-energy crisis

IN THE LAST few years prophets of doom have been predicting that, eventually, population and demand will exceed resources, including food resources. This can already be seen in other countries.

However, with global transportation and the population and economic growth of foreign countries, the U. S. citizen now is competing with people around the world for the food his own farmers grow. The result is fewer types of food available and higher prices. Will this trend continue and grow in the future? Will it lead to nutritional problems in this country? Should we turn back to the land to conserve energy, which is suffering its own crisis? The articles in this last chapter attempt to answer these questions.

The first article, by Paul Ehrlich, the eminent population expert, discusses the crisis of a burgeoning world population and its subsequent demands on food supply. He shows that modern agriculture will not solve the problem in most developing areas which lack capital to build fertilizer plants, construct roads for transportation or buy petroleum for processing and transportation. Ehrlich also discusses the "Green Revolution" in which new genetic varieties of crops were developed to save the world. Unfortunately, most of these new crops need high fertilizer use and irrigation, or are not disease resistant. He also notes that people are reluctant to change food habits and might not accept new foods even if they are free.

Ehrlich considers in depth the problem of bringing more land into use, citing as problems the shortage of water for irrigation and its unreasonable cost for many countries. He also explains the impracticality of relying on the sea to solve our food problems. He points out many of the problems with energy supply, although in 1969 he could not foresee all the problems we now have in energy availability, even in our affluent country. The energy crisis has caused vast problems, which are affecting production around the world.

Without population control, as Ehrlich concludes, technology will not alleviate the food shortage now or in the future. The need for population

423

control is one that few countries are willing to recognize and which causes those concerned to shudder at the consequences.

Altschul and Hornstein present an optimistic picture for the future of food in the United States. They predict the development of more processed foods, more foods consumed away from the home with better nutrition and specific foods to correct dietary problems, such as obesity. Some of these already are on the market, such as the breakfast meal bars and diet bars which supply one-third of the RDA at a low caloric value. These are both nutritious and fairly palatable.

In spite of their optimism, the authors do question the safety of additives used for the formulation and preservation of food. In the next article, Thomas Jukes relates the history of today's problem additives. He examines some presumably toxic materials used in food production, such as DDT, and the contamination of food by industrial pollutants, such as mercury. The decision whether to allow their use is based on the risk involved versus the benefit provided. Dr. Alexander Schmidt, commissioner of the FDA in 1974, discusses this risk-benefit equation in relationship to various food additives used today. The risk is generally that not enough is known about these additives to predict their effects on the human body. The benefits are longer shelf-life, safer food and greater consumer acceptability of the foods.

The last article compares the amount of energy used for food production in the United States to that used in other parts of the world. It is interesting to note that food production accounts for only 12 percent of total energy consumption in the U. S., while heating and lighting account for three times as much. Even so, a look at the energy picture shows how inefficient beef production is for example. Some have recommended that the first step in energy conservation be the elimination of meat; such a suggestion ignores the palatability of meat and the pleasure it provides—an important part of nutrition. Besides, protein from other sources may not be adequate, although soybeans may help alleviate this problem.

The authors of this last article make some interesting recommendations for how to reduce energy use. Although some of them are valid, there is, for example, a danger of microbial contamination from manure use; for this and other reasons, a complete return to organic farming would not be feasible. The authors show some unwarranted prejudice against processed foods, but forget about the increase in shelf-life per unit of energy input, something no one has calculated. They suggest that we change our lifestyle to a less complicated, less appliance-oriented one. Although that would save energy, the argument ignores the intangible benefits of saving time to engage in activities more pleasing than household chores.

39

POPULATION AND PANACEAS
a technological perspective

Paul R. Ehrlich and John P. Holdren *

Today more than one billion human beings are either undernourished or malnourished, and the human population is growing at a rate of 2% per year. The existing and impending crises in human nutrition and living conditions are well-documented but not widely understood. In particular, there is a tendency among the public, nurtured on Sunday-supplement conceptions of technology, to believe that science has the situation well in hand —that farming the sea and the tropics, irrigating the deserts, and generating cheap nuclear power in abundance hold the key to swift and certain solution of the problem. To espouse this belief is to misjudge the present severity of the situation, the disparate time scales on which tech-

* The co-authors are affiliated, respectively, with the department of biological sciences, and with the Institute for Plasma Research and department of aeronautics and astronautics, Stanford University.

We thank the following individuals for reading and commenting on the manuscript: J. H. Brownell (Stanford University); P. A. Cantor (Aerojet General Corp.); P. E. Cloud (University of California, Santa Barbara); D. J. Eckstrom (Stanford University); R. Ewell (State University of New York at Buffalo); J. L. Fisher (Resources for the Future, Inc.); J. A. Hendrickson, Jr. (Stanford University); J. H. Hessel (Stanford University); R. W. Holm (Stanford University); S. C. McIntosh, Jr., (Stanford University); K. E. F. Watt (University of California, Davis). This work was supported in part by a grant from the Ford Foundation.

nological progress and population growth operate, and the vast complexity of the problems beyond mere food production posed by population pressures. Unfortunately, scientists and engineers have themselves often added to the confusion by failing to distinguish between that which is merely theoretically feasible, and that which is economically and logistically practical.

As we will show here, man's present technology is inadequate to the task of maintaining the world's burgeoning billions, even under the most optimistic assumptions. Furthermore, technology is likely to remain inadequate until such time as the population growth rate is drastically reduced. This is not to assert that present efforts to "revolutionize" tropical agriculture, increase yields of fisheries, desalt water for irrigation, exploit new power sources, and implement related projects are not worthwhile. They may be. They could also easily produce the ultimate disaster for mankind if they are not applied with careful attention to their effects on the ecological systems necessary for our survival (Woodwell, 1967; Cole, 1968). And even if such projects are initiated with unprecedented levels of staffing and expenditures, without population control they are doomed to fall far short. No effort to expand the carrying capacity of the Earth can keep pace with unbridled population growth.

To support these contentions, we summarize briefly the present lopsided balance sheet in the population/food accounting. We then examine the logistics, economics, and possible consequences of some technological schemes which have been proposed to help restore the balance, or, more ambitiously, to permit the maintenance of human populations much larger than today's. The most pertinent aspects of the balance are:

1) The world population reached 3.5 billion in mid-1968, with an annual increment of approximately 70 million people (itself increasing) and a doubling time on the order of 35 years (Population Reference Bureau, 1968).

2) Of this number of people, at least one-half billion are undernourished (deficient in calories or, more succinctly, slowing starving), and approximately an additional billion are malnourished (deficient in particular nutrients, mostly protein) (Borgstrom, 1965; Sukhatme, 1966). Estimates of the number actually perishing annually from starvation begin at 4 million and go up (Ehrlich, 1968) and depend in part on official definitions of starvation which conceal the true magnitude of hunger's contribution to the death rate (Lelyveld, 1968).

3) Merely to maintain present inadequate nutrition levels, the food requirements of Asia, Africa, and Latin America will, conservatively, increase by 26% in the 10-year period measured from 1965 to 1975 (Paddock and Paddock, 1967). World food production must double in the period 1965–2000 to stay even; it must triple if nutrition is to be brought up to minimum requirements.

FOOD PRODUCTION

That there is insufficient additional, good quality agricultural land available in the world to meet these needs is so well documented (Borgstrom, 1965) that we will not belabor the point here. What hope there is must rest with increasing yields on land presently cultivated, bringing marginal land into production, more efficiently exploiting the sea, and bringing less conventional methods of food production to fruition. In all these areas, science and technology play a dominant role. While space does not permit even a cursory look at all the proposals on these topics which have been advanced in recent years, a few representative examples illustrate our points.

Conventional agriculture. Probably the most widely recommended means of increasing agricultural yields is through the more intensive use of fertilizers. Their production is straightforward, and a good deal is known about their effective application, although, as with many technologies we consider here, the environmental consequences of heavy fertilizer use are ill understood and potentially dangerous [1] (Wadleigh, 1968). But even ignoring such problems, we find staggering difficulties barring the implementation of fertilizer technology on the scale required. In this regard the accomplishments of countries such as Japan and the Netherlands are often cited as offering hope to the underdeveloped world. Some perspective on this point is afforded by noting that if India were to apply fertilizer at the per capita level employed by the Netherlands, her fertilizer needs would be nearly half the present world output (United Nations, 1968).

On a more realistic plane, we note that although the goal for nitrogen fertilizer production in 1971 under India's fourth 5-year plan is 2.4 million metric tons (Anonymous, 1968a), Raymond Ewell (who has served as fertilizer production adviser to the Indian government for the past 12 years) suggests that less than 1.1 million metric tons is a more probable figure for that date.[2] Ewell cites poor plant maintenance, raw materials shortages, and power and transportation breakdowns as contributing to continued low production by existing Indian plants. Moreover, even when fertilizer is available, increases in productivity do not necessarily follow. In parts of the underdeveloped world lack of farm credit is limiting fertilizer distribution; elsewhere, internal transportation systems are inadequate to the task. Nor can the problem of educating farmers on the advantages and techniques of fertilizer use be ignored. A recent study (Parikh et al., 1968) of the Intensive Agriculture District Program in the Surat district of Gujarat, India (in which scientific fertilizer use was to have been a major ingredient) notes that "on the whole, the performance

[1] Barry Commoner, address to 135th Meeting of the AAAS. Dallas, Texas (28 December 1968).

[2] Raymond Ewell, private communications (1 December 1968).

of adjoining districts which have similar climate but did not enjoy relative preference of input supply was as good as, if not better than, the programme district. . . . A particularly disheartening feature is that the farm production plans, as yet, do not carry any educative value and have largely failed to convince farmers to use improved practices in their proper combinations."

As a second example of a panacea in the realm of conventional agriculture, mention must be given to the development of new high-yield or high-protein strains of food crops. That such strains have the potential of making a major contribution to the food supply of the world is beyond doubt, but this potential is limited in contrast to the potential for population growth, and will be realized too slowly to have anything but a small impact on the immediate crisis. There are major difficulties impeding the widespread use of new high-yield grain varieties. Typically, the new grains require high fertilizer inputs to realize their full potential, and thus are subject to all the difficulties mentioned above. Some other problems were identified in a recent address by Lester R. Brown, administrator of the International Agricultural Development Service: the limited amount of irrigated land suitable for the new varieties, the fact that a farmer's willingness to innovate fluctuates with the market prices (which may be driven down by high-yield crops), and the possibility of tieups at market facilities inadequate for handling increased yields.[3]

Perhaps even more important, the new grain varieties are being rushed into production without adequate field testing, so that we are unsure of how resistant they will be to the attacks of insects and plant diseases. William Paddock has presented a plant pathologist's view of the crash programs to shift to new varieties (Paddock, 1967). He describes India's dramatic program of planting improved Mexican wheat, and continues: "Such a rapid switch to a new variety is clearly understandable in a country that tottered on the brink of famine. Yet with such limited testing, one wonders what unknown pathogens await a climatic change which will give the environmental conditions needed for their growth." Introduction of the new varieties creates enlarged monocultures of plants with essentially unknown levels of resistance to disaster. Clearly, one of the prices that is paid for higher yield is a higher risk of widespread catastrophe. And the risks are far from local: since the new varieties require more "input" of pesticides (with all their deleterious ecological side effects), these crops may ultimately contribute to the defeat of other environment-related panaceas, such as extracting larger amounts of food from the sea.

A final problem must be mentioned in connection with these strains of food crops. In general, the hungriest people in the world are also those with the most conservative food habits. Even rather minor changes such as that from a rice variety in which the cooked grains stick together to

[3] Lester R. Brown, address to the Second International Conference on the War on Hunger, Washington, D. C. (February 1968).

one in which the grains fall apart, may make new foods unacceptable. It seems to be an unhappy fact of human existence that people would rather starve than eat a nutritious substance which they do not recognize as food.[4]

Beyond the economic, ecological, and sociological problems already mentioned in connection with high-yield agriculture, there is the overall problem of time. We need time to breed the desired characteristics of yield and hardiness into a vast array of new strains (a tedious process indeed), time to convince farmers that it is necessary that they change their time-honored ways of cultivation, and time to convince hungry people to change the staples of their diet. The Paddocks give 20 years as the "rule of thumb" for a new technique or plant variety to progress from conception to substantial impact on farming (Paddock and Paddock, 1967). They write: "It is true that a *massive* research attack on the problem could bring some striking results in less than 20 years. But I do not find such an attack remotely contemplated in the thinking of those officials capable of initiating it." Promising as high-yield agriculture may be, the funds, the personnel, the ecological expertise, and the necessary years are unfortunately not at our disposal. Fulfillment of the promise will come too late for many of the world's starving millions, if it comes at all.

Bringing more land under cultivation. The most frequently mentioned means of bringing new land into agricultural production are farming the tropics and irrigating arid and semiarid regions. The former, although widely discussed in optimistic terms, has been tried for years with incredibly poor results, and even recent experiments have not been encouraging. One essential difficulty is the unsuitability of tropical soils for supporting typical foodstuffs instead of jungles (McNeil, 1964; Paddock and Paddock, 1964). Also, "the tropics" are a biologically more diverse area than the temperate zones, so that farming technology developed for one area will all too often prove useless in others. We shall see that irrigating the deserts, while more promising, has serious limitations in terms of scale, cost, and lead time.

The feasible approaches to irrigation of arid lands appear to be limited to large-scale water projects involving dams and transport in canals, and desalination of ocean and brackish water. Supplies of usable ground water are already badly depleted in most areas where they are accessible, and natural recharge is low enough in most arid regions that such supplies do not offer a long-term solution in any case. Some recent statistics will give perspective to the discussion of water projects and desalting which follows. In 1966, the United States was using about 300 billion gal of water per day, of which 135 billion gal were consumed by agriculture and 165 billion gal by municipal and industrial users (Sporn, 1966). The bulk of the agricultural water cost the farmer from 5 to 10 cents/1000 gal; the

[4] For a more detailed discussion of the psychological problems in persuading people to change their dietary habits, see McKenzie, 1968.

highest price paid for agricultural water was 15 cents/1000 gal. For small industrial and municipal supplies, prices as high as 50 to 70 cents/1000 gal were prevalent in the U. S. arid regions, and some communities in the Southwest were paying on the order of $1.00/1000 gal for "project" water. The extremely high cost of the latter stems largely from transportation costs, which have been estimated at 5 to 15 cents/1000 gal per 100 miles (International Atomic Energy Agency, 1964).

We now examine briefly the implications of such numbers in considering the irrigation of the deserts. The most ambitious water project yet conceived in this country is the North American Water and Power Alliance, which proposes to distribute water from the great rivers of Canada to thirsty locations all over the United States. Formidable political problems aside (some based on the certainty that in the face of expanding populations, demands for water will eventually arise at the source), this project would involve the expenditure of $100 billion in construction costs over a 20-year completion period. At the end of this time, the yield to the United States would be 69 million acre feet of water annually (Kelly, 1966), or 63 billion gal per day. If past experience with massive water projects is any guide, these figures are overoptimistic; but if we assume they are not, it is instructive to note that this monumental undertaking would provide for an increase of only 21% in the water consumption of the United States, during a period in which the population is expected to increase by between 25 and 43% (U. S. Dept. of Commerce, 1966). To assess the possible contribution to the *world* food situation, we assume that all this water could be devoted to agriculture, although extrapolation of present consumption patterns indicates that only about one-half would be. Then using the rather optimistic figure of 500 gal per day to grow the food to feed one person, we find that this project could feed 126 million additional people. Since this is less than 8% of the projected world population growth during the construction period (say 1970 to 1990), it should be clear that even the most massive water projects can make but a token contribution to the solution of the world food problem in the long term. And in the crucial short term—the years preceding 1980—*no* additional people will be fed by projects still on the drawing board today.

In summary, the cost is staggering, the scale insufficient, and the lead time too long. Nor need we resort to such speculation about the future for proof of the failure of technological "solutions" in the absence of population control. The highly touted and very expensive Aswan Dam project, now nearing completion, will ultimately supply food (at the present miserable diet level) for less than Egypt's population growth during the time of construction (Borgstrom, 1965; Cole, 1968). Furthermore, its effect on the fertility of the Nile Delta may be disastrous, and, as with all water projects of this nature, silting of the reservoir will destroy the gains in the long term (perhaps in 100 years).

Desalting for irrigation suffers somewhat similar limitations. The desalting plants operational in the world today produce water at individual rates of 7.5 million gal/day and less, at a cost of 75 cents/1000 gal and up, the cost increasing as the plant size decreases (Bender, 1969). The most optimistic firm proposal which anyone seems to have made for desalting with present or soon-to-be available technology is a 150 million gal per day nuclear-powered installation studied by the Bechtel Corp. for the Los Angeles Metropolitan Water District. Bechtel's early figures indicated that water from this complex would be available at the site for 27–28 cents/1000 gal (Galstann and Currier, 1967). However, skepticism regarding the economic assumptions leading to these figures (Milliman, 1966) has since proven justified—the project was shelved after spiralling construction cost estimates indicated an actual water cost of 40–50 cents/1000 gal. Use of even the original figures, however, bears out our contention that the *most* optimistic assumptions do not alter the verdict that technology is losing the food/population battle. For 28 cents/1000 gal is still approximately twice the cost which farmers have hitherto been willing or able to pay for irrigation water. If the Bechtel plant had been intended to supply agricultural needs, which it was not, one would have had to add to an already unacceptable price the very substantial cost of transporting the water inland.

Significantly, studies have shown that the economies of scale in the distilation process are essentially exhausted by a 150 million gal per day plant (International Atomic Energy Agency, 1964). Hence, merely increasing desalting capacity further will not substantially lower the cost of the water. On purely economic grounds, then, it is unlikely that desalting will play a major role in food production by conventional agriculture in the short term.[5] Technological "break-throughs" will presumably improve this outlook with the passage of time, but world population growth will not wait.

Desalting becomes more promising if the high cost of the water can be offset by increased agricultural yields per gallon and, perhaps, use of a single nuclear installation to provide power for both the desalting and profitable on-site industrial processes. This prospect has been investigated in a thorough and well-documented study headed by E. S. Mason (Oak Ridge National Laboratory, 1968). The result is a set of preliminary figures and recommendations regarding nuclear-powered "agro-industrial complexes" for arid and semiarid regions, in which desalted water and fertilizer would be produced for use on an adjacent, highly efficient farm. In underdeveloped countries incapable of using the full excess power output of the reactor, this energy would be consumed in on-site production of industrial materials for sale on the world market. Both near-term (10

---

[5] An identical conclusion was reached in a recent study (Clawson et al., 1969) in which the foregoing points and numerous other aspects of desalting were treated in far more detail than was possible here.

years hence) and far-term (20 years hence) technologies are considered, as are various mixes of farm and industrial products. The representative near-term case for which a detailed cost breakdown is given involves a seaside facility with a desalting capacity of 1 billion gal/day, a farm size of 320,000 acres, and an industrial electric power consumption of 1585 Mw. The initial investment for this complex is estimated at $1.8 billion, and annual operating costs at $236 million. If both the food and the industrial materials produced were sold (as opposed to giving the food, at least, to those in need who could not pay),[6] the estimated profit for such a complex, before subtracting financing costs, would be 14.6%.

The authors of the study are commendably cautious in outlining the assumptions and uncertainties upon which these figures rest. The key assumption is that 200 gal/day of water will grow the 2500 calories required to feed one person. Water/calorie ratios of this order or less have been achieved by the top 20% of farmers specializing in such crops as wheat, potatoes, and tomatoes; but more water is required for needed protein-rich crops such as peanuts and soybeans. The authors identify the uncertainty that crops usually raised separately can be grown together in tight rotation on the same piece of land. Problems of water storage between periods of peak irrigation demand, optimal patterns of crop rotation, and seasonal acreage variations are also mentioned. These "ifs" and assumptions, and those associated with the other technologies involved, are unfortunately often omitted when the results of such painstaking studies are summarized for more popular consumption (Anonymous, 1968b, 1968c). The result is the perpetuation of the public's tendency to confuse feasible and available, to see panaceas where scientists in the field concerned see only potential, realizable with massive infusions of time and money.

It is instructive, nevertheless, to examine the impact on the world food problem which the Oak Ridge complexes might have if construction were to begin today, and if all the assumptions about technology 10 years hence were valid *now*. At the industrial-agricultural mix pertinent to the sample case described above, the food produced would be adequate for just under 3 million people. This means that 23 such plants per year, at a cost of $41 billion, would have to be put in operation merely to keep pace with world population growth, to say nothing of improving the substandard diets of between one and two billion members of the present population. (Fertilizer production beyond that required for the on-site farm is of course a contribution in the latter regard, but the substantial additional costs of transporting it to where it is needed must then be accounted for.)

---

[6] Confusing statements often are made about the possibility that food supply will outrun food demand in the future. In these statements, "demand" is used in the economic sense, and in this context many millions of starving people may generate no demand whatsoever. Indeed, one concern of those engaged in increasing food production is to find ways of increasing demand.

Since approximately 5 years from the start of construction would be required to put such a complex into operation, we should commence work on at least 125 units post-haste, and begin at least 25 per year thereafter. If the technology *were* available now, the investment in construction over the next 5 years, prior to operation of the first plants, would be $315 billion—about 20 times the total U. S. foreign aid expenditure during the past 5 years. By the time the technology *is* available the bill will be much higher, if famine has not "solved" the problem for us.

This example again illustrates that scale, time, and cost are all working against technology in the short term. And if population growth is not decelerated, the increasing severity of population-related crises will surely neutralize the technological improvements of the middle and long terms.

Other food panaceas. "Food from the sea" is the most prevalent "answer" to the world food shortage in the view of the general public. This is not surprising, since estimates of the theoretical fisheries productivity of the sea run up to some 50–100 times current yields (Schmitt, 1965; Christy and Scott, 1965). Many practical and economic difficulties, however, make it clear that such a figure will never be reached, and that it will not even be approached in the foreseeable future. In 1966, the annual fisheries harvest was some 57 million metric tons (United Nations, 1968). A careful analysis (Meseck, 1961) indicates that this might be increased to a world production of 70 million metric tons by 1980. If this gain were realized, it would represent (assuming no violent change in population growth patterns) a small per capita *loss* in fisheries yield.

Both the short- and long-term outlooks for taking food from the sea are clouded by the problems of overexploitation, pollution (which is generally ignored by those calculating potential yields), and economics. Solving these problems will require more than technological legerdemain; it will also require unprecedented changes in human behavior, especially in the area of international cooperation. The unlikelihood that such cooperation will come about is reflected in the recent news (Anonymous, 1968d) that Norway has dropped out of the whaling industry because overfishing has depleted the stock below the level at which it may economically be harvested. In that industry, international controls were tried—and failed. The sea is, unfortunately, a "commons" (Hardin, 1968), and the resultant management problems exacerbate the biological and technical problems of greatly increasing our "take." One suspects that the return per dollar poured into the sea will be much less than the corresponding return from the land for many years, and the return from the land has already been found wanting.

Synthetic foods, protein culture with petroleum, saline agriculture, and weather modification all may hold promise for the future, but all are at present expensive and available only on an extremely limited scale. The research to improve this situation will also be expensive, and, of course, time-consuming. In the absence of funding, it will not occur at all, a fact which occasionally eludes the public and the Congress.

DOMESTIC AND INDUSTRIAL WATER SUPPLIES

The world has water problems, even exclusive of the situation in agriculture. Although total precipitation should in theory be adequate in quantity for several further doublings of population, serious shortages arising from problems of quality, irregularity, and distribution already plague much of the world. Underdeveloped countries will find the water needs of industrialization staggering: 240,000 gal of water are required to produce a ton of newsprint; 650,000 gal to produce a ton of steel (International Atomic Energy Agency, 1964). Since maximum acceptable water costs for domestic and industrial use are higher than for agriculture, those who can afford it are or soon will be using desalination (40–100 + cents/1000 gal) and used-water renovation (54–57 cents/1000 gal [Ennis, 1967]). Those who cannot afford it are faced with allocating existing supplies between industry and agriculture, and as we have seen, they must choose the latter. In this circumstance, the standard of living remains pitifully low. Technology's only present answer is massive externally-financed complexes of the sort considered above, and we have already suggested there the improbability that we are prepared to pay the bill rung up by present population growth.

The widespread use of desalted water by those who *can* afford it brings up another problem only rarely mentioned to date, the disposal of the salts. The product of the distillation processes in present use is a hot brine with salt concentration several times that of seawater. Both the temperature and the salinity of this effluent will prove fatal to local marine life if it is simply exhausted to the ocean. The most optimistic statement we have seen on this problem is that "*smaller plants* (our emphasis) at seaside locations may return the concentrated brine to the ocean if proper attention is paid to the design of the outfall, and to the effect on the local marine ecology" (McIlhenny, 1966). The same writer identifies the major economic uncertainties connected with extracting the salts for sale (to do so is straightforward, but often not profitable). Nor can one simply evaporate the brine and leave the residue in a pile—the 150 million gal/day plant mentioned above would produce brine bearing 90 million lb. of salts daily (based on figures by Parker, 1966). This amount of salt would cover over 15 acres to a depth of one foot. Thus, every year a plant of the billion gallon per day, agro-industrial complex size would produce a pile of salt over 52 ft deep and covering a square mile. The high winds typical of coastal deserts would seriously aggravate the associated soil contamination problem.

ENERGY

Man's problems with energy supply are more subtle than those with food and water: we are not yet running out of energy, but we are being forced to use it faster than is probably healthy. The rapacious depletion of our fossil fuels is already forcing us to consider more expensive mining techniques to gain access to lower-grade deposits, such as the oil shales, and even the status of our high-grade uranium ore reserves is not clear-cut (Anonymous, 1968e).

A widely held misconception in this connection is that nuclear power is "dirt cheap," and as such represents a panacea for developed and under-developed nations alike. To the contrary, the largest nuclear-generating stations now in operation are just competitive with or marginally superior to modern coal-fired plants of comparable size (where coal is not scarce); at best, both produce power for on the order of 4–5 mills (tenths of a cent) per kilowatt-hour. Smaller nuclear units remain less economical than their fossil-fueled counterparts. Underdeveloped countries can rarely use the power of the larger plants. Simply speaking, there are not enough industries, appliances, and light bulbs to absorb the output, and the cost of industrialization and modernization exceeds the cost of the power required to sustain it by orders of magnitude, regardless of the source of the power. (For example, one study noted that the capital requirement to consume the output of a 70,000 kilowatt plant—about $1.2 million worth of electricity per year at 40% utilization and 5 mills/kwh—is $111 million per year if the power is consumed by metals industries, $270 million per year for petroleum product industries [E. A. Mason, 1957].) Hence, at least at present, only those underdeveloped countries which are short of fossil fuels or inexpensive means to transport them are in particular need of nuclear power.

Prospects for major reductions in the cost of nuclear power in the future hinge on the long-awaited breeder reactor and the still further distant thermonuclear reactor. In neither case is the time scale or the ultimate cost of energy a matter of any certainty. The breeder reactor, which converts more nonfissile uranium (^{238}U) or thorium to fissionable material than it consumes as fuel for itself, effectively extends our nuclear fuel supply by a factor of approximately 400 (Cloud, 1968). It is not expected to become competitive economically with conventional reactors until the 1980's (Bump, 1967). Reductions in the unit energy cost beyond this date are not guaranteed, due both to the probable continued high capital cost of breeder reactors and to increasing costs for the ore which the breeders will convert to fuel. In the latter regard, we mention that although crushing granite for its few parts per million of uranium and thorium is possible in theory, the problems and cost of doing so are far from resolved.[7] It is too soon to predict the costs associated with a fusion

[7] A general discussion of extracting metals from common rock is given by Cloud, 1968.

reactor (few who work in the field will predict whether such a device will work at all within the next 15–20 years). One guess puts the unit energy cost at something over half that for a coal or fission power station of comparable size (Mills, 1967), but this is pure speculation. Quite possibly the major benefit of controlled fusion will again be to extend the energy supply rather than to cheapen it.

A second misconception about nuclear power is that it can reduce our dependence on fossil fuels to zero as soon as that becomes necessary or desirable. In fact, nuclear power plants contribute only to the electrical portion of the energy budget; and in 1960 in the United States, for example, electrical energy comprised only 19% of the total energy consumed (Sporn, 1963). The degree to which nuclear fuels can postpone the exhaustion of our coal and oil depends on the extent to which that 19% is enlarged. The task is far from a trivial one, and will involve transitions to electric or fuel-cell powered transportation, electric heating, and electrically powered industries. It will be extremely expensive.

Nuclear energy, then, is a panacea neither for us nor for the underdeveloped world. It relieves, but does not remove, the pressure on fossil fuel supplies; it provides reasonably-priced power where these fuels are not abundant; it has substantial (but expensive) potential in intelligent applications such as that suggested in the Oak Ridge study discussed above; and it shares the propensity of fast-growing technology to unpleasant side effects (Novick, 1969). We mention in the last connection that, while nuclear power stations do not produce conventional air pollutants, their radioactive waste problems may in the long run prove a poor trade. Although the AEC seems to have made a good case for solidification and storage in salt mines of the bulk of the radioactive fission products (Blanko et al., 1967), a number of radioactive isotopes are released to the air, and in some areas such isotopes have already turned up in potentially harmful concentrations (Curtis and Hogan, 1969). Projected order of magnitude increases in nuclear power generation will seriously aggravate this situation. Although it has frequently been stated that the eventual advent of fusion reactors will free us from such difficulties, at least one authority, F. L. Parker, takes a more cautious view. He contends that losses of radioactive tritium from fusion power plants may prove even more hazardous than the analogous problems of fission reactors (Parker, 1968).

A more easily evaluated problem is the tremendous quantity of waste heat generated at nuclear installations (to say nothing of the usable power output, which, as with power from whatever source, must also ultimately be dissipated as heat). Both have potentially disastrous effects on the local and world ecological and climatological balance. There is no simple solution to this problem, for, in general, "cooling" only moves heat; it does not *remove* it from the environment viewed as a whole. Moreover, the Second Law of Thermodynamics puts a ceiling on the efficiency with which we can do even this much, i. e., concentrate and transport heat. In effect, the Second Law condemns us to aggravate the total problem by generating still *more* heat in any machinery we devise for local cooling (consider, for example, refrigerators and air conditioners).

The only heat which actually leaves the whole system, the Earth, is that which can be radiated back into space. This amount steadily is being diminished as combustion of hydrocarbon fuels increases the atmospheric percentage of CO_2 which has strong absorption bands in the infrared spectrum of the outbound heat energy. (Hubbert, 1962, puts the increase in the CO_2 content of the atmosphere at 10% since 1900.) There is, of course, a competing effect in the Earth's energy balance, which is the increased reflectivity of the upper atmosphere to incoming sunlight due to other forms of air pollution. It has been estimated, ignoring both these effects, that man risks drastic (and perhaps catastrophic) climatological change if the amount of heat he dissipates in the environment on a global scale reaches 1% of the incident solar energy at the Earth's surface (Rose and Clark, 1961). At the present 5% rate of increase in world energy consumption,[8] this level will be reached in less than a century, and in the immediate future the direct contribution of man's power consumption will create serious local problems. If we may safely rule out circumvention of the Second Law or the divorce of energy requirements from population size, this suggests that, whatever science and technology may accomplish, population growth must be stopped.

TRANSPORTATION

We would be remiss in our offer of a technological perspective on population problems without some mention of the difficulties associated with transporting large quantities of food, material, or people across the face of the Earth. While our grain exports have not begun to satisfy the hunger of the underdeveloped world, they already have taxed our ability to transport food in bulk over large distances. The total amount of goods of *all* kinds loaded at U. S. ports for external trade was 158 million metric tons in 1965 (United Nations, 1968). This is coincidentally the approximate amount of grain which would have been required to make up the dietary shortages of the underdeveloped world in the same year (Sukhatme, 1966). Thus, if the United States *had* such an amount of grain to ship, it could be handled only by displacing the entirety of our export trade. In a similar vein, the gross weight of the fertilizer, in excess of present consumption, required in the underdeveloped world to feed the additional population there in 1980 will amount to approximately the same figure—150 mil-

[8] The rate of growth of world energy consumption fluctuates strongly about some mean on a time scale of only a few years, and the figures are not known with great accuracy in any case. A discussion of predicting the mean and a defense of the figure of 5% are given in Gúeron et al., 1957.

lion metric tons (Sukhatme, 1966). Assuming that a substantial fraction of this fertilizer, should it be available at all, will have to be shipped about, we had best start building freighters! These problems, and the even more discouraging one of internal transportation in the hungry countries, coupled with the complexities of international finance and marketing which have hobbled even present aid programs, complete a dismal picture of the prospects for "external" solutions to ballooning food requirements in much of the world.

Those who envision migration as a solution to problems of food, land, and water distribution not only ignore the fact that the world has no promising place to put more people, they simply have not looked at the numbers of the transportation game. Neglecting the fact that migration and relocation costs would probably amount to a minimum of several thousand dollars per person, we find, for example, that the entire long-range jet transport fleet of the United States (about 600 planes [Molloy, 1968] with an average capacity of 150), averaging two round trips per week, could transport only about 9 million people per year from India to the United States. This amounts to about 75% of that country's annual population *growth* (Population Reference Bureau, 1968). Ocean liners and transports, while larger, are less numerous and much slower, and over long distances could not do as well. Does anyone believe, then, that we are going to compensate for the world's population growth by sending the excess to the planets? If there were a place to go on Earth, financially and logistically we could not send our surplus there.

CONCLUSION

We have not attempted to be comprehensive in our treatment of population pressures and the prospects of coping with them technologically; rather, we hope simply to have given enough illustrations to make plausible our contention that technology, without population control, cannot meet the challenge. It may be argued that we have shown only that any one technological scheme taken individually is insufficient to the task at hand, whereas *all* such schemes applied in parallel might well be enough. We would reply that neither the commitment nor the resources to implement them all exists, and indeed that many may prove mutually exclusive (e. g., harvesting algae may diminish fish production).

Certainly, an optimum combination of efforts exists in theory, but we assert that no organized attempt to find it is being made, and that our examination of its probable eventual constituents permits little hope that even the optimum will suffice. Indeed, after a far more thorough survey of the prospects than we have attempted here, the President's Science Advisory Committee Panel on the world food supply concluded (PSAC, 1967): "The solution of the problem that will exist after about 1985 *demands* that programs of population control be initiated now." We most emphatically agree, noting that "now" was 2 years ago!

Of the problems arising out of population growth in the short, middle, and long terms, we have emphasized the first group. For mankind must pass the first hurdles—food and water for the next 20 years—to be granted the privilege of confronting such dilemmas as the exhaustion of mineral resources and physical space later.[9] Furthermore, we have not conveyed the extent of our concern for the environmental deterioration which has accompanied the population explosion, and for the catastrophic ecological consequences which would attend many of the proposed technological "solutions" to the population/food crisis. Nor have we treated the point that "development" of the rest of the world to the standards of the West probably would be lethal ecologically (Ehrlich and Ehrlich, 1970). For even if such grim prospects are ignored, it is abundantly clear that in terms of cost, lead time, and implementation on the scale required, technology without population control will be too little and too late.

What hope there is lies not, of course, in abandoning attempts at technological solutions; on the contrary, they must be pursued at unprecedented levels, with unprecedented judgment, and above all with unprecedented attention to their ecological consequences. We need dramatic programs now to find ways of ameliorating the food crisis—to buy time for humanity until the inevitable delay accompanying population control efforts has passed. But it cannot be emphasized enough that if the population control measures are *not* initiated immediately and effectively, all the technology man can bring to bear will not fend off the misery to come.[10] Therefore, confronted as we are with limited resources of time and money, we must consider carefully what fraction of our effort should be applied to the cure of the disease itself instead of to the temporary relief of the symptoms. We should ask, for example, how many vasectomies could be performed by a program funded with the 1.8 billion dollars required to build a single nuclear agro-industrial complex, and what the relative impact on the problem would be in both the short and long terms.

The decision for population control will be opposed by growth-minded economists and businessmen, by nationalistic statesmen, by zealous religious leaders, and by the myopic and well-fed of every description. It is therefore incumbent on all who sense the limitations of technology and the fragility of the environmental balance to make themselves heard above the

[9] Since the first draft of this article was written, the authors have seen the manuscript of a timely and pertinent forthcoming book, *Resources and Man*, written under the auspices of the National Academy of Sciences and edited by Preston E. Cloud. The book reinforces many of our own conclusions in such areas as agriculture and fisheries and, in addition, treats both short- and long-term prospects in such areas as mineral resources and fossil fuels in great detail.

[10] This conclusion has also been reached within the specific context of aid to underdeveloped countries in a Ph.D. thesis by Douglas Daetz: "Energy Utilization and Aid Effectiveness in Nonmechanized Agriculture: A Computer Simulation of a Socioeconomic System" (University of California, Berkeley, May 1968).

hollow, optimistic chorus—to convince society and its leaders that there is no alternative but the cessation of our irresponsible, all-demanding, and all-consuming population growth.

REFERENCES

1. Anonymous. 1968a. India aims to remedy fertilizer shortage. *Chem. Eng. News*, 46 (November 25): 29.

2. _____. 1968b. Scientists Studying Nuclear-Powered Agro-Industrial Complexes to Give Food and Jobs to Millions. *New York Times*, March 10, p. 74.

3. _____. 1968c. Food from the atom. *Technol. Rev.*, January, p. 55.

4. _____. 1968d. Norway—The end of the big blubber. *Time*, November 29, p. 98.

5. _____. 1968e. Nuclear fuel cycle. *Nucl. News*, January, p. 30.

6. Bender, R. J. 1969. Why water desalting will expand. *Power*, 113 (August): 171.

7. Blanko, R. E., J. O. Blomeke, and J. T. Roberts. 1967. Solving the waste disposal problem. *Nucleonics*, 25: 28.

8. Borgstrom, Georg. 1965. *The Hungry Planet*. Collier-Macmillan, New York.

9. Bump, T. R. 1967. A third generation of breeder reactors. *Sci. Amer.*, May, p. 25.

10. Christy, F. C., Jr., and A. Scott. 1965. *The Commonwealth in Ocean Fisheries*. Johns Hopkins Press, Baltimore.

11. Clawson, M., H. L. Landsberg, and L. T. Alexander. 1969. Desalted seawater for agriculture: Is it economic? *Science*, 164: 1141.

12. Cloud, P. R. 1968. Realities of mineral distribution. *Texas Quart.*, Summer, p. 103.

13. Cole, LaMont C. 1968. Can the world be saved? *BioScience*, 18: 679.

14. Curtis, R., and E. Hogan. 1969. *Perils of the Peaceful Atom*. Doubleday, New York. p. 135, 150–152.

15. Ennis, C. E. 1967. Desalted water as a competitive commodity. *Chem. Eng. Progr.*, 63:(1): 64.

16. Ehrlich, P. R. 1968. *The Population Bomb*. Sierra Club/Ballantine, New York.

17. Ehrlich, P. R., and Anne H. Ehrlich. 1970. *Population, Resources and Environment*. W. H. Freeman, San Francisco (In press).

18. Galstann, L. S., and E. L. Currier. 1967. The Metropolitan Water District desalting project. *Chem. Eng. Progr.*, 63,(1): 64.

19. Gúeron, J., J. A. Lane, I. R. Maxwell, and J. R. Menke. 1957. *The Economics of Nuclear Power. Progress in Nuclear Energy*. McGraw-Hill Book Co., New York. Series VIII, p. 23.

20. Hardin, G. 1968. The tragedy of the commons. *Science,* 162: 1243.

21. Hubbert, M. K. 1962. Energy resources, A report to the Committee on Natural Resources. National Research Council Report 1000-D, National Academy of Sciences.

22. International Atomic Energy Agency. 1964. Desalination of water using conventional and nuclear energy. Technical Report 24, Vienna.

23. Kelly, R. P. 1966. North American water and power alliance. In: *Water Production Using Nuclear Energy,* R. G. Post and R. L. Seale (eds.). University of Arizona Press, Tucson, p. 29.

24. Lelyveld, D. 1968. Can India survive Calcutta? *New York Times Magazine,* October 13, p. 58.

25. Mason, E. A. 1957. Economic growth and energy consumption. In: *The Economics of Nuclear Power. Progress in Nuclear Energy.* Series VIII. J. Gúeron et al. (eds.). McGraw-Hill Book Co., New York, p. 56.

26. McIlhenny, W. F. 1966. Problems and potentials of concentrated brines. In: *Water Production Using Nuclear Energy.* R. G. Post and R. L. Seale (eds.). University of Arizona Press, Tucson, p. 187.

27. McKenzie, John. 1968. Nutrition and the soft sell. *New Sci.,* 40: 423.

28. McNeil, Mary. 1964. Lateritic soils. *Sci. Amer.,* November, p. 99.

29. Meseck, G. 1961. Importance of fish production and utilization in the food economy. Paper R11.3, presented at FAO Conference on Fish in Nutrition, Rome.

30. Milliman, J. W. 1966. Economics of water production using nuclear energy. In: *Water Production Using Nuclear Energy.* R. G. Post and R. L. Seale (eds.). University of Arizona Press, Tucson, p. 49.

31. Mills, R. G. 1967. Some engineering problems of thermonuclear fusion. *Nucl. Fusion,* 7: 223.

32. Molloy, J. F., Jr. 1968. The $12-billion financing problem of U. S. airlines. *Astronautics and Aeronautics,* October, p. 76.

33. Novick, S. 1969. *The Careless Atom.* Houghton Mifflin, Boston.

34. Oak Ridge National Laboratory. 1968. Nuclear energy centers, industrial and agro-industrial complexes, Summary Report. ORNL-4291, July.

35. Paddock, William. 1967. Phytopathology and a hungry world. *Ann. Rev. Phytopathol.,* 5: 375.

36. Paddock, William, and Paul Paddock. 1964. *Hungry Nations.* Little, Brown & Co., Boston.

37. ———. 1967. *Famine 1975!* Little, Brown & Co., Boston.

38. Parikh, G., S. Saxena, and M. Maharaja. 1968. Agricultural extension and IADP, a study of Surat. *Econ. Polit. Weekly,* August 24, p. 1307.

39. Parker, F. L. 1968. Radioactive wastes from fusion reactors. *Science,* 159: 83.

40. Parker, H. M. 1966. Environmental factors relating to large water plants. In: *Water Production Using Nuclear Energy,* R. G. Post and R. L. Seale (eds.). University of Arizona Press, Tucson, p. 209.

41. Population Reference Bureau. 1968. Population Reference Bureau Data Sheet. Pop. Ref. Bureau, Washington, D.C.

42. PSAC. 1967. *The World Food Problem.* Report of the President's Science Advisory Committee. Vols. 1–3. U.S. Govt. Printing Office, Washington, D.C.

43. Rose, D. J., and M. Clark, Jr. 1961. *Plasma and Controlled Fusion.* M.I.T. Press, Cambridge, Mass., p. 3.

44. Schmitt, W. R. 1965. The planetary food potential. *Ann. N. Y. Acad. Sci.,* 118: 645.

45. Sporn, Philip. 1963. *Energy for Man.* Macmillan, New York.

46. ———. 1966. *Fresh Water from Saline Waters.* Pergamon Press, New York.

47. Sukhatme, P. V. 1966. Th eworld's food supplies. *Roy Stat. Soc. J.,* 129A: 222.

48. United Nations. 1968. *United Nations Statistical Yearbook for 1967.* Statistical Office of the U.N., New York.

49. U.S. Dept. of Commerce. 1966. *Statistical Abstract of the U.S.* U.S. Govt. Printing Office, Washington, D.C.

50. Wadleigh, C. H. 1968. Wastes in relation to agriculture and industry. USDA Miscellaneous Publication No. 1065. March.

51. Woodwell, George M. 1967. Toxic substances and ecological cycles. *Sci. Amer.,* March, p. 24.

40

FOODS OF THE FUTURE

Aaron M. Altschul and Irwin Hornstein *

Future foods will be handled better, be cleaner, and have better quality and flavor. There will be increased flexibility in the choice of raw materials, including synthetic flavors and new protein sources, for fabricating foods. Computerized selection of food ingredients on a day-to-day basis will produce least cost standard products of high nutritional value and palatability. Foods will be engineered to be nutritionally complete without altering acceptability. Convenience foods will increasingly dominate the institutional and consumer markets. The away-from-home eating market will increase with a concomitant increase in the variety of available foods. Control of diet to prevent certain diseases, including obesity, will become prevalent.

It is, indeed, the height of folly to make predictions in this fast-moving world. We even doubt whether the kind of predictions that Jules Verne fictionalized, many of which came true, would be profitable.

But there is some point in attempting to make predictions. If the prediction extrapolates trends in technology, in social changes, and in the understanding and solution of social problems, one can define the boundary conditions for a variety of solutions. This will be our objective in a lim-

Reprinted from the *Journal of Agricultural and Food Chemistry*, Vol. 20, No. 3, May/June 1972, pp. 532–537. Copyright 1972 by the American Chemical Society and reprinted by permission of the copyright owner.

Presented at the Symposium on Chemical Aspects of Nutritional Needs,–161st ACS meeting, Los Angeles, California, March 30, 1971.

* Office of the Secretary, USDA; present address: Dept. of Community Medicine and International Health, Georgetown University, School of Medicine, Washington, D. C. 20007; and Office of Nutrition, Agency for International Development, Washington, D. C. 20523.

ited sort of a way.   We will not consider foods as an independent outgrowth of the individual efforts of food scientists.   Rather we will regard the nature of future foods as an interaction between social conditions and food science.

What will be the strains on our food supply and our ability to feed everyone in the world adequately?   There are the old strains intensified and a new one, pollution.   The old ones are war, population numbers, and poverty.   War always disrupts food supply and has been a major cause of famine.   Population growth in relation to the ability to produce food has always constituted a threat, but now constitutes a more intense threat. The fact that Malthus was wrong in his day does not free each generation from examining whether Malthus' time has come.   The problem of poverty is being intensified.   Although we are approaching an era of magnificent affluence in certain parts of the world, the spread between the affluent and the poor nations is increasing (Altschul, 1969).   Finally, pollution is not really a new problem but our keen awareness of its existence is new. We are now aware that this is a finite world whose capacity to absorb the indignities of man-made waste is limited.   And this affects the way we can use our land and our natural resources, which, in turn, affects the kinds of foods we can eat.

War and the threat of war always hang over man and his ability to take care of himself.   A new dimension is that war is not the only threat. Even without war the ordinary unchanged course of events with the prevailing growth of population, the increase in the spread between the affluent and the nonaffluent societies, and the increasing problem of pollution could produce stresses of a magnitude which could lead to disaster. We, therefore, have to assume, as the basis for continuance of stable societies, that progress will be made in removing or lessening social and economic strains.   Any predictions on food in the absence of assumed social progress are unrealistic indeed.

In the following sections we will list and discuss major trends and their effect on foods, and then try to take stock of where we might stand 10 to 15 years hence.

MAJOR TRENDS AND THEIR EFFECT ON FOOD

Public and political awareness of nutrition.   It is commonplace to hear that one cannot sell nutrition, that people buy foods primarily for their taste and appearance, and for the enjoyment they provide, rather than for nutrition.   It is probably true that in the order of food priorities caloric requirements are first (man eats to fill his belly), food aesthetics and enjoyment are second, and need to be adequately fed is third.   But the situation is changing.   No one can deny the emerging interest in nutrition not only among all cross-sections of the population in the United States but also in the developing countries. We suggest that the following conditions will become more widespread. There will be an increased willingness on the part of the public and its government to pay the increased cost of good nutrition and to support activities which improve nutrition. There will be increased insistence by the consumer that good nutritional quality be built into foods and that labeling be adequate so that the consumer can evaluate the nutritional quality of the food being purchased. More and more nations will institute regular surveillance procedures to measure food consumption and health as related to nutrition. These surveys will be on a regular basis and will permit corrective measures to be undertaken and later assessed. More examples will be seen of large scale intervention in the food supply to provide deficient nutrients at the lowest possible cost. This will hold equally for societies with poverty-based malnutrition or for affluent societies. Examples of the kinds of intervention already practiced are iodization of salt, fluoridation of water, the fortification of bread and cereal products with amino acids, vitamins, and minerals, the fortification of milk and milk products with vitamins, and the widespread acceptance of nutritional supplements.

It is expected that every country with the burden of supplying enough protein for its population will adopt a cereals policy to maximize the protein content of its major cereal foodstuffs by fortification with amino acids and protein concentrates, by breeding more protein into the cereals, or by a mixture of the two procedures. Thus the major cereal foods will become almost complete foods in themselves (Altschul and Rosenfield, 1970).

Flexibility in raw materials. There will be increased flexibility in the choice of raw materials from which one can fabricate foods. Natural food polymers and other natural complex chemical substances which have been the mainstay of our textured foods, the precursors of many of our flavors, and the basis of most of our beverages will meet increasing competition from man-made cheaper raw materials. Hence we can expect that textured foods from oilseed proteins and other protein sources will take an increasingly large share of the market during the next decade. However, even if their total volume becomes relatively high, their impact on the markets for natural animal foods will probably be small. But it would be folly indeed to predict the slope of the growth curve of these new food ingredients.

The flavor chemist and the food scientist have made impressive strides in incorporating meat-like texture, mouth feel, appearance, and flavor into protein products. Meat analogs from plant protein are a reality. Products resembling beef, ham, and chicken are available (Odell, 1967). In time their quality will improve and their production will increase.

Oilseed proteins can supplement meat protein as well as replace it. It has been estimated that 30 million pounds of soy protein are being used per year to improve processed meats such as chili, spaghetti sauce, Sloppy Joes, and pizza toppings and in bacon-like products.   Five years ago U. S. per capita consumption of soy protein was close to zero, now it is about 0.25 lb per year.   Five years from now it may be 5 lb per year and in 20 years a conservative estimate may be 20 lb per year (Robinson, 1969).

Meat production, too, is undergoing technological changes.   Breeding, animal selection, and feeding are developing animals that mature earlier and have less fat.   Processes have been developed that preform boneless fresh meat to a predetermined fat content.   Selected sections of meat may be reformed into more desirable shapes, such as chops or cubes of lean meat.

With further advances in both oilseed protein and meat technology, and with improvement in the control of texture and flavor, preportioned servings of meat analogs and extended meat products having a predetermined calorie content and protein value will become available.   The label on a future meat purchase might tell not only the weight and price of the item but also the calorie and utilizable protein content.   And, if the chemist's work in flavor and texture "pays off," a meaningful grade related to tenderness and flavor might also be included.

With the variety of meats, meat byproducts, and oilseed proteins that will be available to the processor, programming techniques will calculate on a day-to-day basis ingredient combinations to yield a standard product on a least cost basis.   Thus, uniformity of product and greater price stability will be engineered into this class of foods.

We have limited our remarks to oilseed proteins because their technology is farthest advanced but, obviously, fish protein concentrate (FPC), microbial protein, etc., are potential protein sources.   The probability of widespread commercial use of proteins other than those derived from oilseeds and fish for human food within the time span of the next decade is probably less than 10% (Bird *et al.*, 1968).   But this time scale may be shortened by intensive research and development in countries which lack adequate oilseed supplies.   As for FPC, its competitive position *vis-a-vis* oilseed proteins is not clear.   It may well prove out that fish protein may be a most important contributor to meeting protein needs but perhaps in a form other than FPC.

Just as meat proteins may be replaced by other protein polymers, coffee, tea, or cocoa may bow to the competition of man-made flavors.   Such a development could have immense consequences for the economies of many countries that now depend on these as their major cash crops.   This development can be likened in its economic impact to the effect of synthetic rubber on the existence of rubber plantations.

Engineered foods. The history of the human race is a history of food modification. Hardly any "natural" foods are left. Bread is certainly not a natural food; the invention of bread is probably one of the great inventions of all time. And the invention of texture in protein concentrates is likely, in time, to occupy a similar place in history. Modification of foodstuffs is not new at all. What is new is the engineering or fabrication of foods for special nutritional purposes. And even this concept is not so new. At the beginning of this century the first steps were taken to develop infant food formulas. These have evolved into the sophisticated products available today for all types of infants, with their allergies and specific nutritional needs.

Processed foods intended to be a complete meal will provide all of the nutrients expected from them. Already baked products are available that, together with a glass of milk, supply a complete breakfast. All sorts of combinations will be available to make it easier to provide food easily and at lower cost to such sensitive populations as school children. Bizarre food habits will be converted into adequate food habits by modification of the foods. This will cause no problem to the food industry but will shake the foundations of those who insist on maintaining traditional food patterns.

One panel of the White House Conference (White House Conference, 1970) recommended that major foods should be made as nutritionally complete as is possible without altering acceptability to the consumer. The Panel suggested that each of the basic foods should be fortified with nutrients selected to a level such that if the food were consumed as the sole source of an adequate caloric intake, it would supply complete daily nutrient needs. Since consumption of food is controlled by caloric intake, this concept would prevent either excessive or deficient intake of critical nutrients. This is already being done in a few selected instances for wheat and corn flour in the U. S. domestic Family Food Programs.

Foods which have lesser impact, *i. e.*, provide a smaller proportion of calories in the diet, will likewise be engineered to eliminate malnutrition or to make it easier to do so. For example, it is conceivable that soft drinks will be engineered to be complete foods on the basis of their caloric intake. It may be that the most popular soft drinks of the future will either be those which have no nutritional content, that is will contain no calories for those who desire no calories, or will become close to complete foods for those who need more nutrients. The same rationale may also be applied to snacks, which are assuming a more important role in the diet.

There could be a tendency to over-fortify; this can be controlled by proper government regulations and by exercising good judgment. Fortification will be based on the totality of the food intake in order to take advantage of blending of foods eaten together.

Variety in the classical sense of a variety of food commodities will become less significant as a means of achieving good nutrition in the face of increased consumption of complete meals made up of processed foods. This will provide an added incentive to engineer for better nutrition.

Food processing and preparation.   In general, techniques will resemble those of today.   Conventional and improved methods of canning, freezing, and dehydration will continue to play dominant roles.   Freeze-drying will continue to grow in popularity.   Freeze-dried products need no refrigeration.   In many instances flavor is superior to that of spray-dried or roller-dried products, since the removal of water at low temperature prevents the loss of flavor volatiles.   The reconstituted product is often indistinguishable in taste and smell from the fresh product.   Meats, shellfish, dairy products, eggs, vegetables, fruits, desserts, even salads can be freeze-dried and later rehydrated to yield products of excellent acceptability (Bird *et al.*, 1968).   The commercial success of freeze-dried coffee is a forerunner of things to come (Bird, 1969).

Currently freeze-drying is expensive, but more efficient methods and improved equipment and handling procedures will lower costs (Brockmann, 1970).   There are built-in economic advantages to freeze-drying that counterbalance higher processing costs, *e. g.*, fruits and vegetables may be produced under ideal growing conditions, freeze-dried near the growing site, and transported cheaply to faroff population centers since 70% or more of the product in the form of water may be left at the point of origin.

Boil-in-bag food (Bird *et al.*, 1968) is an example of convenience plus improved acceptability.   Centrally-processed vegetables are precooked, surrounded by a medium such as a precisely formulated, flavorful cream sauce, and packaged in a sealed plastic bag.   The vegetable is cooked by immersing the bag in hot or boiling water.   Since the pouch is sealed, cooking odors are eliminated; further, the product is not burnt or overheated. The technique is of course not limited to vegetables; the consumer buys, in addition to the fully prepared food, extra flavor, cleanliness, and convenience.   Some problems of stability of the products in-the-bag may require further technological improvements and very careful quality control.

Thus, as a result of improved techniques in packaging and in the preprocessing of foods prior to their final preparation step, we can expect our future foods to be more complete and to be more easily processed at home.

Legislation to minimize pollution of our environment and our food will have an impact on food processing and food utilization.   Obvious examples are solid waste disposal associated with feed lot operations and clean-up of effluents associated with canneries, dairies, slaughterhouses, etc.   Techniques to remove organic colloids and solutes from aqueous media need to be improved, and, equally important, techniques to utilize the recovered waste products need to be developed.   One can foresee that such cleanup procedures need not prove costly.   Just as the electrolytic refining of copper pays for itself in the gold and silver recovered as byproducts, the cleanup of plant wastes may also yield valuable byproducts.

Built-in services. Food companies, to increase product sales, have been building more services into the foods which they market. And the consumer for reasons of convenience and because of requirements of new life styles is accepting them. There is little doubt that increase convenience and variety will characterize the new generation of foods. "Convenience" foods will increasingly dominate the institutional and consumer markets. Convenience foods will be equally important in the developing world. A homemaker in the United States, if that is her sole job, may enjoy spending some time on food preparation. A woman in a less developed country, beset with an endless number of daily chores, may find any degree of labor- and time-saving in food preparation, even at some added cost, to be more than welcome.

Convenience foods for the affluent countries and for the developing world are as far apart as their technologies. In the U. S. it may mean "popping" an entire meal into a microwave oven. In Guatemala it may mean the purchase of a preground and prepackaged tortilla mix made from high lysine or fortified corn. In both instances convenience is equally welcome.

One countertrend to convenience foods may well emerge. As affluence and leisure time play an increasing role in our lives, more people will seek pastimes combining play and utility. Gourmet cooking is developing into one such endeavor. Specialty shops and organizations designed to bring exotic foods and drinks from around the world to amateur clients may become an expanding leisure-time business. And time spent in food preparation, home cooking, and concocting of flavorful sauces and desserts may become an all-absorbing avocation for at least some.

Institutional feeding. There will be an increase in the "away from home" eating market. With increasing affluence, more and more meals are consumed in restaurants, cafeterias, hotels, etc. One estimate is that by 1975 thirty-five billion dollars will be spent within the U. S. for food away from home (Bird *et al.*, 1968). And if the growth rate in population and income increase as in the past 10 years, a 50% increase can be anticipated by 1985. With so great a market, incentives for innovation abound.

It is not difficult to envision a completely automated restaurant of the future. The customer will indicate his food choices by proper notation on a data card. The data will be analyzed by computer, preportioned items will be selected, cooked, then assembled and delivered to the proper table in a time sequence determined by the customer as the meal proceeds; all steps will be automated and free of human intervention.

Institutions, where the final preparation of thousands of meals per hour is required demand more of innovation than the home. It is not merely a difference in the number of meals served that differentiates the home from the institution.   The institution presents an entirely different concept.   The institution must provide meals as attractive and nutritious as individually-prepared and served home meals.   Yet for most institutions, except high-priced restaurants, individual preparation is no longer practicable.   This puts a serious demand on technology to preserve flavor, color, and texture throughout the chain of events in institutional foods: factory-made, stored, delivered (often over long distances), reconstituted, and reheated.   But there are some advantages: there is a greater flexibility in choice of food ingredients over home-made foods.   And there is a greater flexibility in the choice of nutrients and control of cooking conditions to minimize damage during preparation.   Hence, foods in institutions could approximate the best nutrition achievable by current practice and knowledge.

We will look on institutional feeding, whether it is private or public, as a natural outgrowth of our way of life, of increased population, of increased urbanization, and of increased modernization.   Rather than rail against it and wish for the good old times, the better policy will be to utilize food dispensing institutions as a means of providing food and eliminating malnutrition under the best possible circumstances achievable.   There should be no excuse for malnutrition among any school age population exposed to school lunches.   And school lunches will not only be a simple way of providing a meal but will be part of intervention programs to furnish any deficient nutrients revealed by surveillance.

Sophisticated selection of foods.   Flexibility in ingredient composition and the trend toward production of complete foods will allow greater use of computers.   Such techniques are indispensable for producing low-cost nutritional meals and for developing specifically tailored diets.   Miller and Mumford (1970) described an approach to both of these problems.

Thus, to develop diets high or low in nitrogen, sodium, fat, and carbohydrates, appropriate foods are selected by the computer from basic data from food composition tables such as those published by the U. S. Department of Agriculture (Watt and Merrill, 1963) or by FAO (1970). Not all combinations make for an appetizing meal.   To formulate a palatable diet from a listing such as this, there must be an interaction between the dietitian and the computer.   The dietitian roughly constructs a diet from the selected foods to meet the individual's requirement.   The items are then fed into the computer which, in turn, calculates the exact nutrient content, notes deficiencies or excesses, and suggests foods to correct these.   The dietitian then amends the diet accordingly and thus builds up a palatable mixture of desired composition.   The entire process can be carried out at the computer keyboard.

Least cost diets can be prepared by a similar approach (Miller and Mumford, 1970).   As might be expected the major expenditures are for calories and protein; vitamin and mineral requirements can be met for a few pennies a day. Nutritionally satisfactory least cost diets must be modified to achieve consumer acceptability. At a conservative estimate, 25% of the cost even of the most economical diet is for nutrients and 75% is for palatability.

One major medical advance will be the increasing importance attached to preventive medicine. Insofar as knowledge permits, control of diet to prevent certain diseases will become more prevalent. It will be possible for a person to select a diet from specially engineered foods to meet any nutrition-engendered disease. For example, obesity is a major problem of the affluent society. It should be possible to control obesity by providing low calorie foods with built-in texture and flavor. In fact, it should prove possible to separate the enjoyment of food from nutrition—just as the enjoyment of sex can now be separated from procreation.

Properly tailored diets should provide control of metabolic defects involving nutrition. Here the problem involves limiting the intake of specific substances which cannot be metabolized, but at the same time supplying a relatively satisfactory diet. In some instances this can be done relatively simply, in others such as phenylketonuria (PKU), where phenylalanine must be restricted, the problem becomes more difficult.

It is difficult to define a normal diet. In addition to metabolic defects and allergies, we have individuals with anemias, malabsorption problems, diabetes, renal malfunctions, high cholesterol, etc. For each one of these individuals specific nutritional requirements must be met. The more we learn about the relationship between nutrition and disease the more specific we can be in defining the nutritional needs of the individual (Hegsted, 1970).

Better professional practice of nutrition and food science. We suppose that included in a discussion of new foods should be what might be expected of the people who are responsible for the new foods. It is quite clear that greater sophistication will be required in the practice of both nutrition and food science. The demands for the kinds of activities listed above can only be met by the highest type of professionalism in both of these areas. Much more information will be necessary in order to make possible the proper intervention and control of our food supply. One example is the need for better methods of testing populations for existence of protein deficiency problems.

Entirely new concepts of testing additives for safety are needed to replace the time-consuming and expensive methodologies now employed, which make it almost impossible to think of developing new kinds of foods or new concepts in foods without enormous expense. Moreover, the present methods are not always satisfactory in predicting what might happen in the human being. More fundamental studies will be required to determine the metabolism of new foods and food additives, and to try to relate this information to possible metabolic effects in the human.   There will need to be better methods for total surveillance of population and for monitoring new foods and additives so that changes can be made in accordance with new knowledge.   Everyone rejects the notion of experimentation on human beings.   Yet, in spite of all efforts taken to anticipate what might happen to humans from experience with prior experiments on animals (and sometimes with volunteers), the final experimental animal on a new food or for that matter on an old food under new conditions is the human being himself.   More attention will have to be given to the epidemiology of new foods and of old foods so that, continuously, information will be made available on what foods are doing for humans under real-life conditions.   All this requires new knowledge and new technology.

More knowledge is needed on the role of nutrition in improving performance of humans of various ages, and much more is needed on the role of nutrition in the etiology of specific diseases.

Food scientists will have to learn more about design of texture and flavor so as to be able to increase flexibility and utilize to the fullest extent the new raw materials that will become available for incorporation into foods.

DISCUSSION

There is no question that our foods have improved, no matter how you look at it.   The handling is better; they are cleaner, quality and flavor are better; uniformity is greater; quality standards and quality assurance are better.   The cost of foods has risen less rapidly than other costs of goods or services.

There have been regressions.   Flavors of certain artificially-ripened fruits and vegetables do not compare with the same products harvested under ideal conditions.   For those who preferred the stronger flavors of farm-fed poultry of 50 years ago to the bland and uniform flavor of the computer-fed and factory-produced poultry of today, this might be a regression.   Nero Wolf (a favorite gourmet of one of the authors) once extolled the virtues of ham made from peanut-fed hogs.   But this is a delicacy available to just a few.   And there will be other regressions forced by higher labor costs, increased problems of pollution control, and increased problems of transportation and marketing.

But balanced against these, for example, is the disappearance of seasonal foods.   Fruits and vegetables are available all year around from all parts of the world, preserved by advanced techniques, and flown to the market.   The acceptability and pleasurability of foods is in a dynamic state.   Advances in breeding and in agricultural practice, and newer knowledge about ripening, will improve our ability to market perishable items with least deterioration. We must not rule out the possibilities that flavors can be improved over what we now have or what we assume to be "natural" (Hornstein and Teranishi, 1967). We conclude that food science can cope with the increasing problems superimposed by a more complex society, and even get ahead.

Complaints are being voiced about nutritive quality of some classes of foods. Some foods which at first provided an insignificant proportion of the caloric intake have become, for certain age groups at least, important foods so that their nutritive value becomes an important consideration. There have been complaints about overstatement of virtues of certain foods. And there have been complaints about inadequate information on the labels. Above all these activities are symbolic of the greater awareness and interest in nutrition by the consumer, which we cited earlier. With this greater awareness will come more frequent expressions of satisfaction and dissatisfaction with the procedures and products of the food industry.

It is not our function to weigh the pros and cons of the arguments. But it is worth mentioning that the positive response of the American food industry to the challenges of the White House Conference on Food, Nutrition, and Health (1970) is an impressive social phenomenon and may be one of the important social developments of the last few years. An entire industry publicly recognized its share of responsibility for the nutrition and health of the American community and took specific steps, each company according to its ability and interests. In the Follow-up Conference held in February, Mr. James P. McFarland, (1971) speaking for the industry, summed up as follows: "As I look over the past year, I am impressed by what has been accomplished. It has been innovative, it has been constructive, and it has been substantial. And as I view where we are today, I am once again impressed—this time by how much more demands to be done. None of us in industry views today's session as anything more than a brief respite, a breathing spell that gives us the chance to make a progress report. Tomorrow, like yesterday, we'll be back on the firing line and working toward the full attainment of those goals we set for ourselves one year ago."

The present climate encourages the cooperation of government and industry to stimulate food innovation for social benefit. This uniquely favorable situation is a challenge to the leadership of both government and industry.

What will the foods of the future look like? We cannot rule out the appearance of entirely new and novel forms and flavors. These have appeared in soft drinks, breakfast foods, and in snacks. But, by and large, the appearance will be the same and the tastes or flavors more or less the same, even if the composition, processing, handling, stability, and packaging will differ.

Nutrition will become less a matter of chance.   One anthropologist, when asked about foods of the future said "A person will take a pill in the morning and eat whatever he likes the rest of the day."   This observation reflects an important and accepted part of our modern food culture: micronutrients are not just found in natural surroundings; they are equally available in pills, capsules, wafers, or liquid concentrates and the like. Affluent malnutrition which arises from lower calorie intakes, less variety in the nutritional sense, and a greater proportion of food eaten as processed food will be overcome by proper design of foods and food systems.   The strategies will include utilization of nutritional supplements, proper engineering of foods, and fortification.   And control of poverty-based malnutrition will be more easily attained, and at lower cost.

One could possibly be wildly optimistic that we are approaching a relationship of food to society undreamed of.

But this could all be a dream.   The time has passed that technology alone can overwhelm and transform societies regardless of other trends or conditions.   No longer is there automatic acceptance of technological innovation.   And food is no exception.

The public climate must be responsible and understanding.   Violent fluctuations in interest and position, and religious devotion to food fads could delay progress for years or decades.   One committee at the follow-up conference to the original White House Conference was moved to express itself as follows: "A.   *Balance between Knowledge and Action*.   In all of the food and health problems facing our society, we should recognize the need for a national balance between action and knowledge.   We do not know all we need to know about nutrition or safety, yet we must make decisions about new foods, old foods, additives, pesticides and environmental contaminants.   At any moment, our decisions should be balanced and sophisticated, recognizing that our knowledge is incomplete and that we must, therefore, choose among risks that cannot fully be known.   (For example: Shall we choose at the moment persistent pesticides or current supplies of food and fiber?)   We should recognize the relation between decisions on food and nutrition and other elements of our social fabric and should be reluctant to make extreme decisions of acceptance or abandonment without full and informed consideration of the consequences of such decisions" (White House Conference, 1971).

The ever-widening gulf between the affluent and poor nations continues to be a major cause of world instability; localized differences within a country contribute to national instability.   Technological improvements alone could further widen the gulf and exacerbate the instability. Whether or not we come closer to achieving the zenith of nutrition and food enjoyment that we can expect on the basis of knowledge and technology will depend on how well we solve all the rest of our problems.   It is not likely that society can get too far ahead of itself in any one aspect.

Conversely, new technology can stimulate new social effort and instill a sense of optimism. Surely, most of the food problems cannot be solved without the intervention of new technologies. When the new technologies appear, they stimulate hope and action. This influences action and rhetoric by governments in the field of the particular technology, but there is also some spillover to the other fields and problems.

New food technologies could be a generator of general social action and hope. And this might be the most important contribution of all.

LITERATURE CITED

1. Altschul, A. M., *Chem. Eng. News* 47, 68 (Nov. 24, 1969).
2. Altschul, A. M., Rosenfield, D., *Progress, The Unilever Quarterly* 54, 76 (1970).
3. Bird, K., *Food Technol.* 23, 1159 (1969).
4. Bird, K., Arthur, H., Goldberg, R., The Technological Front in the Food and Fiber Economy, Harvard Univ. Sch. Business Administration, Boston, Mass., June 1968.
5. Brockmann, M. C., *Chem. Eng. Progr. Symp. Ser.* 66, 51 (1970).
6. Food and Agriculture Organization, "Amino Acid Composition of Foods: Nutritional Studies No. 24," Rome, Italy (1970).
7. Hegsted, D. M., *J. Amer. Diet. Ass.* 56, 303 (1970).
8. Hornstein, I., Teranishi, R., *Chem. Eng. News* 45, 92 (April 3, 1967).
9. McFarland, J. P., White House Conference on Food, Nutrition and Health, Report of Follow-up Conference, p 14 (1971).
10. Miller, D. S., Mumford, P., *Proc. Nutr. Soc.* 29, 116 (1970).
11. Odell, A. D. Proceedings of International Conference on Soybean Protein Foods, Agricultural Research Service, USDA, ARS 71–35, May 1967, p 163.
12. Robinson, H. E., Swift and Co., Chicago, Ill., personal communication, 1969.
13. Watt, B. K., Merrill, A. L., "Composition of Foods," Agr. Handbook No. 8, U. S. Dept. of Agriculture, Washington, D.C. (1963).
14. White House Conference on Food, Nutrition and Health, Final Report, U.S. Gov't Printing Office 1970, p 118.
15. White House Conference on Food, Nutrition and Health, Report of Follow-up Conference, p 36 (1971).

41

FACT AND FANCY IN NUTRITION AND FOOD SCIENCE

Thomas H. Jukes *

The theme of this convention, I was told, is "The Dietitian in the Age of Aquarius." This seems a highly appropriate title, reflecting as it does the current preoccupation with the signs of the Zodiac—a turning back of the clock to the age of mysticism and superstition. I recently saw a cartoon which showed two loan desks in a public library, one for astronomy and the other for astrology. The astronomy desk was deserted, but many readers were crowded around the other desk. I am reasonably convinced that we stand on the threshold of a new Dark Age, which we shall enter unless, perhaps, enough of us can keep the light of scientific knowledge burning—for, without science and technology, our food supply will soon dwindle and few things cause human beings to break down as rapidly as an insufficiency of food.

Much publicity has been given to the announcement that a majority of students preferred organically-grown foods, when offered a choice in a campus restaurant on the Santa Cruz campus of the University of California. Either no one has told them, or they don't believe, that there is no such thing as organic plant nutrition. Plants utilize only inorganic forms of plant food. Compost and manure are broken down by bacteria to components, such as nitrate, potassium ion, and phosphate, before they

Reprinted from *Journal of The American Dietetic Association*, Vol. 59, No. 3, September 1971. © The American Dietetic Association. Printed in U.S.A.

Presented at the joint meeting of the California and Nevada Dietetic Associations in Las Vegas on April 19, 1971.

* Division of Medical Physics, Donner Laboratory, University of California, Berkeley.

are assimilated.   Hydroponics, in which plants are grown inorganically without soil, leads to the production of vegetables and fruits with the same protein, carbohydrate, vitamin, and mineral content as when the same strains of plants are grown in the ground with lots of manure.   An important difference is that organically grown vegetables are more likely to carry Salmonella, which leads to a common form of food poisoning.   Salmonella has recently been reported to be present in vegetables in Holland, grown with the organic benefits of sewage effluent (1).

The book, *Silent Spring* (2), which contained pleasant statements, such as "We are in little better position than the guests of the Borgias," is used in many public and high schools as an authoritative text.   Many imitators have followed the same approach in fomenting alarm against agricultural chemicals, and, as a result, the public is questioning the quality of our abundant and nutritious food supply, the safest, cheapest, most diverse and best in the history of the world.   I say cheapest in terms of hours of work necessary for the average person to exchange for his daily food supply when purchased in the open market.   Only within the past forty years or so has it become possible to buy numerous delicious fruits, vegetables, meats and dairy products free from contamination, fresh, canned or frozen, at any time of the year.   Remember that we are only two generations away from the days when food was frequently polluted with cockroaches, rat filth, insect parts, tuberculosis bacteria, meal-worms, weevils, and molds.   The fungus, *Phytophthoria infestans*, that destroyed the potato crop in Ireland and caused the famine, is still around.   A sample of what could happen on a large scale was seen last year when another blight swept through many corn fields in the eastern United States.   As a result of scientific agriculture, in 1971, a broiler chicken costs less in *actual, inflated* cents per pound than it did in cents per pound in the depth of the Depression.

Unless we are vigilant, however, all this will vanish, dissipated by a destructive and vociferous few who have grown up to think that food comes right out of the floor of the supermarket.   Two years ago, I said in a talk in Seattle: "Perhaps man cannot understand how precious food is unless he has to toil to produce it himself, fighting against drought, blight, and insects for the privilege of getting something to eat.   Can we learn without repeating such bitter experiences?"   I believe that dietitians have a great responsibility to instruct and lead the new urban generation in the facts of nutrition and food science.

SOME TOXICOLOGIC PRINCIPLES

Let me emphasize certain fundamental points regarding measurement of the effects of chemicals.   First, tests carried out by injecting a chemical are usually meaningless in terms of residues present in foods.   Injecting sodium glutamate, or DDT, or distilled water into baby rats will injure or kill them, especially if the quantity is large.   Therefore, the first rule is that the route of administration must be by mouth.

Next comes the quantity used.   It is astonishing to see, repeatedly, newspaper articles with scare headlines describing the toxic effects of some enormous dose of a chemical such as 2,4,5–T, inferring that this incriminates tiny amounts in food.   Several essential nutrients or metabolites are recognized poisons at levels that do not greatly exceed the daily requirement or the amount naturally in the body.   Examples are copper, iodine, selenium (which is a carcinogen), table salt, hydrochloric acid, and hydroxyl ion.

The next point, which is frequently raised when it is pointed out that the dosage is small, is the cumulative effect.   Alarmists often say that traces of any residue will be retained by the body and will build up to dangerous levels.   Actually no completely cumulative effect exists.   There is always some excretion, and the total amount stored represents the balance between intake and excretion.   Let me quote Professor Wayland Hayes, Jr. (3):

> Compounds which are absorbed tend to reach a steady state of storage and for each compound the storage at equilibrium corresponds to dosage. People not trained in the biological sciences are usually unfamiliar with these facts and suppose that compounds are of two distinct sorts, those that are stored and those that are not.   They suppose that compounds that are stored at all continue to accumulate indefinitely with no tendency to reach a steady state in which the amount lost each day is equal to the amount absorbed.   It may seem odd to mention this folklore . . . but the views of the public are a most important factor, which must be taken into account in any long-term effort to achieve general public acceptance of a particular usage or course of action.

The balance or reservoir of a chemical in the body will depend on the species of animal, the rate of metabolism of the substance, and its chemical properties.   One compound that is most frequently under attack as being stored in the body from food residues is DDT.   DDT is not cumulative.   It is stored in the fat and is steadily broken down and excreted in the urine.   If the daily intake goes down, the level in the fat drops.   There is a straight line relationship which has been worked out in several careful experiments, as shown by Hayes (3).   The average amount of DDT in the fat of the general American population is progressively dropping, year by year because the amount used in agriculture has been reduced (Table 1).

The next point is one that I should probably have mentioned first: How reliable is the test method?   There is a delicate analytical procedure called gas liquid chromatography with electron capture.   Sometimes I wonder whether this method, in the hands of inexpert people, has done more harm than good.   There has been a great hue and cry over alleged traces of DDT in Antarctic penguins, amounts of the order of 1 or 2 parts per billion. I have not yet been convinced of the validity of the results. A few months ago, at the University of Wisconsin, some soil samples that had been sealed since 1910 were tested for synthetic organo-chlorine pesticides by the latest and most delicate gas chromatographic procedure. Several pesticides were detected in thirty-two of the thirty-four samples (5). The only flaw was that these pesticides not only were not used in 1910, they didn't even exist until after 1940! Another complication is that residues of a class of modern compounds called polychlorinated biphenyls (PCB's) interfere with the DDT test (5). The PCB's are used in water-proofing compounds, asphalt, waxes, synthetic adhesives, hydraulic fluids, electrical apparatus, and generally in plastics. They are widely distributed in the fat of wildlife species, in which they have originated as industrial wastes taken up by aquatic species. They overlap in the test with DDT and its metabolic breakdown products, DDD and DDE. PCB's are sufficiently toxic to kill fish in hatcheries (5). To sum up, PCB's are not used as pesticides, but they interfere with pesticide residue analysis, and they are toxic.

Thus, I don't believe the stories of "newspaper scientists" about pesticide residues until they have been published in the scientific literature, scrutinized, and reliably confirmed.

MERCURY

This brings us to the current concern over mercury: Has it always been there anyway? In this case: Yes.

Sources of mercury may be either industrial and technologic or natural (6). The industrial sources include coal smoke, chlor-alkali plants which use mercury electrodes, plastic manufacture, fungicides (such as methyl mercury dicyanodiamide, used as a seed dressing), slimicides (used in the paper industry), and electrical equipment. About 200 gm. mercury may be used per ton of chlorine manufactured, and it has been estimated to add up to a total of 300,000 lb. mercury annually in Canada and 500,000 in the United States. A large amount of this got into the Great Lakes and information on mercury in fish was published in Canada after eighteen months of government investigation. It was disclosed that unacceptably high levels of mercury were present in many fish caught in inland waters where they had ingested methyl mercury formed by bacteria in bottom muds. The industrial use of mercury in Sweden appears to have led to decreases in bird populations, together with paralytic symptoms in the birds, which, of course, were blamed on DDT. However, the most tragic incident of mercury pollution was in Japan, where more than fifty people, including babies, died in the 1950's from "Minamata disease," caused by eating fish and shellfish contaminated with mercury in the effluent of a chemical plant. Some of the shellfish sampled from 1956 to 1958 contained 9 to 24 p.p.m. (wet basis); a level of 5 to 6 p.p.m. in the diet is regarded as potentially lethal.

The second source of mercury is natural. Interest in this was triggered by industrial contamination, following which some samples of canned tuna were found to contain about 1 p.p.m. mercury. This set off a shock wave of publicity, and 12.5 million cans of tuna were removed from the market. It was then reported that mercury concentrations in tuna caught ninety years ago are about the same as those in recently caught fish (6). It was also found that swordfish commonly contained 1 or 2 p.p.m. mercury, even when they were caught in ocean waters hundreds of miles from possible industrial contamination.

The presence of mercury in sea water has been known and measured ever since 1777. All the metals known in the earth's crust, including gold, are present in sea water. Some marine organisms concentrate them from sea water; for example, shrimp concentrate arsenic to a level "higher than the government allows." Seaweed picks up iodine. And apparently, swordfish and tuna frequently concentrate natural mercury to a point higher than the tolerance set by the Food and Drug Administration. The residues are higher in older fish. The following statement was in the *Marine Pollution Bulletin* for January 1971 (7):

> If one considers that there is a natural occurrence of mercury in the sea of between 0.03 and 0.3 parts per billion and that tuna fish has a higher respiration rate than most other edible fish, swimming continuously and passing large quantities of water over its gill surfaces, and that it can accumulate metals in its tissues at concentrations thousands of times greater than those in the water, it could be that the phenomenon we are observing is caused not by levels of mercury increased by pollution, but by the unusual susceptibility of the tuna fish to the naturally occurring mercury.

Such a situation is quite difficult for regulatory authorities to accept mentally. For example, FDA Commissioner Charles C. Edwards was quoted (8) as follows:

> *Q.* What about the mercury content in swordfish?
>
> *A.* We're wrestling with that. We're not quite as far along as with tuna, but I think before too long we'll be able to say that all swordfish left on the market is clean.
>
> *Q.* Is there some on the market now that isn't?
>
> *A.* I suspect there is. Again, we're working with the industry. Some 85 to 90 per cent of the swordfish that we've been testing has been running over our guideline.
>
> *Q.* How much over?
>
> *A.* Quite a little more than tuna. Some samples have been running over 1 part per million. But swordfish is a somewhat different problem than tuna because the consumption in the U. S. is considerably less.

This remarkable piece of semantic gymnastics should be examined in the light of the facts that mercury is toxic, regardless of its origin, that "natural" mercury in swordfish is commonly above the "safe" level set by the FDA and that this level (0.5 p.p.m.) is ten times as high as that proposed to the World Health Organization (0.05 p.p.m.), which would effectively remove most fish as an article of human diet. Deposits of mercury ores, such as cinnabar, are present in the coastal and foothill ranges of northern California, where mercury is mined, and inevitably mercury gets into the streams. On May 2, 1971, for example, the fish in Almaden reservoir, California, were found to contain up to 4 or 5 p.p.m. mercury. The pollution was believed to result from "numerous ancient mercury mines in the area."

Is the FDA tolerance for mercury too strict? It is one tenth of the potentially lethal level. Compare the mercury tolerance with the DDT level (0.05 p.p.m.) permitted in milk and note that levels of DDT thousands of times as high as this have been consumed for prolonged periods without any evidence of harm (Table 1).

Table 1: Dosage response of DDT in man *

Dosage	Remarks
mg./kg./day	
? † ‡	Fatal
16–286 †	Prompt vomiting at higher doses (all poisoned, convulsions in some)
10 †	Moderate poisoning in some
6 †	Moderate poisoning in one man
0.5	Tolerated by volunteers for 21 months
0.5	Tolerated by workers for 6.5 yr.
0.25	Tolerated by workers for 19 yr.
0.004	Dosage of Indians, 1964; combined intake from living in sprayed houses and from food
0.0025	Dosage of general population of U.S., 1953–1954
0.0004	Current dosage of general population of U.S.

* From WHO statement, January 22, 1971 (4).
† One dose only.
‡ Dosage unknown.

The reason for this incongruity is, of course, that condemning nature is unpopular. The dogma of the environmentalists seems to be that "only man is vile." Puffer fish, blowfish, loco weed, and rattlesnake bites are all both "natural" and toxic. Mercury poisoning is especially unpleasant because it causes brain damage and affects unborn babies.

What are we going to do about it? We will have to establish a tolerance for mercury and make a mental adjustment to it, for mercury, like all the elements, is naturally present in all living organisms, including fish. It is most interesting that mercury residues were first shown to come from industrial pollution; then, as a result of this discovery, levels of mercury in fish, arising from natural sources, were shown to reach potentially toxic proportions.

THE "DELANEY CLAUSE"

Our next point is the celebrated Delaney anti-cancer clause in the federal Food, Drug and Cosmetic Act. The effect of this is to require the removal from interstate commerce of any food which contains analytically detectable amounts of a food additive shown to be capable of inducing cancer in experimental animals (9).

This law is impossible to enforce and impossible to repeal. Rivers of ink have been spilled on it. Many naturally occurring food ingredients are known to be carcinogenic (10) and at least one essential nutrient, selenium, is a carcinogen (11). Iodine *deficiency* will produce tumors in experimental animals. All the steroid sex hormones are carcinogenic in animals, and so is cholesterol. The barbecuing of meat products identifiable carcinogens.

The Delaney clause does not permit tolerances; thus any detectable amount, even one molecule, comes within the meaning of the Act. It is sometimes argued that there is no threshold level for a stimulus that produces cancer, but this concept cannot be true for the tumors produced by iodine deficiency. Nor can it be true for selenium. Furthermore, the dose-response curves plotted against time sometimes show that at low levels of a carcinogen, the predictable occurrence of cancer would take more than a lifetime to be reached.

Similar problems exist with respect to mutagenic and teratogenic substances because these are always present in foods, and mutations are a normal process of all life. Evolution cannot take place without the constant occurrence of mutations.

DDT AND MALARIA—PRESENT STATUS

DDT is specifically needed to protect millions of people in tropical countries from death by malaria. This has repeatedly been made plain by the World Health Organization, for example (12):

> The withdrawal of DDT would mean the interruption of most malaria programs throughout the world . . .   DDT used as a residual spray of the interior surfaces of houses . . . led to the idea of nation-wide malaria control campaigns including the whole of the rural areas of a country. The success of these campaigns resulted in the con-

cept of malaria eradication which was adopted . . . for the world by the World Health Assembly in May, 1955.

Since then DDT has been the main weapon in the world-wide malaria eradication program. Research has continued for the development of other methods of attack against malaria and for the development of alternative insecticides. To date, there is no insecticide that could effectively replace DDT which would permit the continuation of the eradication program or maintain the conquests made so far.

The withdrawal of DDT will represent a regression to a malaria situation similar to that in 1945. The reestablishment of malaria endemicity would be probably attained following a period of large scale outbreaks and epidemics which would be accompanied by high morbidity and mortality due to loss of immunity by populations previously protected by eradication programs.

This prediction has been fulfilled in Ceylon (4). To continue (12):

Toxicological observations of spraymen working for a number of years in malaria eradication and even in formulation plants, has not revealed toxic manifestations in them. Neither has there been any evidence of toxicologic manifestations in people residing in houses that have been repeatedly sprayed at six-month intervals.

We therefore believe that a great harm will result from the unqualified withdrawal of DDT. We feel that selective use of DDT is justified and warranted.

This is what the argument is all about. If the manufacture and export of DDT are banned in the United States, the world-wide anti-malarial program will collapse. Most of the DDT manufactured domestically is for this program. Furthermore, a ban in the United States would lead to prejudice against the use of DDT elsewhere.

The substitute insecticides are more expensive and more profitable than DDT. These substitutes can be used, with varying degrees of lower efficiency, against the agricultural pests controlled by DDT. But, there is no effective substitute for DDT in the world campaign against malaria. The other compounds either decompose rapidly, produce resistance too fast, or they are too poisonous to people.

Malaria is caused by a microscopic parasite of the genus *Plasmodium*. These parasites spend part of their life-cycle in mosquitoes, but the cycle is not complete without going through several stages in man, where they reach maturity in the red blood cells and reproduce, in enormous numbers, into a form called *merozoites*. These change into the sexual stage which enters the body of a blood-sucking mosquito. Other stages of the life-cycle then take place, and the parasite reaches the salivary gland of the mosquito, from which it is inoculated into the next victim to be bitten. The cycle then continues from man to mosquito and mosquito to man. The principal method for breaking this pernicious chain is to kill mosquitoes with DDT by spraying the interior walls of human dwellings.

Public health authorities in the tropics commonly use a figure of 1 per cent per year to estimate the mortality from malaria; thus the 75 million cases in India were calculated to be responsible for 750,000 deaths annually (33). The survivors in many cases are severely debilitated and unable to work. The effects aimed for in the mosquito control program are based on the following conditions: The mosquitoes rest on the walls by day and attack sleeping people at night. The DDT on the walls kills the mosquitoes, and for this purpose, an insecticide must be *persistent* because it is not possible for spray teams to go into the same house frequently.

As a result of international cooperation, WHO has had a world-wide malaria eradication program so that (14):

> Today more than 960 million people who a few years ago were subject to malaria endemicity are now free of malaria; another 288 million live in areas where the disease is being vigorously attacked and transmission is coming to an end. Because much of Africa remains highly malarious and because about 288 million people live in malarious areas not yet subject to eradication measures, it is logical that the United States should maintain an active interest in this disease.

These estimates indicate that the U. S. contribution to saving lives from malaria has paid off quite well in terms of human welfare. As I said recently, however, "Some Americans, by demanding a ban on DDT, are reversing the traditional role of their country in relieving the sufferings of others" (15).

DDT IN HUMAN MILK

One of the organizations leading the fight on DDT is the Environmental Defense Fund (EDF). A recent newspaper article on the EDF stated:

> The turning point came when Cameron decided to spend $5,000 of the organization's total remaining assets of $23,000 on an advertisement in the New York *Times* on Sunday, March 29, headlined 'Is Mother's Milk Fit for Human Consumption?' It referred to the amounts of DDT in the human body.
>
> The ad appealed for members, starting at $10 for a basic membership. It produced $7,000, a profit, and the EDF turned to a direct mail campaign and now has 10,000 members, a stable financial base and a chance at major foundation support.

This is most interesting. The EDF appealed to the public on the basis of the DDT content of human milk. As a means of arousing alarm concerning DDT, the EDF and the National Audubon Society have both stated that DDT causes cancer. The implication that DDT in breast milk may cause cancer in babies is superlatively sensational copy. The following lurid passage appeared in *Purple Martin Capital News*, July 29, 1970, as a quotation from an article by Ed Chaney, Information Director of National Wildlife Federation, in *Conservation News*, June 15, 1970:

> A five-day-old human being lies asleep in the other room. His name is Eric. His tiny, wiggly, red body contains DDT passed on to him from his mother's placenta. And every time he sucks the swollen breasts, he gets more DDT than is allowed in cow's milk at the supermarket. Be objective? Forget it. Objective is for fence posts. How can you be objective in the face of a global insanity that is DDT? In the face of abdicated responsibility by the men the public pays to protect its interests? Are the anarchists right? Are ashes the only fertile seed bed for growing new responsiveness to the public interest? Picture a swarm of angry citizens bathed in the light of flames engulfing the Agriculture Department.

It is distressing that an official of a large organization should discard objectivity and purpose anarchy in its stead. It is also distressing to read such absolute rubbish when DDT has saved the lives of hundreds of thousands of babies who otherwise would have died from one of the most lethal of diseases, infantile malaria, which Sir Macfarlane Burnet in 1953 called "the main agent of infantile mortality in the tropics." In the years following 1953, this disease was stopped in many countries by DDT.

Let us examine the factual and scientific background for the propaganda campaign regarding DDT in human milk. Improvements in technology have made it possible to detect fantastically small quantities of DDT. But, such extremely delicate tests can easily give "false positive" readings because of accidental contamination of the equipment or lack of expertise by the tester. Next, cow's milk has occupied an unusual position among foods with respect to regulations. "Zero tolerance" has been the policy with respect to additives to milk, except for vitamin D. The improvements in testing procedures made it necessary to re-examine the definition of zero, since every chemist knows that zero content, in molecular terms, does not exist. More than ten years ago, it was evident that the entire stocks of canned milk in the United States gave positive tests for DDT. It was, therefore, necessary to face facts, and two choices were available: to ban cow's milk from interstate commerce or to set a tolerance.

The latter choice was taken, and the tolerance set was 0.05 p.p.m. This was a far lower level than the 7 p.p.m. which was permitted for most agricultural products. A rule-of-thumb for tolerance levels is 1 per cent of the toxic dose which is lethal to 50 per cent of a group of experimental animals. Obviously, if 7 p.p.m. had been estimated to be non-injurious, a tolerance of 0.05 p.p.m. provided an unusually large margin of safety. The low tolerance was possible primarily because cows effectively metabolize and break down DDT, and also because great attention was paid to avoiding the use of DDT on crops, such as alfalfa, which are consumed by dairy cattle. In contrast, human beings are less efficient than cows in metabolizing DDT, and they do not eat hay. There is a straight-line relationship between DDT intake and DDT level in body fat.

The DDT in human beings enters the fat of breast milk. This was noted in 1950 by Laug and co-workers (16), who found an average concentration of DDT of 0.13 p.p.m. in thirty-two samples taken in Washington, D. C., with a range from undetectable ("zero") to 0.77 p.p.m. Several similar reports have since appeared.

The level of DDT in human milk is about twice as high as the FDA tolerance allowed in cow's milk. This statement needs an explanation of its background and meaning in terms of toxicology. Using the unexplained statement to alarm the public, particularly nursing mothers, is a scientifically irresponsible act.

The World Health Organization and the Food and Agricultural Organization of the United Nations set a permissible rate of intake of 0.01 mg. DDT per kilogram body weight for breast-fed infants. The DDT intake of breast-fed babies in the United States may be higher than this; estimates range from 0.014 to 0.02 mg. per kilogram per day at birth, if the infant consumes 600 ml. (about 1⅓ pt.) of breast milk daily. As the infant grows, the intake of milk on a per-kilogram basis decreases because food intake per unit of body weight lessens when the size of an animal increases and because breast-fed infants usually receive supplementary feeding with other foods.

The "permissible rate" set by the WHO–FAO, according to the chairman of the meeting that established the value, is highly conservative, and he points out (13):

> It offers a safety factor of about 25 compared with what workers in a DDT manufacturing plant have tolerated for 19 years without any detectable clinical effect (see Laws *et al.*, Arch. Environ. Health 15:766–775, 1967). The safety factor of the WHO-FAO permissible rate is 150 compared to the dosage of DDT given daily for 6 months to a patient with congenital unconjugated jaundice without producing any side effects (Thompson *et al.*, Lancet II [7610] :2–6, July 5, 1969.)

> Infants are more susceptible than adults to some compounds, but the difference is seldom great—usually about 2 to 3 times. In a study of 49 different compounds, newborn rats were found to vary from 5 times less susceptible to 10 times more susceptible than adults. Although there is no information on the relative susceptibility of human infants and adults to DDT, it was shown by Lu *et al.* (Food and Cosmetic Toxic. 3:591–596, 1965) that weanling rats are slightly more resistant than adult rats to this compound, and that preweanling rats are more than twice as resistant and newborn rats are over 20 times more resistant than adults.

Evidently it is possible for breast-fed infants to obtain DDT from the milk at a level up to twice the WHO–FAO "permissible rate." Again, the voluminous and carefully-documented background information indicates that no toxic effects have been detected or could be anticipated at this level, in babies, children, or adults. The levels of DDT encountered in various conditions and the effects of some of these levels are summarized in Table 1.

ANTIOXIDANTS

Several workers have found that mice and rats fed diets with large amounts of added antioxidants live longer than those fed standard laboratory diets (17–20). The antioxidants include vitamin E, 2-mercaptoethylamine, ethoxyquin, butylated hydroxytoluene (BHT), and nordihydroguaiaretic acid (NDGA). The rationale for the effect is that natural and radiation-induced aging may be accompanied by a free-radical attack on lipids, including mitochondrial lipids, and this effect may be buffered by antioxidants (17). In a longevity experiment with mice fed a diet containing 0.5 per cent ethyoxyquin, the mice fed the antioxidant had an 18 per cent increase in average life span over the controls (20). The authors suggest as one explanation that many antioxidants are powerful enzyme inducers; ethyoxyquin may cause liver enlargement. They suggest that "experiments with other potent enzyme inducers, such as DDT or barbiturates, seem to be necessary."

ANTIBIOTICS IN ANIMAL FOODS

Antibiotics have been used successfully in feeding farm animals for twenty years. The procedure results in lower morbidity, lower mortality, more rapid gains in body weight, and an increase in the efficiency with which livestock feed is converted into human foods, such as meat and eggs. The value of antibiotics in feeds is due to the fact that domestic animals live in an environment that is universally contaminated with harmful microorganisms, many of which are susceptible to antibiotics.

The use of antibiotic supplements in commercial feeds was rapidly and widely adopted, starting in 1950 to 1952, as a means of improving the growth of poultry, pigs and calves (21). The levels used were low, usually 10 gm. or less of antibiotic per ton of feed. The practice gave satisfactory results over prolonged periods, and investigations soon turned to the use of higher levels in the treatment or prevention of certain endemic diseases of livestock.

Many members of the public are asking questions about antibiotic residues in their food. What quantities of such residues are present in food produced from domestic animals and what are their pharmacologic as well as their bacteriologic effects? These points will be discussed with chlortetracycline as an example, in view of its wide use in animal feeds.

The amounts present in chicken tissues following the feeding of chlortetracycline were measured by Broquist and Kohler (22) as summarized in Table 2. The antibiotic was not detectable in the muscle meat until a

Table 2: Chlortetracycline (CTC) in tissues of chickens *

CTC in diet	CTC in tissue		
	Blood serum	Liver	Muscle
		Experiment 1	
		p.p.m.	
0	0	0	0
200	0 −0.01	0	0
600	0.011–0.024	0 −0.10	0
2,000	0.039–0.024	0.14–0.30	0.05–0.16
		Experiment 2	
0	0	0	0
2,000	0.06 −0.10	0.15–0.49	0.05–0.10
6,000	0.09 −0.35	0.18–0.39	0.08–0.33

* From Broquist and Kohler (22). Five replicate groups of 5 chickens each used at each level.

level was fed that is about ten times as high as any that is used continuously in practice. Additional experiments with an even more sensitive method using *Bacillus mycoides* spores showed that the muscle meat of chickens fed 50 p.p.m. chlortetracycline for twelve weeks contained less than 1 part per 100 million of the antibiotic as a residue. More recent experiments by Shor, Abbey, and Gale (23) have produced essentially similar findings (Table 3). For example, chickens fed 2,000 gm. chlortetracycline per ton of feed, which is about ten times as much as is used in practice, had 0.63 p.p.m. antibiotic in their flesh. To get an average dose of chlortetracycline, a dose commonly prescribed for home use for patients by physicians, a person would have to eat 1 ton of raw chicken meat at a sitting! If the chickens were taken off feed for a day, the amount of raw chicken would have to be 10 tons, and if the meat were cooked, the antibiotic would be destroyed. Truly, the public in 1971 is being encouraged to get worried about nonsense.

The effect of cooking on chlortetracycline residues in beef, fish, and chicken meat was studied during extensive studies of chlortetracycline in the prevention of food spoilage. Broquist and Kohler found (22) that chlortetracycline disappeared from poultry meat on roasting (Table 4). The degradation product during cooking was identified as isochlortetracycline (24) which has an oral LD_{50}[1] in mice greater than 10 gm. per kilogram and has no known antibacterial effect.

Table 3: Chlortetracycline (CTC) residues in chicken tissues after oral administration for 5 days*

Time after withdrawal	Average CTC tissue concentration			
	Muscle	Liver	Kidney	Fat
	800 Gm. CTC per Ton in Diet			
days		— *mcg./gm.* —		
0	0.38	0.90	6.44	0.09
1	0.01	0.02	0.16	neg †
3	neg †	0.01	0.12	neg †
	2,000 Gm. CTC per Ton in Diet			
0	0.63	1.55	11.8	0.17
1	0.05	0.07	0.49	0.01
3	neg †–0.02	0.02	0.20	neg †
6	neg †	neg †	0.11	neg †

* From Shor *et al.* (23).

† No activity or less than 0.025 mcg. per gram.

For several years, chlortetracycline and oxytetracycline were used for delaying spoilage of poultry meat and fresh fish. The application to fish was especially useful in Japan and in Canada, where it was developed by Tarr at the Canadian Government Laboratories in British Columbia (25). No side effects of public health problems arose, but the FDA authorization for this use was withdrawn about three years ago, as a result of theoretical considerations raised by bacteriologists, who suggested that bacterial resistance might develop.

Table 4: Effect of roasting at 230° F. on chlortetracycline (CTC) in chicken breast muscle *

Cooking time	Residual CTC in muscle			
	0.03 mg. CTC/ml. dipping solution	0.1 mg. CTC/ml. dipping solution	0.3 mg. CTC/ml. dipping solution	1.0 mg. CTC/ml. dipping solution
min.		— *p.p.m.* —		
0	8.25 †	25.0	60.0	120.0
15	none	none	0.33	1.15
30	none	none	none	0.31

* From Broquist and Kohler (22).

† A level of 8.25 p.p.m. CTC is about 13 times as high a level in meat as resulted from feeding CTC at 2,000 p.p.m. in the diet (23). This, in turn, is about 5 times as high as any level used in feeding animals.

[1] LD_{50} indicated level of dosage that is lethal to 50 per cent of the test group.

Tarr found (25) that heating salmon or lingcod flesh containing 5 to 10 p.p.m. chlortetracycline was followed by destruction of at least 80 to 90 per cent of antibiotic. Similarly Tomiyama *et al.* reported (26) that chlortetracycline disappeared from bonito fillets heated for 60 min. at 93°. The fillets originally contained 21 p.p.m. of the antibiotic.

Chlortetracycline is an unstable substance and decomposes fairly rapidly in meat even at refrigerator temperatures. Goldberg *et al.* found (27) that 2 p.p.m. added to ground beef disappeared after 96 hr. of storage at 10°.

Chlortetracycline (CTC) was in extensive commercial use as a food additive for a number of years in Canada for delaying spoilage in poultry meat. The raw meat was dipped in a solution of the antibiotic. This practice was valuable because it enabled the effects of residues to be studied at a higher level than that occurring in the meat of chickens fed the antibiotic as an animal feed ingredient. Thatcher and Loit of the Canadian Food and Drug Directorate carried out microbiologic examinations of commercial poultry meat samples, both untreated and treated with chlortetracycline, for various microbial categories (28). Salmonella was isolated from only one specimen of treated poultry meat, but was present in sixteen untreated samples. Four serotypes were recognized, including *S. typhimurium.* Cell isolates grew in broth containing 0.21 p.p.m. of CTC, but none grew at 0.43 p.p.m. Thatcher and Loit commented that "no data to indicate an increased health hazard as a result of the use of CTC as a poultry preservative were obtained. No evidence was revealed for modification of hazard due to the presence of staphylococci, enterococci, coliforms, or pathogenic yeasts."

The effects of prolonged feeding of antibiotics to human subjects were investigated during 1950 to 1955 (29). Reports in the medical literature reviewed up to 1956 described the long-term administration of chlortetracycline to 889 patients, all under close medical supervision, and drawn from all age groups: Approximately half were subjected to extensive clinical tests, including blood and bone marrow examinations and liver function tests. No evidence of toxicity from the antibiotic was found. In one study (30), two patients received 3 to 4 gm. chlortetracycline daily over twenty-one- and eleven-month periods, respectively. Initially, and every three months, liver biopsy and sternal marrow samples were examined. A peripheral blood study and urinalysis were done weekly, blood non-protein nitrogen monthly, electrocardiograms every two months, and also urinary ketosteroids, liver function tests, and glucose tolerance tests. No toxic manifestations were detected. It is unusual for a chemotherapeutic substance to be administered to human subjects for so long a period at so high a level without side effects.

Of particular interest are the results with infants and children. A total of 423 children received chlortetracycline, 20 to 500 mg. per day, by mouth for two to thirty-six months. In addition, there were findings on 120 premature infants who received 20 to 50 mg. per kilogram body weight per day for five to fifty-six days. Among the results in this group were lower mortality, more rapid gain in weight and lower incidence of diarrhea. There were no reports of any signs of toxicity or of outbreaks of disease due to resistant pathogens (29).

In one study (31), chlortetracycline was given at 60 mg. per kilogram body weight per day. All treated infants survived, and five of the fifteen controls died. In another investigation (32), in which 50 mg. chlortetracycline were fed daily, there was one death in forty-seven premature infants who received the antibiotic and eight deaths among the forty-eight controls.

SUMMARY

The public reaction towards the use of chemical technology in the production and processing of food has been greatly heightened by the environmentalist movement. Much misinformation has been circulated in the news media. I have selected a few examples of residue problems for discussion, each illustrating a different point of importance.

The propaganda against DDT served to create distrust of all pesticides. Yet DDT is one of the safest compounds ever to be placed in contact with human beings. It has saved more lives and made more people healthy than any chemical in the history of the world. Its effects on wildlife are largely unknown, because wild animals pick up other contaminants from the environment, including polychlorinated biphenyls, lead, and mercury.

Of these, mercury is a natural ingredient of the ocean. According to Hammond (6), the total input of mercury into the seas from man's activities is between one-hundredth and one-thousandth of the hundred million tons of mercury in the ocean. He estimates that "except for coastal and estuarial areas, it does not seem likely that man could have increased concentrations in the sea by as much as 1 per cent." Clearly, the mercury present in fish of the deep oceans, including tuna, swordfish, sailfish, and albacore, is of natural origin. The Food and Drug Administration should make this clear to the public.

The addition of synthetic antioxidants to processed foods will no doubt draw the wrath of the natural food enthusiasts. Yet a typical antioxidant has been shown to prolong the life of mice to a highly significant extent.

The major antibiotics used in animal feeds were thoroughly tested for safety more than fifteen years ago. Their use has improved the health of farm animals and has increased the yields of animal products for human food, including beef, pork, poultry, and eggs. The residues in these products are a tiny fraction of the amounts of antibiotics used routinely in medicine, and the residues are destroyed by cooking.

These examples illustrate the tendency to exaggerate and misinterpret the food residue problem. Adequate and accurate scientific information, especially on toxicology, is needed before decisions are taken.

REFERENCES

1. Guinee, P.: Bacterial drug resistance in animals. Trans. N. Y. Acad. Sci., in press.

2. Carson, R.: Silent Spring. Boston: Houghton Mifflin Co., 1962.

3. Hayes, W. J., Jr.: Toxicity of pesticides in man. Proc. Roy. Soc. B 167: 101, 1967.

4. The place of DDT in operations against malaria and other vector-borne diseases. WHO statement, EB 47/WP/14, 22 Jan. 1971.

5. Frazier, B. E., Chesters, G., and Lee, G. B.: "Apparent" organochlorine insecticide content of soil, sampled in 1910. Pesticides Monitoring J. 4: 67, 1970.

6. Hammond, A. L., Mercury in the environment: Natural and human factors. Science 171: 788, 1971.

7. Tuna scare: Was pollution to blame? Marine Pollution Bull. 2: 2 (Jan.), 1971.

8. How safe is your food? Interview with C. C. Edwards. U. S. News & World Rept. 70: 50 (Apr. 19), 1971.

9. Report of the Secretary's Commission on Pesticides and Their Relation to Environmental Health. Pts. 1 & 2. Washington, D. C.: Dept. Health, Education, & Welfare, Dec. 1969.

10. Miller, J. A.: Tumorigenic and carcinogenic natural products. *In* Toxicants Occurring Naturally in Foods. Natl. Acad. Sci.-Natl. Research Council Pub. No. 1354, 1967.

11. Cherkes, L. A., Aptfkar, S. G., and Volgarev, M. N.: Hepatic tumors induced by selenium. Bull. Exp. Biol. Med. 53: 313, 1963.

12. Garcia-Martin, G. (WHO): Personal communication to S. Rotrosen, June 19, 1969.

13. Hayes, W. J., Jr.: Personal communication, 1970.

14. Russell, P. F.: The United States and malaria: Debits and credits. Bull. N. Y. Acad. Med. 44: 623, 1968.

15. Jukes, T. H.: DDT: The chemical of social change. Clin. Toxicol. 2: 359, 1969.

16. Laug, E. P., Kunze, F. M., and Prickett, C. S.: Occurrence of DDT in human fat and milk. Arch. Industr. Hyg. 3: 245, 1951.

17. Pryor, W. A.: Free radical pathology. Chem. Engin. News, June 7, 1971, p. 34.

18. Harman, D.: Free radical theory of aging: Effect of free radical reaction inhibitors on the mortality rate LAF mice. J. Gerontol. 23: 476, 1968.

19. Buu-Hoi, N. P., and Ratsimamanga, A. R.: Action retardante de l'acide nordi-hydroguairèteque sur le vieillissement chez le rat. Compt. Rend. Soc. Biol. 153: 1180, 1959.

20. Comfort, A., Youhotsky-Gore, I., and Pathmanathan, K.: Effect of ethoxyquin on the longevity of C3H mice. Nature 229: 254, 1971.

21. Jukes, T. H.: Antibiotics in Nutrition. N. Y.: Medical Encyclopedia, Inc., 1955.

22. Broquist, H. P., and Kohler, A. R.: Studies of the antibiotic potency in the meat of animals fed chlortetracycline. *In* Antibiotics Annual, 1953–54. N. Y.: Medical Encyclopedia, Inc., 1954.

23. Shor, A. L., Abbey, A., and Gale, G. O.: Disappearance of chlortetracycline residues from edible tissues. 2. Chickens and turkeys. *In* Antimicrobial Agents and Chemotherapy. Washington, D. C.: Amer. Soc. for Microbiol., 1967, p. 757.

24. Shirk, R. J., Whitehill, A. R., and Hines, L. J.: A degradation product in cooked chlortetracycline-treated poultry. *In* Antibiotics Annual. N. Y.: Medical Encyclopedia, Inc., 1957, p. 843.

25. Tarr, H. L. A.: Control of Bacterial Spoilage of Fish with Antibiotics. Canad. Natl. Acad. Sci. Pub. 397, 1956, p. 199.

26. Tomiyama, T., Yone, Y., and Mikajiri, K.: Uptake of aureomycin chlortetra-cycline by fish and its heat inactivation. Food Tech. 11: 290, 1957.

27. Goldberg, H. S., Weiser, H. H., and Deatherage, F. E.: Aureomycin in the prevention of spoilage of beef. Food Tech. 7: 165, 1953.

28. Thatcher, F. S., and Loit, A.: Comparative microflora of chlortetracycline-treated and nontreated poultry with special reference to public health aspects. Appl. Microbiol. 9: 39, 1961.

29. Hines, L. R.: Appraisal of effects of long-term chlortetracycline administra-tion. Antibiot. Chemother. 6: 623, 1956.

30. McVay, L. V., and Carroll, D. S.: Aureomycin treatment of systemic North American blastomycosis. Amer. J. Med. 12: 289, 1952.

31. Robinson, P.: Control trial of aureomycin in premature twins and triplets. Lancet 1: 52, 1952.

32. Snelling, C. E., and Johnson, R.: Value of aureomycin in prevention of cross infection in hospital for sick children. Canad. Med. Ass. J. 66: 6 (Jan), 1952.

33. Pal, R.: Contributions of insecticides to public health in India. World Rev. Pest Control 1: 6, 1962.

42

THE BENEFIT–RISK EQUATION

Alexander Schmidt*

One common thread runs through the entire fabric of FDA activity, and that thread is what we all know as the benefit-risk equation.

Consciously or subconsciously, each of us makes a benefit-to-risk judgment each time he crosses a busy intersection or steps into his car. Such judgments are a common part of daily living. There is even a finite risk in taking a bath or choking on a tough piece of meat.

In FDA decisions as in all aspects of human endeavor, we must accept the probability of nonexistence of absolute safety. We usually make our regulatory judgments based on an accommodation between benefits and risks.

The benefit-to-risk equation is most clearly applied by the FDA when evaluating New Drug Applications.

Under clear and present law, FDA must evaluate each new drug on a basis of the best available science, and approve the drug for use in humans only after careful judgment by experts that the good of its use outweighs the bad.

Such benefit-to-risk judgments range from the very easy to the very difficult. An antacid product may present a relatively easy choice—simple biochemistry, measurable benefit, and minimum risk. But a powerful steroid or complex drugs like L-dopa or propranolol present well-defined and sometimes serious risks in usage.

Reprinted from *FDA Consumer*, May 1974, by permission of the publisher.

Paper based on speech before the American Association for the Advancement of Science's Symposium on Food Additives in San Francisco, February 25, 1974.

* Commissioner of Food and Drugs, FDA.

It takes no special sophistication to recognize that if a product poses an unusual or serious risk to the user, then its benefits must be proportionately high and urgently required.

It is less well understood that the benefit-to-risk equation applies to some degree in most matters under FDA purview. This includes the safety of foods, cosmetics, and all other products that we regulate.

When we turn from drugs to foods and other products, we may encounter different dimensions to the benefit-to-risk equation. But the equation is still there. And, again, the decisions range from easy to near-impossible.

For example, when FDA was responsible for toy safety, it was generally easy to decide that all possible risk of injury posed by a child's toy must be avoided. We always acted on that basis.

On the other hand, we have such complicated questions as the use of nitrites and nitrates in preserving meats. These chemicals in some form have been used for generations to form the flavor, color, and texture of cured meat products. Even more important to FDA, the chemicals also act to prevent contamination of the meat by *Clostridium botulinum*.

Yet, some investigators now have evidence that nitrite residues in cured meat may combine in the human gut to form nitrosamines, some of which are known carcinogens.

A similar problem exists with the artificial sweeteners. Cyclamate is now banned as a food additive, but on the basis of new evidence, FDA has been petitioned to reaccept the chemical as an approved food additive.

Saccharin presently is allowed in the food supply with minimum restrictions. But at least one scientific study has presented evidence that requires FDA to relook at its regulation of this substance. We are now doing so, with the help of the National Academy of Sciences.

In such cases as these, just where and when does one draw the line in weighing demonstrable benefit against theoretical risk? And who is to draw the line? Government? Industry? The individual consumer?

Such questions loom larger every day. In fact, the entire history of food and drug legislation is a reflection of society's growing sense of the uncertainties that go hand in hand with the benefits of scientific progress. The evolution of the FDA law in some cases mirrors not only society's concern, but its confusion.

In an earlier, less technical, and less sophisticated age, the law required only that food and drugs be "pure."

Later, the law specified that pharmaceuticals as well as foods be proven "safe."

In 1962, the first full benefit-to-risk accommodation was written into law with a requirement that pharmaceuticals be effective—that is to say "beneficial"—as well as safe. Thus, we were put into the benefit-risk business.

Today, the application of the benefit vs. risk equation is readily applied and generally—not universally, but generally—accepted as the proper criterion for FDA evaluation of pharmaceuticals.

The same cannot be said for foods. In 1958, the Congress first added a specific anticancer clause to the laws governing food safety. This is the so-called Delaney Clause in the Food Additive Amendments to the Food, Drug, and Cosmetic Act. It says that any material found to induce cancer when fed to test animals is flatly forbidden in the food supply.

In 1962, the anticancer clause was amended by the Congress to require FDA to approve a cancer-causing drug for use in food-producing animals as long as there were do detectable residues in an edible portion of the food animal.

The anticancer clauses affecting food safety present two major difficult issues, for which we have no satisfactory answer at this time.

First, they seem to reject all accommodation between benefit and risk. Literally interpreted, they leave no room for scientific judgment. They call for zero risks from all new food ingredients. The unhappy alternative, of course, advocated by some, is the establishment of tolerances for "safe" levels of a carcinogen.

Second, the rationale for the 1958 and 1962 amendments was based on the technology of that time. Methods for detecting trace chemicals then were far less sensitive than they are today.

The legislative history shows that Congress in 1958 regarded 50 parts per million as the practical equivalent of "zero." Detection methods today can find trace chemical residues below 2 parts per billion (ppb), and at times, a few parts per trillion.

In other words, today's "zero" is far lower than the "zero" of 1958, and today's "zero" is not likely to remain constant in the years ahead.

The fact is that our scientific capacities to detect chemical residues have in many cases outstripped our scientific ability to interpret their meaning.

The case of the carcinogen diethylstilbestrol (DES) as a growth promotant in food animals is an example of the difficulty inherent in administering the congressional mandate on carcinogens in the food supply.

Between 1962 and 1972, testing methods for DES became increasingly sensitive—from 50 ppb to 20 ppb to 10 ppb to 2 ppb. Finally, the 1972–73 testing methods were used which could detect parts per trillion of DES, and we began finding residues where we had not found them before—in livers of animals fed DES as a growth promotant.

FDA then banned the product from use in food animals, on the basis of its never having been demonstrated as safe. That ban, of course, has now been declared invalid by the courts, on the basis of procedure, as we denied a hearing on our original ban. The court has ordered us to hold a hearing on the ban before taking any further action.

The dilemma faced by FDA on DES again makes the point that while detection methods increase in sensitivity, the ability of scientists to relate these findings to human health are not keeping pace.

It seems clear to me that we will never correct this situation by chasing a series of constantly receding "zeros." The more practical course is to try to find out if it makes any difference to human health that minute traces of various chemicals exist in human food—and if so, at what levels.

This tack requires low-dose, long-term toxicological testing in animals, and better ways to extrapolate these findings to the human situation. And that's a job for science. Only after that job is done can the legislators and the regulators make benefit-to-risk judgments that will let us get on with the business of protecting the public safety and still meet the nutritional needs of an ever greater population.

The Delaney Clause is a legitimate legislative expression of society's increasing concern with technologic advances in the food industry and its reluctance to accept less than absolute safety in the food supply.

Carcinogenesis is getting a lot of attention today, but equally serious are questions of mutagenesis (abnormalities) and teratogenesis (birth defects). Yet, the pressures in the future for increased food production for increased nutritive value of the increasing amount of manufactured food, will lead to greater problems of food safety. It is clear that we must continue to seek new ways to increase our supply of food. And new ways include chemical fertilizers as well as chemical preservatives and growth promotants.

But in our search for progress, our goal remains the same. For FDA and the consumer, no less than industry, that goal should be an absolutely safe food supply. That has been our goal all along. It will continue to be so.

But, we live in a world of probabilities; few human decisions are based on absolutes. This applies to food safety as well as to most other problems.

Right now we are in a situation in which science has not provided a sufficient data base to let us speak intelligently about the risk side of the benefit-to-risk equation as it affects food safety.

The benefit side is easy. A food is good or not good according to public demand. It is nutritionally useful or valueless according to well-developed scientific and empirical criteria. Industry usually judges the benefit side of the equation well before it decides to produce and market any given product.

But the risk side is neither as easy nor as well defined. I take it as an FDA responsibility to speak to this issue and to urge upon science a greater concern with the risk side of the equation. I know this is not the most exciting prospect for science, but we simply are not going to get the answers we must have without more low-dose, long-term, animal testing combined with new emphasis on extrapolating animal results to the human condition. This must somehow become an urgent national priority!

Many of you are aware that FDA is now engaged in a multimillion dollar effort to assess the safety of all food additives, both new and old.

We recognize that a revised system for food additive regulations, coupled with our best benefit-to-risk judgments, will only be as good as the state of scientific knowledge at any given moment. And, we are determined not to sit back and wait on others to give us still better answers. Within the reach of our own resources, we are doing what we can to aid the search.

One hopeful enterprise in this direction is now underway at FDA's new National Center for Toxicological Research at Jefferson, Arkansas.

There, we are gearing up the technical and scientific machinery to help us better understand the effects of a growing array of chemicals that find their way into the human body—not only through the foods we eat and the beverages we drink, but through the drugs we take and the environment in which we live.

At the National Center for Toxicological Research, we have four specific goals:

• To determine through animal tests the adverse effects of low-dose, long-term exposure to chemical toxicants.

• To determine how these toxicants affect animal organisms.

• To develop better tests to evaluate the limits of safe use of toxic chemicals in animal systems.

• And, finally, to develop data to help extrapolate test results from animals to man.

In a closely related effort, FDA has set up specific criteria for administering the congressional requirement that drugs, such as diethylstilbestrol, be approved for use in food animals provided there is no residue left in the edible meat.

The new FDA procedures provide for evaluating the hazard potential of each drug used in food animals and then requiring an analytical detection system sensitive enough to measure appropriately low levels of residues. The method of analysis will help us keep residues below the point of potential risk in humans. If such a detection system cannot be developed, the drug cannot be approved. If a system can be devised, it can be improved as technology allows, without invalidating the drug approval.

In addition to new drugs offered for marketing approval, FDA's proposal also includes procedures for reviewing drugs approved in years past, when detection methodology was not as sensitive as it is today.

The research in Arkansas and the new procedures to establish appropriately sensitive methods for detecting chemicals likely to reach the food supply—both of these are examples of FDA's own attempts to expand the scientific basis for making reasonable judgments on the relative safety of foods, drugs, and other products.

But our need for answers goes far beyond FDA's own resources. We need all the help we can get. Let me close by asking:

- How do we get greater attention to the kinds of narrowly targeted research that we in FDA need if we are to make our benefit-risk decisions on adequate scientific assessment of risks inherent in ingesting small amounts of chemicals?
- Who is to sponsor the research? Who pays?
- If much of the research needed for better regulation must be sponsored by the regulated industries, how do we guard against duplication and still maintain fair competition?
- What should be the perspective of Government on trade secrets and competitive advantage when considered in a field as vital to national health and stamina as a safe and nutritious food supply?
- How do we deal with the problem of having to make regulatory decisions at times without being able to wait until science gets around to doing needed research?
- How do we ensure that when regulatory action is needed that we mobilize all available scientific knowledge to support our decision for action?
- In the face of public doubt and skepticism, how do we in Government, in the scientific community, and in industry improve public understanding of and public confidence in our decision-making?
- And, finally, how do we together gain broader public understanding of the limits imposed upon both science and Government in facing the kinds of issues that I have discussed?

For it is undoubtedly true that science and scientific regulation can only go so far. We can find facts, measure results, define probabilities, and purpose limits. Beyond this, there are moral and ethical considerations with which society and its social institutions must contend.

At some point, the amount of risk a society is willing to assume in order to achieve a certain benefit becomes a matter for the public at large to decide. It thus is imperative for scientists to educate the public in these matters, and to serve as expert witnesses for our social institutions.

At this point, I have more questions than answers. I know only that at foods and drugs and all conditions of the human environment grow more complex, as the techniques of analysis push against the limits of our ability to understand what we detect, as the human population and its demands expand—as these forces move ever forward—and often not in harmony—it is essential that we look more closely, and as a total society, at these and related issues so important to the future of society.

43

ENERGY USE IN THE U.S. FOOD SYSTEM

John S. Steinhart and Carol E. Steinhart *

In a modern industrial society, only a tiny fraction of the population is in frequent contact with the soil, and an even smaller fraction of the population raises food on the soil. The proportion of the population engaged in farming halved between 1920 and 1950 and then halved again by 1962. Now it has almost halved again, and more than half of these remaining farmers hold other jobs off the farm (1). At the same time the number of work animals has declined from a peak of more than 22×10^6 in 1920 to a very small number at present (2). By comparison with earlier times, fewer farmers are producing more agricultural products and the value of food in terms of the total goods and services of society now amounts to a smaller fraction of the economy than it once did.

Energy inputs to farming have increased enormously during the past 50 years (3), and the apparent decrease in farm labor is offset in part by the growth of support industries for the farmer. With these changes on the farm have come a variety of other changes in the U. S. food system, many of which are now deeply embedded in the fabric of daily life. In the past 50 years, canned, frozen, and other processed foods have become the principal items of our diet. At present, the food processing industry

Reprinted courtesy of the authors and *Science* 184:307–316, April 1974. Copyright © 1974 by the American Association for the Advancement of Science. Condensed from *Energy: Sources, Use and Role in Human Affairs*, by Carol and John Steinhart, Duxbury Press, North Scituate, Mass., 1974.

* Dr. J. S. Steinhart is professor of geology and geophysics, and professor in the Institute for Environmental Studies, University of Wisconsin–Madison. Dr. C. E. Steinhart, formerly a biologist with the National Institutes of Health, is now a science writer and editor.

is the fourth largest energy consumer of the Standard Industrial Classification groupings (4). The extent of transportation engaged in the food system has grown apace, and the proliferation of appliances in both numbers and complexity still continues in homes, institutions, and stores. Hardly any food is eaten as it comes from the fields. Even farmers purchase most of their food from markets in town.

Present energy supply problems make this growth of energy use in the food system worth investigating. It is our purpose in this article to do so. But there are larger matters at stake. Georgescu-Roegen notes that "the evidence now before us—of a world which can produce automobiles, television sets, etc., at a greater speed than the increase in population, but is simultaneously menaced by mass starvation—is disturbing" (5). In the search for a solution to the world's food problems, the common attempt to transplant a small piece of a highly industrialized food system to the hungry nations of the world is plausible enough, but so far the outcome is unclear. Perhaps an examination of the energy flow in the U. S. food system as it has developed can provide some insights that are not available from the usual economic measures.

MEASURES OF FOOD SYSTEMS

Agricultural systems are most often described in economic terms. A wealth of statistics is collected in the United States and in most other technically advanced countries indicating production amounts, shipments, income, labor, expenses, and dollar flow in the agricultural sector of the economy. But, when we wish to know something about the food we actually eat, the statistics of farms are only a tiny fraction of the story.

Energy flow is another measure available to gauge societies and nations. It would have made no sense to measure societies in terms of energy flow in the 18th century when economics began. As recently as 1940, four-fifths of the world's population were still on farms and in small villages, most of them engaged in subsistence farming.

Only after some nations shifted large portions of the population to manufacturing, specialized tasks, and mechanized food production, and shifted the prime sources of energy to move society to fuels that were transportable and usable for a wide variety of alternative activities, could energy flow be used as a measure of societies' activities. Today it is only in one-fifth of the world where these conditions are far advanced. Yet we can now make comparisons of energy flows even with primitive societies. For even if the primitives, or the euphemistically named "underdeveloped" countries, cannot shift freely among their energy expenditures, we *can* measure them and they constitute a different and potentially useful comparison with the now traditional economic measures.

What we would like to know is: How does our present food supply system compare, in energy measures, with those of other societies and with our own past?   Perhaps then we can estimate the value of energy flow measures as an adjunct to, but different from, economic measures.

ENERGY IN THE U.S. FOOD SYSTEM

A typical breakfast includes orange juice from Florida by way of the Minute Maid factory, bacon from a midwestern meat packer, cereal from Nebraska and General Mills, eggs and milk from not *too* far away, and coffee from Colombia.   All of these things are available at the local super-market (several miles each way in a 300-horse-power automobile), stored in a refrigerator-freezer, and cooked on an instant-on stove.

The present food system in the United States is complex, and the at-tempt to analyze it in terms of energy use will introduce complexities and questions far more perplexing than the same analysis carried out on sim-pler societies.   Such an analysis is worthwhile, however, if only to find out where we stand.   We have a food system, and most people get enough to eat from it.   If, in addition, one considers the food supply problems present and future in societies where a smaller fraction of the people get enough to eat, then our experience with an industrialized food system is even more important.   There is simply no gainsaying that many nations of the world are presently attempting to acquire industrialized food sys-tems of their own.

Food in the United States is expensive by world standards.   In 1970 the average annual per capita expenditure for food was about $600 (3). This amount is larger than the per capita gross domestic product of more than 30 nations of the world which contain the majority of the world's people and a vast majority of those who are underfed.   Even if we con-sider the diet of a poor resident of India, the annual cost of his food at U. S. prices would be about $200—more than twice his annual income (3). It is crucial to know whether a piece of our industrialized food system can be exported to help poor nations, or whether they must become as indus-trialized as the United States to operate an industrialized food system.

Our analysis of energy use in the food system begins with an omis-sion.   We will neglect that crucial input of energy provided by the sun to the plants upon which the entire food supply depends.   Photosynthesis has an efficiency of about 1 percent; thus the maximum solar radiation captured by plants is about 5×10^3 kilocalories per square meter per year (3).

Seven categories of energy use on the farm are considered here.   The amounts of energy used are shown in Table 1.   The values given for farm machinery and tractors are for the manufacture of new units only and do not include parts and maintenance for units that already exist.   The amounts shown for direct fuel use and electricity consumption are a bit too high because they include some residential uses of the farmer and his family.   On the other hand, some uses in these categories are not reported

Table 1: Energy use in the United States food system. All values are multiplied by 10¹² kcal.

Component	1940	1947	1950	1954	1958	1960	1964	1968	1970	References
On farm										
Fuel (direct use)	70.0	136.0	158.0	172.8	179.0	188.0	213.9	226.0	232.0	(13–15)
Electricity	0.7	32.0	32.9	40.0	44.0	46.1	50.0	57.3	63.8	(14, 16)
Fertilizer	12.4	19.5	24.0	30.6	32.2	41.0	60.0	87.0	94.0	(14, 17)
Agricultural steel	1.6	2.0	2.7	2.5	2.0	1.7	2.5	2.4	2.0	(14, 18)
Farm machinery	9.0	34.7	30.0	29.5	50.2	52.0	60.0	75.0	80.0	(14, 19)
Tractors	12.8	25.0	30.8	23.6	16.4	11.8	20.0	20.5	19.3	(20)
Irrigation	18.0	22.8	25.0	29.6	32.5	33.3	34.1	34.8	35.0	(21)
Subtotal	124.5	272.0	303.4	328.6	356.3	373.9	440.5	503.0	526.1	
Processing industry										
Food processing industry	147.0	177.5	192.0	211.5	212.6	224.0	249.0	295.0	308.0	(13, 14, 22)
Food processing machinery	0.7	5.7	5.0	4.9	4.9	5.0	6.0	6.0	6.0	(23)
Paper packaging	8.5	14.8	17.0	20.0	26.0	28.0	31.0	35.7	38.0	(24)
Glass containers	14.0	25.7	26.0	27.0	30.2	31.0	34.0	41.9	47.0	(25)
Steel cans and aluminum	38.0	55.8	62.0	73.7	85.4	86.0	91.0	112.2	122.0	(26)
Transport (fuel)	49.6	86.1	102.0	122.3	140.2	153.3	184.0	226.6	246.9	(27)
Trucks and trailers (manufacture)	28.0	42.0	49.5	47.0	43.0	44.2	61.0	70.2	74.0	(28)
Subtotal	285.8	407.6	453.5	506.4	542.3	571.5	656.0	787.6	841.9	
Commercial and home										
Commercial refrigeration and cooking	121.0	141.0	150.0	161.0	176.0	186.2	209.0	241.0	263.0	(13, 29)
Refrigeration machinery (home and commercial)	10.0	24.0	25.0	27.5	29.4	32.0	40.0	56.0	61.0	(14, 30)
Home refrigeration and cooking	144.2	184.0	202.3	228.0	257.0	276.6	345.0	433.9	480.0	(13, 29)
Subtotal	275.2	349.0	377.3	416.5	462.4	494.8	594.0	730.9	804.0	
Grand total	685.5	1028.6	1134.2	1251.5	1361.0	1440.2	1690.5	2021.5	2172.0	

in the summaries used to obtain the values for direct fuel and electricity usage. These and similar problems are discussed in the references. Note the relatively high energy cost associated with irrigation. In the United States less than 5 percent of the cropland is irrigated (1). In some countries where the "green revolution" is being attempted, the new high-yield varieties of plants require irrigation where native crops did not. If that were the case in the United States, irrigation would be the largest single use of energy on the farm.

Little food makes its way directly from field and farm to the table. The vast complex of processing, packaging, and transport has been grouped together in a second major subdivision of the food system. The seven categories of the processing industry are listed in Table 1. Energy use for the transport of food should be charged to the farm in part, but we have not done so here because the calculation of the energy values is easiest (and we believe most accurate) if they are taken for the whole system.

After the processing of food there is further energy expenditure. Transportation enters the picture again, and some fraction of the energy used for transportation should be assigned here. But there are also the distributors, wholesalers, and retailers, whose freezers, refrigerators, and very establishments are an integral part of the food system. There are also the restaurants, schools, universities, prisons, and a host of other institutions engaged in the procurement, preparation, storage, and supply of food. We have chosen to examine only three categories: the energy required for refrigeration and cooking, and for the manufacture of the heating and refrigeration equipment (Table 1). We have made no attempt to include the energy used in trips to the store or restaurant. Garbage disposal has also been omitted, although it is a persistent and growing feature of our food system; 12 percent of the nation's trucks are engaged in the activity of waste disposal (1), of which a substantial part is related to food. If there is any lingering doubt that these activities—both the ones included and the ones left out—are an essential feature of our present food system, one need only ask what would happen if everyone should attempt to get on without a refrigerator or freezer or stove? Certainly the food system would change.

Table 1 and the related references summarize the numerical values for energy use in the U. S. food system, from 1940 to 1970. As for many activities in the past few decades, the story is one of continuing increase. The totals are displayed in Fig. 1 along with the energy value of the food consumed by the public. The food values were obtained by multiplying the daily caloric intake by the population. The differences in caloric intake per capita over this 30-year period are small (1), and the curve is primarily an indication of the increase in population in this period.

OMISSIONS AND DUPLICATIONS FOR FOOD SYSTEM ENERGY VALUES

Several omissions, duplications, and overlaps have been mentioned. We will now examine the values in Table 1 for completeness and try to obtain a crude estimate of their numerical accuracy.

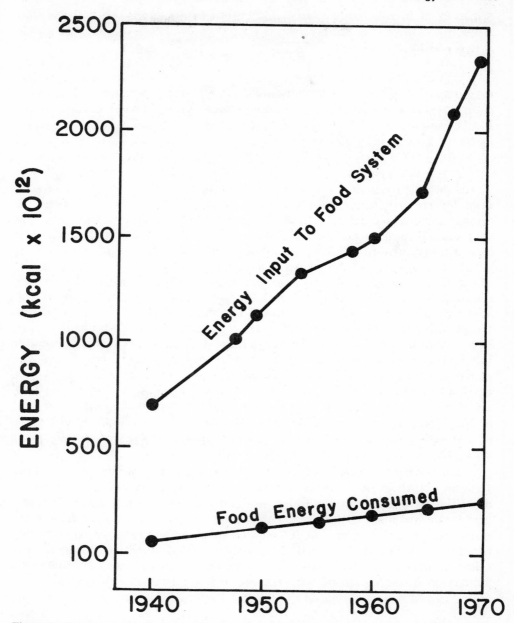

Figure 1: Energy use in the food system, 1940 through 1970, compared to the caloric content of food consumed.

The direct fuel and electricity usage on the farm may be overstated by some amounts used in the farmer's household, which, by our approach, would not all the chargeable to the food system. But about 10 percent of the total acreage farmed is held by corporate farms for which the electrical and direct fuel use is not included in our data. Other estimates of these two categories are much higher [see Table 1 (15, 16)].

No allowance has been made for food exported, which has the effect of overstating the energy used in our own food system. For the years prior to 1960 the United States was at times a net importer of food, at times an exporter, and at times there was a near balance in this activity. But during this period the net flow of trade was never more than a few percent of the total farm output. Since 1960 net exports have increased to about 20 percent of the gross farm product (1, 3). The items comprising the vast majority of the exports have been rough grains, flour, and other plant products with very little processing. Imports include more processed food than exports and represent energy expenditure outside the United States. Thus the overestimate of energy input to the food system might be 5 percent with an upper limit of 15 percent.

The items omitted are more numerous. Fuel losses from the wellhead or mineshaft to end use total 10 to 12 percent (6). This would represent a flat addition of 10 percent or more to the totals, but we have not included this item because it is not customarily charged to end uses.

We have computed transport energy for trucks only. Considerable food is transported by train and ship, but these items were omitted because the energy use is small relative to the consumption of truck fuel. Small amounts of food are shipped by air, and, although air shipment is energy-intensive, the amount of energy consumed appears small. We have traced support materials until they could no longer be assigned to the food system. Some transportation energy consumption is not charged in the transport of these support materials. These omissions are numerous and hard to estimate, but they would not be likely to increase the totals by more than 1 or 2 percent.

A more serious understatement of energy usage occurs with respect to vehicle usage (other than freight transport) on farm business, food-related business in industry and commercial establishments, and in the supporting industries. A special attempt to estimate this category of energy usage for 1968 suggests that it amounts to about 5 percent of the energy totals for the food system. This estimate would be subject to an uncertainty of nearly 100 percent. We must be satisfied to suggest that 1 to 10 percent should be added to the totals on this account.

Waste disposal is related to the food system, at least in part. We have chosen not to charge this energy to the food system, but, if one-half of the waste disposal activity is taken as food-related, about 2 percent must be added to the food system energy totals.

We have not included energy for parts and maintenance of machinery, vehicles, buildings, and the like, or lumber for farm, industry, or packaging uses. These miscellaneous activities would not constitute a large addition in any case. We have also excluded construction. Building and replacement of farm structures, food industry structures, and commercial establishments are all directly part of the food system. Construction of roads is in some measure related to the food system, since nearly half of all trucks transport food and agricultural items [see Table 1 (27)]. Even home construction could be charged in part to the food system since space, appliances, and plumbing are, in part, a consequence of the food system. If 10 percent of housing, 10 percent of institutional construction (for institutions with food service), and 10 percent of highway construction is included, about 10 percent of the total construction was food-related in 1970. Assuming that the total energy consumption divides in the same way that the Gross National Product does (which overstates energy use in construction), the addition to the total in Table 1 would be about 10 percent or 200×10^{12} kcal. This is a crude and highly simplified calculation, but it does provide an estimate of the amounts of energy involved.

The energy used to generate the highly specialized seed and animal stock has been excluded because there is no easy way to estimate it. Pimentel *et al.* (3) estimate that 1800 kcal are required to produce 1 pound (450 grams) of hybrid corn seed. But in addition to this amount, some energy use should be included for all the schools of agriculture, agricultural experiment stations, the far-flung network of county agricultural agents [one local agent said he traveled over 50,000 automobile miles (80,000 kilometers) per year in his car], the U. S. Department of Agriculture, and the wide-ranging agricultural research program that enables man to stay ahead of the new pest and disease threats to our highly specialized food crops. These are extensive activities but we cannot see how they could add more than a few percent to the totals in Table 1.

Finally, we have made no attempt to include the amount of private automobile usage involved in the delivery system from retailer to home, or other food-related uses of private autos. Rice (7) reports 4.25×10^{15} kcal for the energy cost of autos in 1970, and shopping constitutes 15.2 percent of all automobile usage (8). If only half of the shopping is food-related, 320×10^{12} kcal of energy use is at stake here. Between 8 and 15 percent should be added to the totals of Table 1, depending on just how one wishes to apportion this item.

It is hard to take an approach that might calculate smaller totals but, depending upon point of view, the totals could be much larger. If we accumulate the larger estimates from the above paragraphs as well as the reductions, the total could be enlarged by 30 to 35 percent, especially for recent years. As it is, the values for energy use in the food system from Table 1 account for 12.8 percent of the total U. S. energy use in 1970.

PERFORMANCE OF AN INDUSTRIALIZED FOOD SYSTEM

The difficulty with history as a guide for the future or even the present lies not so much in the fact that conditions change—we are continually reminded of that fact—but that history is only one experiment of the many that might have occurred.   The U. S. food system developed as it did for a variety of reasons, many of them not understood.   We would do well to examine some of the dimensions of this development before attempting to theorize about how it might have been different, or how parts of this food system can be transplanted elsewhere.

ENERGY AND FOOD PRODUCTION

Figure 2 displays features of our food system not easily seen from economic data.   The curve shown has no theoretical basis but is suggested

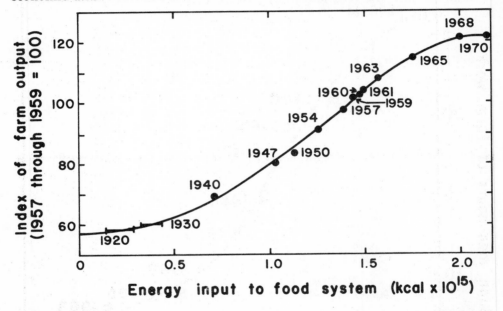

Figure 2: Farm output as a function of energy input to the U. S. food system, 1920 through 1970.

by the data as a smoothed recounting of our own history of increasing food production.   It is, however, similar to most growth curves and suggests that, to the extent that the increasing energy subsidies to the food system have increased food production, we are near the end of an era.   Like the logistic growth curve, there is an exponential phase which lasted from 1920 or earlier until 1950 or 1955.   Since then, the increments in production have been smaller despite the continuing growth in energy use.   It is likely that further increases in food production from increasing energy inputs will be harder and harder to come by.   Of course, a major change in the food system could change things, but the argument advanced by the technological optimist is that we can always get more if we have enough energy, and that no other major changes are required. Our own history—the only one we have to examine—does not support that view.

ENERGY AND LABOR IN THE FOOD SYSTEM

One farmer now feeds 50 people, and the common expectation is that the labor input to farming will continue to decrease in the future. Behind this expectation is the assumption that the continued application of technology—and energy—to farming will substitute for labor. Figure 3 shows

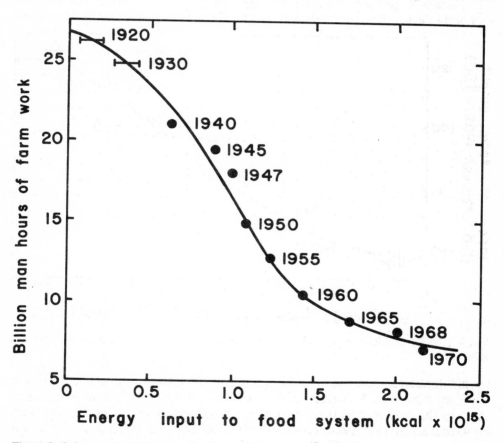

Figure 3: Labor use on farms as a function of energy use in the food system.

this historic decline in labor as a function of the energy supplied to the food system, again the familiar S-shaped curve. What it implies is that increasing the energy input to the food system is unlikely to bring further reduction in farm labor unless some other, major change is made.

The food system that has grown in this period has provided much employment that did not exist 20, 30, or 40 years ago. Perhaps even the idea of a reduction of labor input is a myth when the food system is viewed as a whole, instead of from the point of view of the farm worker only. When discussing inputs to the farm, Pimentel *et al.* (3) cite an estimate of two farm support workers for each person actually on the farm. To this must be added employment in food-processing industries, in food wholesaling and retailing, as well as in a variety of manufacturing enterprises that support the food system. Yesterday's farmer is today's canner, tractor mechanic, and fast food carhop. The process of change has been painful to many ordinary people. The rural poor, who could not quite compete in the growing industrialization of farming, migrated to the cities. Eventually they found other employment, but one must ask if the change was worthwhile. The answer to that question cannot be provided by energy analysis anymore than by economic data, because it raises fundamental questions about how individuals would prefer to spend their lives. But if there is a stark choice between long hours as a farmer or shorter hours on the assembly line of a meat-packing plant, it seems clear that the choice would not be universally in favor of the meat-packing plant. Thomas Jefferson dreamed of a nation of independent small farmers. It was a good dream, but society did not develop in that way. Nor can we turn back the clock to recover his dream. But, in planning and preparing for our future, we had better look honestly at our collective history, and then each of us should closely examine his dreams.

THE ENERGY SUBSIDY TO THE FOOD SYSTEM

The data in Fig. 1 can be combined to show the energy subsidy provided to the food system for the recent past. We take as a measure of the food supplied the caloric content of the food actually consumed. This is not the only measure of the food supplied, as the condition of many protein-poor peoples of the world clearly shows. Nevertheless, the comparison between caloric input and output is a convenient way to compare our present situation with the past, and to compare our food system with others. Figure 4 shows the history of the U. S. food system in terms of the number of calories of energy supplied to produce 1 calorie of food for actual consumption. It is interesting and possibly threatening to note that there is no real suggestion that this curve is leveling off. We appear to be increasing the energy input even more. Fragmentary data for 1972 suggest that the increase continued unabated. A graph like Fig. 4 could approach zero. A natural ecosystem has no fuel input at all, and those primitive people who live by hunting and gathering have only the energy of their own work to count as input.

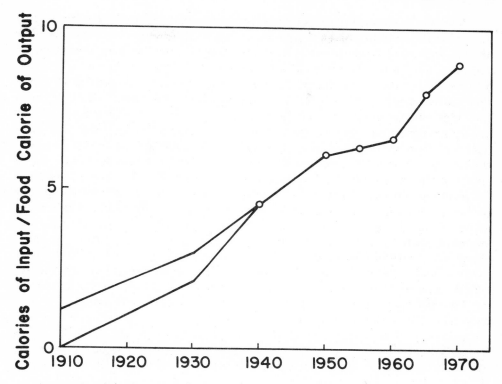

Figure 4: Energy subsidy to the food system needed to obtain 1 food calorie.

SOME ECONOMIC FEATURES OF THE U.S. FOOD SYSTEM

The markets for farm commodities in the United States come closer than most to the economist's ideal of a "free market." There are many small sellers and many buyers, and thus no individual is able to affect the price by his own actions in the marketplace. But government intervention can drastically alter any free market, and government intervention in the prices of agricultural products (and hence of food) has been a prominent feature of the U. S. food system for at least 30 years. Between 1940 and 1970, total farm income has ranged from $4.5 to $16.5 billion, and the National Income originating in agriculture (which includes indirect income from agriculture) has ranged from $14.5 to $22.5 billion (1). Meanwhile, government subsidy programs, primarily farm price supports and soil bank payments, have grown from $1.5 billion in 1940 to $6.2 billion in 1970. In 1972 these subsidy programs had grown to $7.3 billion, despite foreign demand of agricultural products. Viewed in a slightly different way, direct government subsidies have accounted for 30 to 40 percent of the farm income and 15 to 30 percent of the National Income attributable to agriculture for the years since 1955. This point emphasizes once again the striking gap between the economic description of society and the economic models used to account for that society's behavior.

This excursion into farm price supports and economics is related to energy questions in this way: first, so far as we know, government intervention in the food system is a feature of all highly industralized countries (and despite the intervention, farm incomes still tend to lag behind national averages); and, second, reduction of the energy subsidy to agriculture (even if we could manage it) might decrease the farmer's income. One reason for this state of affairs is that the demand for food quantity has definite limits, and the only way to increase farm income is then to increase the unit price of agricultural products. Consumer boycotts and protests in the early 1970's suggest that there is considerable resistance to this outcome.

Government intervention in the functioning of the market in agricultural products has accompanied the rise in the use of energy in agriculture and the food supply system, and we have nothing but theoretical suppositions to suggest that any of the present system can be deleted.

SOME ENERGY IMPLICATIONS FOR THE WORLD FOOD SUPPLY

The food supply system of the United States is complex and interwoven into a highly industrialized economy. We have tried to analyze this system on account of its implications for future energy use. But the world is short of food. A few years ago it was widely predicted that the world would suffer widespread famine in the 1970's. The adoption of new high-yield varieties of rice, wheat, and other grains has caused some experts to predict that the threat of these expected famines can now be averted, perhaps indefinitely. Yet, despite increases in grain production in some areas, the world still seems to be headed toward famine. The adoption of these new varieties of grain—dubbed hopefully the "green revolution"—is an attempt to export a part of the energy-intensive food system of the highly industrialized countries to nonindustrialized countries. It is an experiment, because, although the whole food system is not being transplanted to new areas, a small part of it is. The green revolution requires a great deal of energy. Many of the new varieties of grain require irrigation where traditional crops did not, and almost all the new crops require extensive fertilization.

Meanwhile, the agricultural surpluses of the 1950's have largely disappeared. Grain shortages in China and Russia have attracted attention because they have brought foreign trade across ideological barriers. There are other countries that would probably import considerable grain, if they could afford it. But only four countries may be expected to have any substantial excess agricultural production in the next decade. These are Canada, New Zealand, Australia, and the United States. None of these is in a position to give grain away, because each of them needs the foreign trade to avert ruinous balance of payments deficits. Can we then export energy-intensive agricultural methods instead?

ENERGY–INTENSIVE AGRICULTURE ABROAD

It is quite clear that the U. S. food system cannot be exported intact at present. For example, India has a population of 550×10^6 persons. To feed the people of India at the U. S. level of about 3000 food calories per day (instead of their present 2000) would require more energy than India now uses for all purposes. To feed the entire world with a U. S. type food system, almost 80 percent of the world's annual energy expenditure would be required just for the food system.

The recourse most often suggested to remedy this difficulty is to export methods of increasing crop yield and hope for the best. We must repeat as plainly as possible that this is an experiment. We know that our food system works (albeit with some difficulties and warnings for the future). But we cannot know what will happen if we take a piece of that system and transplant it to a poor country, without our industrial base of supply, transport system, processing industry, appliances for home storage, and preparation, and, most important of all, a level of industrialization that permits higher costs for food.

Fertilizers, herbicides, pesticides, and in many cases machinery and irrigation are needed for success with the green revolution. Where is this energy to come from? Many of the nations with the most serious food problems are those nations with scant supplies of fossil fuels. In the industrialized nations, solutions to the energy supply problems are being sought in nuclear energy. This technology-intensive solution, even if successful in advanced countries, poses additional problems for underdeveloped nations. To create the bases of industry and technologically sophisticated people within their own countries will be beyond the capability of many of them. Here again, these countries face the prospect of depending upon the goodwill and policies of industrialized nations. Since the alternative could be famine, their choices are not pleasant and their irritation at their benefactors—ourselves among them—could grow to threatening proportions. It would be comfortable to rely on our own good intentions, but our good intentions have often been unresponsive to the needs of others. The matter cannot be glossed over lightly. World peace may depend upon the outcome.

CHOICES FOR THE FUTURE

The total amount of energy used on U. S. farms for the production of corn is now near 10^3 kcal per square meter per year (3), and this is more or less typical of intensive agriculture in the United States. With this application of energy we have achieved yields of 2×10^3 kcal per square meter per year of usable grain—bringing us to almost half of the photosynthetic limit of production. Further applications of energy are likely to yield little or no increase in this level of productivity. In any case, no amount of research is likely to improve the efficiency of the photosynthetic process itself. There is a further limitation on the improvement of yield. Faith in technology and research has at times blinded us to the basic limitations of the plant and animal material with which we work. We have been able to emphasize desirable features already present in the gene pool and to suppress others that we find undesirable. At times the cost of the increased yield has been the loss of desirable characteristics— hardiness, resistance to disease and adverse weather, and the like. The farther we get from characteristics of the original plant and animal strains, the more care and energy is required. Choices need to be made in the directions of plant breeding. And the limits of the plants and animals we use must be kept in mind. We have not been able to alter the photosynthetic process or to change the gestation period of animals. In order to amplify or change an existing characteristic, we will probably have to sacrifice something in the overall performance of the plant or animal. If the change requires more energy, we could end with a solution that is too expensive for the people who need it most. These problems are intensified by the degree to which energy becomes more expensive in the world market.

WHERE NEXT TO LOOK FOR FOOD?

Our examination in the foregoing pages of the U. S. food system, the limitations on the manipulation of ecosystems and their components, and the risks of the green revolution as a solution to the world food supply problem suggests a bleak prospect for the future. This complex of problems should not be underestimated, but there are possible ways of avoiding disaster and of mitigating the severest difficulties. These suggestions are not very dramatic and may be difficult of common acceptance.

Figure 5 shows the ratio of the energy subsidy to the energy output for a number of widely used foods in a variety of times and cultures. For comparison, the overall pattern for the U. S. food system is shown, but the comparison is only approximate because, for most of the specific crops, the energy input ends at the farm. As has been pointed out, it is a long way from the farm to the table in industrialized societies. Several things are immediately apparent and coincide with expectations. High-protein

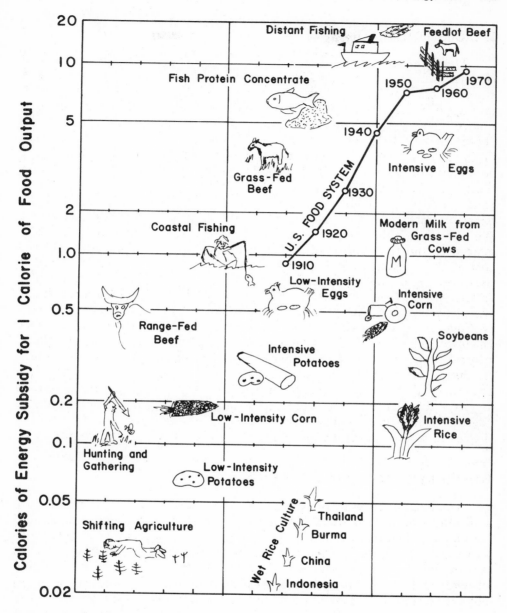

Figure 5: Energy subsidies for various food crops. The energy history of the U. S. food system is shown for comparison. [Source of data: (31)]

foods such as milk, eggs, and especially meat, have a far poorer energy return than plant foods. Because protein is essential for human diets and the amino acid balance necessary for good nutrition is not found in most of the cereal grains, we cannot take the step of abandoning meat sources altogether. Figure 5 does show how unlikely it is that increased fishing or fish protein concentrate will solve the world's food problems. Even if we leave aside the question of whether the fish are available—a point on which expert opinions differ somewhat—it would be hard to imagine, with rising energy prices, that fish protein concentrate will be anything more than a by-product of the fishing industry, because it requires more than twice the energy of production of grass-fed beef or eggs (9). Distant fishing is still less likely to solve food problems. On the other hand, coastal fishing is relatively low in energy cost. Unfortunately, without the benefit of scholarly analysis fishermen and housewives have long known this, and coastal fisheries are threatened with overfishing as well as pollution.

The position of soybeans in Fig. 5 may be crucial. Soybeans possess the best amino acid balance and protein content of any widely grown crop. This has long been known to the Japanese who have made soybeans a staple of their diet. Are there other plants, possibly better suited for local climates, that have adequate proportions of amino acids in their proteins? There are about 80,000 edible species of plants, of which only about 50 are actively cultivated on a large scale (and 90 percent of the world's crops come from only 12 species). We may yet be able to find species that can contribute to the world's food supply.

The message of Fig. 5 is simple. In "primitive" cultures, 5 to 50 food calories were obtained for each calorie of energy invested. Some highly civilized cultures have done as well and occasionally better. In sharp contrast, industrialized food systems require 5 to 10 calories of fuel to obtain 1 food calorie. We must pay attention to this difference—especially if energy costs increase. If some of the energy subsidy for food production could be supplied by on-site, renewable sources—primarily sun and wind— we might be able to continue an energy-intensive food system. Otherwise, the choices appear to be either less energy-intensive food production or famine for many areas of the world.

ENERGY REDUCTION IN AGRICULTURE

It is possible to reduce the energy required for agriculture and the food system. A series of thoughtful proposals by Pimentel and his associates (3) deserves wide attention. Many of these proposals would help ameliorate environmental problems, and any reductions in energy use would provide a direct reduction in the pollutants due to fuel consumption as well as more time to solve our energy supply problems.

First, we should make more use of natural manures. The United States has a pollution problem from runoff from animal feedlots, even with the application of large amounts of manufactured fertilizer to fields. More than 10^6 kcal per acre (4×10^5 kcal per hectare) could be saved by substituting manure for manufactured fertilizer (3) (and, as a side benefit, the soil's condition would be improved). Extensive expansion in the use of natural manure will require decentralization of feedlot operations so that manure is generated closer to the point of application. Decentralization might increase feedlot costs, but, as energy prices rise, feedlot operations will rapidly become more expensive in any case. Although the use of manures can help reduce energy use, there is far too little to replace all commercial fertilizers at present (10). Crop rotation is less widely practiced than it was even 20 years ago. Increased use of crop rotation or interplanting winter cover crops of legumes (which fix nitrogen as a green manure) would save 1.5×10^6 kcal per acre by comparison with the use of commercial fertilizer.

Second, weed and pest control could be accomplished at a much smaller cost in energy. A 10 percent saving in energy in weed control could be obtained by the use of the rotary hoe twice in cultivation instead of herbicide application (again with pollution abatement as a side benefit). Biologic pest control—that is, the use of sterile males, introduced predators, and the like—requires only a tiny fraction of the energy of pesticide manufacture and application. A change to a policy of "treat when and where necessary" pesticide application would bring a 35 to 50 percent reduction in pesticide use. Hand application of pesticides requires more labor than machine or aircraft application, but the energy for application is reduced from 18,000 to 300 kcal per acre (3). Changed cosmetic standards, which in no way affect the taste or the edibility of foodstuffs, could also bring about a substantial reduction in pesticide use.

Third, plant breeders might pay more attention to hardiness, disease and pest resistance, reduced moisture content (to end the wasteful use of natural gas in drying crops), reduced water requirements, and increased protein content, even if it should mean some reduction in overall yield. In the longer run, plants not now widely cultivated might receive some serious attention and breeding efforts. It seems unlikely that the crops that have been most useful in temperate climates will be the most suitable ones for the tropics where a large portion of the undernourished peoples of the world now live.

A dramatic suggestion, to abandon chemical farming altogether, has been made by Chapman (11). His analysis shows that, were chemical farming to be ended, there would be much reduced yields per acre, so that most land in the soil bank would need to be put back into farming. Nevertheless, output would fall only 5 percent and prices for farm products would increase 16 percent. Most dramatically, farm income would rise 25 percent, and nearly all subsidy programs would end. A similar set of propositions treated with linear programming techniques at Iowa State University resulted in an essentially similar set of conclusions (12).

The direct use of solar energy farms, a return to wind power (modern windmills are now in use in Australia), and the production of methane from manure are all possibilities. These methods require some engineering to become economically attractive, but it should be emphasized that these technologies are now better understood than the technology of breeder reactors. If energy prices rise, these methods of energy generation would be attractive alternatives, even at their present costs of implementation.

ENERGY REDUCTION IN THE U.S. FOOD SYSTEM

Beyond the farm, but still far from the table, more energy savings could be introduced. The most effective way to reduce the large energy requirements of food processing would be a change in eating habits toward less highly processed foods. The current aversion of young people to spongy, additive-laden white bread, hydrogeneated peanut butter, and some other processed foods could presage such a change if it is more than just a fad. Technological changes could reduce energy consumption, but the adoption of lower energy methods would be hastened most by an increase in energy prices, which would make it more profitable to reduce fuel use.

Packaging has long since passed the stage of simply holding a convenient amount of food together and providing it with some minimal protection. Legislative controls may be needed to reduce the manufacturer's competition in the amount and expense of packaging. In any case, recycling of metal containers and wider use of returnable bottles could reduce this large item of energy use.

The trend toward the use of trucks in food transport, to the virtual exclusion of trains, should be reversed. By reducing the direct and indirect subsidies to trucks we might go a long way toward enabling trains to compete.

Finally, we may have to ask whether the ever-larger frostless refrigerators are needed, and whether the host of kitchen appliances really means less work or only the same amount of work to a different standard.

Store delivery routes, even by truck, would require only a fraction of the energy used by autos for food shopping. Rapid transit, giving some attention to the problems with shoppers with parcels, would be even more energy-efficient. If we insist on a high-energy food system, we should consider starting with coal, oil, garbage—or any other source of hydrocarbons—and producing in factories bacteria fungi, and yeasts. These products could then be flavored and colored appropriately for cultural tastes. Such a system would be more efficient in the use of energy, would solve waste problems, and would permit much or all of the agricultural land to be returned to its natural state.

ENERGY, PRICES, AND HUNGER

If energy prices rise, as they have already begun to do, the rise in the price of food in societies with industrialized agriculture can be expected to be even larger than the energy price increases. Slesser, in examining the case for England, suggests that a quadrupling of energy prices in the next 40 years would bring about a sixfold increase in food prices (9). Even small increases in energy costs may make it profitable to increase labor input to food production. Such a reversal of a 50-year trend toward energy-intensive agriculture would present environmental benefits as a bonus.

We have tried to show how analysis of the energy flow in the food system illustrates features of the food system that are not easily deduced from the usual economic analysis. Despite some suggestions for lower intensity food supply and some frankly speculative suggestions, it would be hard to conclude on a note of optimism. The world drawdown in grain stocks which began in the mid-1960's continues, and some food shortages are likely all through the 1970's and early 1980's. Even if population control measures begin to limit world population, the rising tide of hungry people will be with us for some time.

Food is basically a net product of an ecosystem, however simplified. Food production starts with a natural material, however modified later. Injections of energy (and even brains) will carry us only so far. If the population cannot adjust its wants to the world in which it lives, there is little hope of solving the food problem for mankind. In that case the food shortage will solve our population problem.

REFERENCES AND NOTES

1. *Statistical Abstract of the United States* (Government Printing Office, Washington, D.C., various annual editions).
2. *Historical Statistics of the United States* (Government Printing Office, Washington, D.C., 1960).
3. D. Pimentel, L. E. Hurd, A. C. Bellotti, M. J. Forster, I. N. Oka, O. D. Scholes, R. J. Whitman, *Science* 182, 443 (1973).
4. A description of the system may be found in: *Patterns of Energy Consumption in the United States* (report prepared for the Office of Science and Technology, Executive Office of the President, by Stanford Research Institute, Stanford, California, Jan. 1972), appendix C. The three groupings larger than food processing are: primary metals, chemicals, and petroleum refining.
5. N. Georgescu-Roegen, *The Entropy Law and the Economic Process* (Harvard Univ. Press, Cambridge, 1971), p. 301.
6. *Patterns of Energy Consumption in the United States* (report prepared for the Office of Science and Technology, Executive Office of the President, by Stanford Research Institute, Stanford, Calif., Jan. 1972).
7. R. A. Rice, *Technol. Rev.* 75, 32 (Jan. 1972).
8. Federal Highway Administration, Nationwide Personal Transportation Study Report No. 1 (1971) [as reported in Energy Research and Development, hearings before the Congressional Committee on Science and Astronautics, May 1972, p. 151].

9. M. Slesser, *Ecologist* 3 (No. 6), 216 (1973).

10. J. F. Gerber, personal communication (we are indebted to Dr. Gerber for pointing out that manures, even if used fully, will not provide all the needed agricultural fertilizers).

11. D. Chapman, *Environment (St. Louis)* 15 (No. 2), 12 (1973).

12. L. U. Mayer and S. H. Hargrove [*CAED Rep. No. 38* (1972)] as quoted in Slesser (*9*).

13. We have converted all figures for the use of electricity to fuel input values, using the average efficiency values for power plants given by C. M. Summers [*Sci. Am.* 224 (No. 3), 148 (1971)]. Self-generated electricity was converted to fuel inputs at an efficiency of 25 percent after 1945 and 20 percent before that year.

14. Purchased material in this analysis was converted to energy of manufacture according to the following values derived from the literature or calculated. In doubtful cases we have made what we believe to be conservative estimates: steel (including fabricated and castings), 1.7×10^7 kcal/ton (1.9×10^4 kcal/kg); aluminum (including castings and forgings), 6.0×10^7 kcal/ton; copper and brass (alloys, millings, castings, and forgings), 1.7×10^6 kcal/ton; paper, 5.5×10^6 kcal/ton; plastics, 1.25×10^6 kcal/ton; coal, 6.6×10^6 kcal/ton; oil and gasoline, 1.5×10^4 kcal/barrel (9.5×10^3 kcal/liter); natural gas, 0.26×10^3 kcal/cubic foot (9.2×10^3 kcal/m³); petroleum wax, 2.2×10^6 kcal/ton; gasoline and diesel engines, 3.4×10^6 kcal/engine; electric motors over 1 horsepower, 45×10^3 kcal/motor; ammonia, 2.7×10^7 kcal/ton; ammonia compounds, 2.2×10^6 kcal/ton; sulfuric acid and sulfur, 3×10^6 kcal/ton; sodium carbonate, 4×10^6 kcal/ton; and other inorganic chemicals, 2.2×10^6 kcal/ton.

15. Direct fuel use on farms: Expenditures for petroleum and other fuels consumed on farms were obtained from *Statistical Abstracts (1)* and the *Census of Agriculture* (Bureau of the Census, Government Printing Office, Washington, D.C., various recent editions) data. A special survey of fuel use on farms in the 1964 *Census of Agriculture* was used for that year and to determine the mix of fuel products used. By comparing expenditures for fuel in 1964 with actual fuel use, the apparent unit price for this fuel mix was calculated. Using actual retail prices and price indices from *Statistical Abstracts* and the ratio of the actual prices paid to the retail prices in 1964, we derived the fuel quantities used in other years. Changes in the fuel mix used (primarily the recent trend toward more diesel tractors) may understate the energy in this category slightly in the years since 1964 and overstate it slightly in years before 1964. S. H. Schurr and B. C. Netschert [*Energy in the American Economy, 1850–1975* (Johns Hopkins Press, Baltimore, 1960), p. 774], for example, using different methods, estimate a figure 10 percent less for 1955 than that given here. On the other hand, some retail fuel purchases appear to be omitted from all these data for all years. M. J. Perelman [*Environment (St. Louis)* 14 (No. 8), 10 (1972)] from different data, calculates 270×10^{12} kcal of energy usage for tractors alone.

16. Electricity use on farms: Data on monthly usage on farms were obtained from the "Report of the Administrator, Rural Electrification Administration" (U.S. Department of Agriculture, Government Printing Office, Washington, D.C., various annual editions). Totals were calculated from the annual farm usage multiplied by the number of farms multiplied by the fraction electrified. Some nonagricultural uses are included which may overstate the totals slightly for the years before 1955. Nevertheless, the totals are on the conservative side. A survey of on-farm electricity usage published by the Holt Investment Corporation, New York, 18 May 1973, reports values for per farm usage 30 to 40 percent higher than those used here, suggesting that the totals may be much too small. The discrepancy is probably the result of the fact that the largest farm users are included in the business and commercial categories (and excluded from the U.S. Department of Agriculture tabulations used).

17. Fertilizer: Direct fuel use by fertilizer manufacturers was added to the energy required for the manufacture of raw materials purchased as inputs for fertilizer manufacture. There is allowance for the following: ammonia and related compounds, phosphatic compounds, phosphoric acid, muriate of potash, sulfuric acid, and sulfur. We made no allowance for other inputs (of which phosphate rock, potash, and "fillers" are the largest), packaging, or capital equipment. Source: *Census of Manufacturers* (Government Printing Office, Washington, D.C., various recent editions).

18. Agricultural steel: Source, *Statistical Abstracts for various years* (1). Converted to energy values according to (*14*).

19. Farm machinery (except tractors): Source, *Census of Manufacturers*. Totals include direct energy use and the energy used in the manufacture of steel, aluminum, copper, brass, alloys, and engines converted according to (*14*).

20. Tractors: numbers of new tractors were derived from *Statistical Abstracts* and the *Census of Agriculture* data. Direct data on energy and materials use for farm tractor manufacture was collected in the *Census of Manufacturers* data for 1954 and 1947 (in later years these data were merged with other data). For 1954 and 1947 energy consumption was calculated in the same way as for farm machinery. For more recent years a figure of 2.65 $\times$ 10^6 kcal per tractor horsepower calculated as the energy of manufacture from 1954 data (the 1954 energy of tractor manufacture, 23.6 $\times$ 10^{12} kcal, divided by sales of 315,000 units divided by 28.7 average tractor horsepower in 1954). This figure was used to calculate energy use in tractor manufacture in more recent years to take some account of the continuing increase in tractor size and power. It probably slightly understates the energy in tractor manufacture in more recent years.

21. Irrigation energy: Values are derived from the acres irrigated from *Statistical Abstracts* for various years; converted to energy use at 10^6 kcal per acre irrigated. This is an intermediate value of two cited by Pimentel *et al.* (*3*).

22. Food processing industry: Source, *Census of Manufacturers*; direct fuel inputs only. No account taken for raw materials other than agricultural

products, except for those items (packaging and processing machinery) accounted for in separate categories.

23. Food processing machinery: Source, *Census of Manufactures* for various years. Items included are the same as for farm machinery [see (*13*)].

24. Paper packaging: Source, *Census of Manufactures* for various years. In addition to direct energy use by the industry, energy values were calculated for purchased paper, plastics, and petroleum wax, according to (*14*). Proportions of paper products having direct food usage were obtained from *Containers and Packaging* (U.S. Department of Commerce, Washington, D.C., various recent editions). [The values given include only proportional values from Standard Industrial Classifications 2651 (half), 2653 (half), 2654 (all).]

25. Glass containers: Source, *Census of Manufactures* for various years. Direct energy use and sodium carbonate [converted according to (*14*)] were the only inputs considered. Proportions of containers assignable to food are from *Containers and Packaging*. Understatement of totals may be more than 20 percent in this category.

26. Steel and aluminum cans: Source, *Census of Manufacturers* for various years. Direct energy use and energy used in the manufacture of steel and aluminum inputs were included. The proportion of cans used for food has been nearly constant at 82 percent of total production (*Containers and Packaging*).

27. Transportation fuel usage: Trucks only are included in the totals given. After subtracting trucks used solely for personal transport (all of which are small trucks), 45 percent of all remaining trucks and 38 percent of trucks larger than pickup and panel trucks were engaged in hauling food or agricultural products, or both, in 1967. These proportions were assumed to hold for earlier years as well. Comparison with ICC analyses of class I motor carrier cargos suggests that this is a reasonable assumption. The total fuel usage for trucks was apportioned according to these values. Direct calculations from average mileage per truck and average number of miles per gallon of gasoline produces agreement to within ±10 percent for 1967, 1963, and 1955. There is some possible duplication with the direct fuel use on farms, but it cannot be more than 20 percent considering on-farm truck inventories. On the other hand, inclusion of transport by rail, water, air, and energy involved in the transport of fertilizer, machinery, packaging, and other inputs of transportation energy could raise these figures by 30 to 40 percent if ICC commodity proportions apply to all transportation. Sources: *Census of Transportation* (Government Printing Office, Washington, D.C., 1963, 1967); *Statistical Abstracts (1); Freight Commodity Statistics of Class I Motor Carriers* (Interstate Commerce Commission, Government Printing Office, Washington, D.C., various annual editions).

28. Trucks and trailers: Using truck sales numbers and the proportions of trucks engaged in food and agriculture obtained in (*27*) above, we calculated the energy values at 75×10^6 kcal per trucks for manufacturing and delivery energy [A. B. Makhijani and A. J. Lichtenberg, *Univ. Calif. Berkeley Mem. No. ERL-M310* (revised) (1971)]. The results were checked against the *Census of Manufactures* data for 1967, 1963, 1958, and 1939 by proportioning motor vehicles categories between automobiles and trucks. These checks

suggest that our estimates are too small by a small amount. Trailer manufacture was estimated by the proportional dollar value to truck sales (7 percent). Since a larger fraction of aluminum is used in trailers than in trucks, these energy amounts are also probably a little conservative. Automobiles and trucks used for personal transport in the food system are omitted. Totals here are probably significant, but we know of no way to estimate them at present. Sources: *Statistical Abstracts, Census of Manufacturers,* and *Census of Transportation* for various years.

29. Commercial and home refrigeration and cooking: Data from 1960 through 1968 (1970 extrapolated) from *Patterns of Energy Consumption in the United States* (*6*). For earlier years sales and inventory in-use data for stoves and refrigerators were compiled by fuel and converted to energy from average annual use figures from the Edison Electric Institute [*Statistical Year Book* (Edison Electric Institute, New York, various annual editions] and American Gas Association values [*Gas Facts and Yearbook* (American Gas Association, Inc., Arlington, Virginia, various annual editions] for various years.

30. Refrigeration machinery: Source, *Census of Manufacturers.* Direct energy use was included and also energy involved in the manufacture of steel, aluminum, copper, and brass. A few items produced under this SIC category for some years perhaps should be excluded for years prior to 1958, but other inputs, notably electric motors, compressors, and other purchased materials should be included.

31. There are many studies of energy budgets in primitive societies. See, for example, H. T. Odum [*Environment, Power and Society* (Wiley, Interscience, New York, 1970)] and R. A. Rappaport [*Sci. Am.* 224 (No. 3), 104 (1971)]. The remaining values of energy subsidies in Fig. 5 were calculated from data presented by Slesser (*9*), Table 1.

32. This article is modified from C. E. Steinhart and J. S. Steinhart, *Energy: Sources, Use, and Role in Human Affairs* (Duxbury Press, North Scituate, Mass., in press) (used with permission). Some of this research was supported by the U.S. Geological Survey, Department of the Interior, under grant No. 14–08–0001–G–63. Contribution 18 of the Marine Studies Center, University of Wisconsin—Madison. Since this article was completed, the analysis of energy use in the food system of E. Hirst has come to our attention ["Energy Use for Food in the United States," *ONRL–NSF–EP–57* (Oct. 1973)]. Using different methods, he assigns 12 percent of total energy use to the food system for 1963. This compares with our result of about 13 percent in 1964.

Epilogue

This book has presented articles from critical areas of nutrition in a form which allows one to examine the nutrition crisis. This information also provides the basis for a prudent diet which not only can be enjoyable, but can aid in disease prevention. Following are diet guidelines based on these articles:

1. The use of multi-vitamin pills is not necessary unless recommended after a medical examination that includes biochemical data. The "placebo effect," however, might make one feel better, especially during times of stress; therefore, the use of vitamin pills is not totally discouraged. If one's diet provides wide variety, however, vitamin pills are not necessary.

2. The fiber content of the diet should be increased. Perhaps the easiest way is to eat "an apple a day," which would help regulate bowel movement and help prevent colon disease.

3. Drinking at least two glasses of milk a day, preferably skim or lowfat, will help to produce a more desirable calcium-phosphorus ratio, especially important if carbonated beverages are consumed regularly.

4. Women of child-bearing age should check with a doctor to determine if an iron supplement is needed.

5. Breakfast should be an important meal, but it need not be eaten immediately upon rising. Cereal with milk is an excellent breakfast, but items such as a lunchmeat sandwich and salad also are acceptable. If neither is eaten, some form of the new meal bars which supply at least one-third of the RDA should be substituted.

6. Snacks such as potato chips and pop should be reduced or replaced with fruits and vegetables.

7. The amount of protein in the average diet could be reduced by 50 percent with no adverse effects. This means smaller portions of meats, fish, eggs, etc. The bulk should be made up by vegetables or salads.

8. From a heart disease standpoint, reducing consumption of fatty protein foods may be beneficial. This should be accompanied by reductions in sugar and salt.

9.   Any preventive medicine regimen should include some form of vigorous exercise.

10.   The intake of high doses of single vitamins such as C or E to prevent disease conditions is useless and may be harmful.

11.   Crash or unusual diets should not be followed; rather a gradual weight loss is best.   This could be accomplished by going on a 1000 to 1200 calorie diet every other day and eating 2000 to 3000 calories on the alternate days.   This type of diet, besides causing the desired weight loss, also teaches new eating habits.

12.   A diet of organic foods may reduce the consumption of additives. But the advantage of eating organic foods is questionable, not only because they cost more than processed foods, but also because of the minimal toxicological risk of additives.

Index

†